THE CLASSICAL DOCTRINE OF INDIAN MEDICINE

THE CLASSICAL DOCTRINE OF INDIAN MEDICINE

ITS ORIGINS AND ITS GREEK PARALLELS

By

J. FILLIOZAT

COSMO PUBLICATIONS
2011 New Delhi

THE CLASSICAL DOCTRINE OF INDIAN MEDICINE

Published by
Cosmo Publications, 2011

ISBN 978-81-307-1216-1

Published by
COSMO PUBLICATIONS
for
GENESIS PUBLISHING PVT. LTD.
24-B, Ansari Road, Darya Ganj,
New Delhi-110 002,
INDIA

Printed and Bound in India

TABLE OF CONTENTS

Translator's Note

PROF. FILLIOZAT'S work on Indian medicine was published in French in 1949 and became immediately thereafter a classic in this field. The author had first qualified as a medical practitioner and had set up practice in Paris. Being, however, deeply interested in Indology, he had been devoting all his spare time and energy to a study of ancient Indian society with especial emphasis on medicine. The present work is the result of years of hard work done in this domain—years marked by the publication of a number of research articles and books such as the *Kumāra-tantra*. His training in European classical languages as also in Avestan, Tibetan, Chinese, etc. enabled him to take a comparative view in regard to the development of medical doctrines in this country.

The work proper starts with a discussion about the legends concerning Ayurveda and after dealing with the traditions of the two major texts, those of Caraka and Suśruta, sums up the essential doctrines of all the texts available today. This is followed by a discussion on the pre-Aryan and Indo-Aryan data on medicine, juxtaposed with similar data from the *Avesta*. The next three chapters deal with the Vedic data on Pathology, Anatomy and Physiology leading, in the next chapter, to a discussion of the relationship between the Veda and Ayurveda. In the seventh chapter the author makes a comparative study of the doctrine of wind as adumbrated in India and as found in a Greek text. This is followed by a critical examination, from the point of view of medical doctrine, of the *Timaeus* and corresponding data found in Indian medical texts. The last chapter takes up the specific question of contacts between India and Greece, before Alexander, wherein Persia was the intermediary. This is confirmed in a striking manner by showing that these contacts had also been maintained with the Accadian civilisation.

Although written primarily as a treatise on the development of Indian medical doctrine, the work had been undertaken with a much wider vision and a student of ancient Indian society in general is also sure to benefit from a perusal of this book. Prof. Filliozat's findings on India's contacts with Persia and Greece before Alexander as also with the Accadian civilisation are bound to evoke deep interest in our country.

We hope that this classic, now available to a large number of our countrymen, will help focus their attention on the essentials of a science, which, though quite ancient, is equally modern, as it is still being widely practised in our country as also in neighbouring countries like Ceylon.

The printing of such a text, with many words of Chinese, Tibetan, Avestan, Greek and Latin, in addition to those of ancient Indian languages, has proved to be quite a difficult task and has considerably delayed its publication. For the same reason, a number of accented types, as in the case of Avestan words, had to be dispensed with and in certain cases they have not been used throughout the book. As the choice was between non-publication and publication with these technical shortcomings, we have had to opt for the latter, believing that the learned reader will forgive this lapse as also others that he may notice.

We are grateful to Prof. Filliozat for his permission to undertake this translation and for evincing, despite his extremely busy work-schedule, continuous interest in its progress. At our request, he has also contributed a special introduction to this edition. Our thanks are also due to Dr. Romila Thapar for having gone through the entire manuscript. Without the editorial help of Shri S. Balu Rao the book would not have been what it is now. Shri Shambhu Datt Sharma has very kindly prepared the bibliography and the index.

Inst. of Post-Grad. (eve.) Studies, University of Delhi, Delhi.

DEV RAJ CHANANA

PREFACE FOR THE ENGLISH VERSION

THE WORK ON HIPPOCRATIC MEDICINE which continues actively and has, during the last few years, helped produce the thesis of Mr. Bourgey at Paris and Mr. R. Joly at Liege is chiefly interesting for the history of the scientific spirit of the Antiquity and for ancient Greek Philology. On its side, the history of the Ayurveda reaches into the same Antiquity but concerns something always modern. The Ayurvedic medicine is still alive. Some attack it as the anachronic survival of a once glorious past but unworthy of being ranked with new scientific achievements. Others defend it with a conviction and ingeniousness which do harm to its cause. In fact, some support the view that it is fully worthy of figuring in the front rank of modern medicines and even that it is the only one worthy of the front rank. In their view it already contains all the useful discoveries of not only the present-day medicine but also of medicine in future. It is the complete science, revealed once for all for the good of the feeble humanity and does not require any research and trials of present-day science. All that the latter discovers with a great deal of effort, had not only been foreshadowed but had been written down in its books. It is because we cannot understand them properly and cannot understand their formulae because of the condensed expression of the truth, that we always look for the detailed solutions of physiological and therapeutic problems which had been, in general, fully solved by Ayurveda.

Moved by this spirit, a number of the partisans of Ayurveda have written about the identification of modern concepts with those of Ayurveda. This is how it is desired to recognise in certain organic elements mentioned by the Ayurvedic texts, the elements defined by present-day physiology and geological Chemistry. For instance, as the action of *prāṇa* is invoked by Ayurveda for explaining the physiological movements of the organs, and as modern Nerurology talks about nervous influx, some have claimed that *prāṇa* is that nervous influx and that modern Nerurology has merely rediscovered what Ayurveda had already taught. This is how, once again, a substance like *ojas*, which plays an important rôle in the organism, according to the Physiology of Ayurveda, has been identified with albumin, because albumin appears as playing a rôle of fundamental importance in the same organism. Numerous other identifications in detail or identifications of theories explaining the same phenomena proposed on both sides by the Ayurvedic authors and modern medical men have, once again, been recently put forward. But it should be evident to everybody that the majority of these identifications cannot be defended because the elements mistakenly held to be the same, as they serve to explain the same functions, are altogether differently defined on the two sides. It is certainly much more important to note that the Ayurvedic authors have recognised numerous problems posed by life and by the inter-play of pathological functions or by their alterations and that they have sought to solve them by means of rational explanations, on the basis of data obtained from observations available to them, as can always be done by the Physiologists, Biologists and the Pathologists with the help of data gathered by them. But it is absolutely unwarranted to claim that the explanations thus offered are equivalent and that the more ancient ones had already the value of the latter ones; indeed they have an absolute and definitive value. Now in the European science of the Middle Ages the maintenance of any liquid in a tube, first filled and then turned upside down on a vat containing the same liquid, had been sought to be explained by means of the property of nature having *horror* of the vacuum. Later on Physics, having discovered atmospheric pressure, has explained the same phenomenon because of the atmospheric pressure. But no one has, however, come to the conclusion that mediaeval science had already known the atmospheric pressure and had named it, "horror of the vaccum".

The same should have been the case with regard to Ayurvedic explanations. It gives evidence of a rational scientific spirit, rarely seen in other civilisations of the world. But these explanations have for their basis a knowledge, as yet rudimentary and incomplete in so far as the real conditions of the production of these phenomena were concerned; they cannot, therefore, prevail against those which today rest on much more detailed information and which will not be valid before those of the future, the latter being based on much more complete knowledge. Making claims to the contrary is not only to naively mix up concepts and theories which, though applicable to the same phenomena, have altogether different bases, but is also to give to the detractors of Ayurveda a chance of denigrating its partisans as making unjustifiable claims for the same. One should not plead a good cause with bad arguments.

In the history of universal scientific development, Ayurveda has an eminent place, which should be conceded to the same and we will refer to it a little later, but its theories of yesterday do not supercede those of today. It retains its importance for other reasons.

From another side, the extremely widespread persistence of the usage of Ayurvedic remedies and treatments does not, by itself, prove their value. It is known that in the absence of a sufficient number of practitioners of modern medicine, a large number of Indian people have no other choice save that of having recourse to Ayurvedic medicine, the only one available in a large number of localities. Often when modern medicine is represented by perfectly qualified practitioners, it remains inaccessible because of the high cost of its therapeutics or because of the complexity of the installations required by the same.

Even when inferior in efficacity, Ayurvedic medicine will be able to maintain itself, regardless of the fact that it is traditional, because it is at the same time cheap. This is an important practical problem, regarding whose solution opinion is divided.

Certain persons think that it is useful, even necessary, while waiting for a more complete propagation of modern universal medicine, which India, besides, possesses and to whose progress its research-workers are contributing and which alone should be spread all over and installed over its entire territory. While waiting for this propagation and only for this propagation, Ayurvedic medicine must be encouraged. But in that case it must be correctly practised by the Ayurvedic practitioners, with verified competence, instead of being, sometimes, practised at the hands of healers who use it ill and render it inefficacious or dangerous.

But this presupposes that its value be well-established and

that a distinction be clearly made between those cases where it can be usefully applied and those which can be treated only by modern methods. In other words it will be necessary that its competence be proved and defined. It will also be necessary that its teaching-programmes be properly established.

In the absence of decisive research concerning the value and the scope of its methods, others think that its teaching should not be encouraged and must not be officially sanctioned by means of diplomas. In their view, official sanction would perpetuate worn-out methods and this would lead to delay in the complete medical equipment of the country and the replacement of Ayurvedic medicine by inferior techniques.

The former retort that as it is impossible to carry out this replacement in a very short time, no matter how desirable, there is a danger in abandoning it to private initiative, generous but sometimes ignorant or imprudent. For example, mercurial medicines, used by the practitioners of the *rasāyana*-tradition, are toxic. Administered by a prudent practitioner, closely in touch with indications and dosages, they can be salutary. Otherwise, as is unfortunately proved by experience, they can give rise to grave nephritis or can be immediately fatal. As a precautionary measure their use can be prohibited, but they will still be sometimes used either surreptitiously or in ignorance of their real nature and the danger will not be entirely removed. Even medicines, made from non-toxic plants or from plants which are only a little toxic, can be harmful when not administered in proper measure. The most harmless can also, unduly prescribed, make one lose precious time which could, otherwise, have been utilised for efficacious treatment, which a more competent doctor, even Ayurvedic, could have begun. In brief, as Ayurvedic medicine exists without being immediately replaced, it should be better practised and not at random.

During these arguments from both the sides, at least the difficulty of the problem comes to the surface. It is a social problem because the existence of Ayurvedic medicine, being actually practised in Indian society, is a fact, the health and life of a part of this society depend on it and on the manner in which it is practised. Now this problem can only be resolved by a clear determination of what is Ayurvedic medicine and what it can become.

Under these conditions, it appears that, first of all, it must be deeply studied. The interest in its study is, therefore, not simply retrospective, as if it were a mere historical fact without any importance for the present, like the medicine of Greek or Egyptian or Mesopotamian antiquity. It is also, and above all, practical as it has a social presence, which cannot be overlooked.

In the present work, written in France and outside the domain of practical Ayurvedic medicine, we have only tried to examine its doctrinal bases, examine the nature and foundations of its theories. They have appeared to us to be highly respectable because of the spirit of rational comprehension of vital and pathological phenomena they reveal. Upto now, after studying the ancient medical systems, we have found proofs of an original rational effort only among the Greeks and the Chinese (not counting the medical systems which are only derived from those of Greece and China)—an effort analogous to that of India, which is shown in the Ayurveda.

Thus we observe that Ayurveda is definitely in the front rank of the scientific realisations of ancient time, when its doctrines were constituted. But it is for the Indian practitioners of today, for Biologists, for Pharmocologists, for Dieteticians, to find out the practical results which can be obtained from the practice of Ayurveda, whose theories and accumulated treasure of observations are remarkable but whose power of investigation has been by-passed by present-day research, always going ahead.

It is an immense and difficult but necessary task. It will have been necessary even if there were no need of justifying or condemning the methods which are, rightly or wrongly, applied at present. In fact, the data of the Ayurvedic texts refer to real diseases, to dietetic measures effectively applied, to largely applied remedies. It constitutes a considerable mass of information relating to Pathology, to nutrition and to the effect of drugs and all this information should be gathered and verified by modern research.

Already numerous Ayurvedic drugs have been examined from the point of view of their pharmocological properties. The cases of their application are not equally well-known, because of the difficulties often present in the identification of diseases, enumerated by modern nosology, in the descriptions furnished by Ayurvedic texts. These texts have, in fact, classified a large number of diseases in a different manner, according to the analogy of the symptoms, confusing, for example, under the nomenclature of *jvara*, "fever", different diseases, in which fever is only a secondary manifestation. On other occasions, and quite frequently, these texts distinguish several varieties in a single disease, according to whether certain symptoms are attributed to the predominance of one of the three morbid elements *(tridoṣa)*, theoretically and hypothetically distinguished by them but whose real presence cannot be found by modern medicine.

Besides, the extremely rich dietetic indications of Ayurveda, necessarily based on observations over long periods, cannot but have interest for us, both from the practical view-point and for the study of the problems of nutrition. Systems of ancient medicine always attached a great deal of importance to regimen and to behaviour whether for the preservation of health or for the treatment of diseases. They often explained diseases as being due to a departure from regimen or to inadequate hygiene. In this regard their prescriptions were extremely thorough. The medicine of the nineteenth century, following its great discoveries and notably after the work of Pasteur concerning the pathogenic role of bacteria, has undermined many of their hypotheses. This has tended to relegate to the second rank the preoccupation concerning the regimen of diseases, exception however being made in the case of diseases of nutrition, as Diabetes. Alimentation and behaviour, being no longer considered as the essential causes of diseases, have lost a great deal of their importance in the eyes of doctors and are now considered among the favourable circumstances or among the accessory means of therapeutics. At present, however, a deeper study of the biological conditions, particularly the biochemical conditions of normal equilibria and of minor pathological perturbations is once again drawing attention to the effects of alimentation and to the mode of life, to the influence of climates, of seasons and to environmental conditions. For example, in regard to alimentation, observations have been made and experimental verifications are being made *in vitro*, concerning the influence of rice on the development and activity of pathogenic amoeba, which lose this activity when the proportion of rice in the contents of the digestive tube becomes too high. Therefore, in this respect the data of the Ayurveda deserve examination and verification. They can help many lines of research.

A number of Indian doctors, in the know of both modern medicine and Ayurveda, have understood this point. Some editions of ancient texts accompanied by interpretations made in the double light of tradition and of present-day clinical conditions have been published. Among them we may mention the edition of *Caraka-samhitā*, published by the Gulabkunwarba Ayurvedic Society, under the direction of Dr. Mehta.

Ayurveda need neither be exalted beyond measure nor condemned either for its antiquity or for the failure of those who practise it without prudence. It should be studied as an original system of science and as an exceptional source of medical experience.

College de France,
Paris.

J. FILLIOZAT

INTRODUCTION

THE HISTORY of Indian science is ordinarily not considered important either by the Indologist or by the historian of sciences. For the former, it is only of secondary importance as India has been great more because of her various schools of philosophy than because of her learning. For the latter, it is an aberration because it does not put itself on the continuous line of scientific evolution which starting from Greek science continues right into modern science. Both of them suspect her to be lacking in originality, to be based in a number of its branches on borrowings firstly from Greek science, then from the Arab world and even from that of China. But it is a fact that it has been studied, with prodigious activity in India, where it has given rise, not to one, but to many immense literatures and also throughout the Indianised parts of Asia and Insulindia.

This fact alone should attract attention. In the absence of all other interest, Indian science, the element of the expansion of one of the greatest world cultures, does have evident historical importance. Its diffusion outside India is exactly parallel to that of Greek science outside the Hellenic world. Mentioning merely the chief facts, it may be observed that Indian science has been adopted in Tibet, in Central Asia, in certain Chinese and Japanese circles, in the entire Indo-China and in Indonesia. The Tibetans communicated it to the Mongols. And it is not only the empirical notions or the techniques of India which have thus spread among so many distant and diverse peoples; have equally spread among these peoples texts teaching the theories, which, like those of the Greeks, attempted to explain the Universe. The Tibetans, chiefly, have translated the Sanskrit texts with extreme care and with full understanding of the teachings. Their translations cannot be surpassed in precision aud faithfulness, because the Indians did not merely give them their learning and the practical knowledge of Sanskrit. They also gave them their precise analysis of this language, which is the means of understanding it better and is the model for a clear comprehension of the resources of their own language. They also taught them their logic, the totality of their reflections on the criteria of truth and on the legitimacy of reasoning. Indian science has thus spread itself giving at the same time, both its methods and its results. Therefore it is not merely because of the extent of the geographical area wherein it spread itself, but more because of its learned mode of transmission, that it is comparable to Hellenic science. This parallelism ceases to be valid only during the recent epochs, when suddenly in Europe starts, among the inheritors of Hellenism, the modern scientific growth, because ancient Indian science has produced nothing comparable to the same. But this growth is definitely not the exclusive result of and the natural consequence of the scientific Greek tradition. Upto this exceptional growth, on the one hand Greek science and its derivatives in Christianity and Islam and on the other Indian science and its derivatives in the form of exported Brahmanism and Buddhism have, between themselves, shared the world. Outside these, only the Chinese science kept a domain for itself, extended in sooth, but without distant expansion and often mixed with Indian influence.

Someone can, however, object that it is not legitimate to put in this manner Indian science on a par with Greek science and it may be preferable to compare the former with that of Islam. The prevalent opinion which feels that Indian science is lacking in originality, supposes that it has been derived from Greek science and as a consequence is a sister of Islamic science. In this case, even when regard is to be had to the great historical role of Indian science as also to its intrinsic value, the problem of its originality re-appears—the problem dominating all the ideas that must be had thereof.

This problem has been very early resolved by the authors who had taken it up. In India, because of National pride, certain persons make it a principle to claim that in early antiquity the science of their country had gone much farther than that of the present occident. On the other hand, in the occident many claim that the spirit of scientific research could not arise but among them and that India could have had only that much in science, which she could have borrowed. In both cases, only certain examples, thought to be the characteristics, are offered as proofs; these examples are immediately generalised, with hypotheses supplementing the missing data, without making any effort for acquiring the latter. In truth, judgement is given on the basis of racial or rational prejudice rather than on that of a profound comparative study of the two great scientific traditions, on whose respective values pronouncements are made. It can be easily observed that those who settle this question with greater certainty are familiar only with the tradition in whose favour they give the decision and know the other only by means of fragmentary data or through studies they cannot appreciate. This is the least to be said in the most favourable case, because, clearly, we do not have to consider those who know neither of the two sciences, with which they deal.

The greatest historians of science have not always been able to escape this inconvenience of unilateral knowledge when they had to compare the Greek and Indian data. A. Paul Tannery, so justly famous for his studies in the field of ancient Mathematics, has been himself an example of the same. It is known that the trigonometric sinus is not mentioned by the Greek Mathematicians and Astronomers, that it has been in use in India since the Gupta period, as the *Sūrya-siddhānta* of the fourth or the fifth century A.D. gives a table of sinus, that the Arab Astronomers who borrowed from India had known the sinus and that its usage came to the occident in the twelfth century A.D., when the astronomical work of Al-Battani was translated into Latin. From this, the conclusion should have been drawn that the sinus had been invented, not by the Greeks but by the Indians whose tradition on this point had been taken up by the Arabs for completing that of the Greeks. But, being sure that the Indians could not have invented anything in Mathematics and believing that this science had no place among them, Tannery has preferred to suppose, without any basis whatsoever, that the sinus could have been the response to a Greek idea, not adopted by Hipparchos, who had merely established a table of chords. The mere fact that Indians had known the sinus sufficed to persuade Tannery that the Greeks had known it and had then taught its concept to the Indians.[1]

1. P. Tannery, *Recherche sur l'histoire de l'astronomie ancienne*, Paris, 1893, p. 66.

Reasoning in this way, we have only the Greek science left in the world and the great problem of knowing whether scientific spirit is the exclusive product of the Greek miracle, whether scientific invention has taken place only among the Greeks, is solved in advance. That is to say that it is not at all resolved because the expression of a prejudice is not a solution. Only a profound study of Indian science in parallel with the contemporary sciences, especially with corresponding Greek science, will enable us to recognise if it has some originality or not and in such a case, to measure the same, to truly judge the role of India in the history of science, to determine whether she has been only a propagator or also a creator.

In his great series of works on science in Antiquity, interrupted too soon, the late Abel Rey, centring his research on the originality and the genius of Hellenic science, has objectively tried to give due share to foreign science which had surrounded the same.[2] The method, which for this purpose had appeared to him to be the surest, consisted in making a list of documents which introduce these sciences to us, in dating them to the best of ability and in comparing their dates with those of the corresponding Greek documents. This was a strict application of the historical and comparative method. When a foreign scientific work was surely anterior to the Greek texts containing analogous teaching, he made a comparative analysis of the tenor of teaching given on both sides. When, on the contrary, it was found to be posterior, he did not think it necessary to take note of the same. In this way he had come to the conclusion that, in the present state of our documentation,—in sooth extremely fragmentary in so far as the ancient sciences of Egypt and classical Orient are concerned —the Orient, before the Greeks had merely furnished a *proto-science,* chiefly of a practical nature and that it was only after the growth of Greek science that the later Oriental peoples had known a more developed science. But in certain cases, particularly while examining the data of Indian science, Abel Rey has much too exclusively considered the chronology of

2. Collection *L' Evolution de l' Humanité* : I. *La science orientale avant les Grecs,* Paris, 1930; II. *La jeunesse de la science grecque,* 1933; III. *La maturité de la pensé scientifique en Gréce,* 1939; IV and V. *L' apogée de la science technique grecqne,* 1946 and 1948.

works, whereas the full application of the historical method would demand the determination of a chronology of ideas.

The special texts of Indian medicine, which have reached us, are didactic works of relatively late date. In the majority of cases, they are not the original compositions of initiators, they are only the manuals of schools, which have, at a certain moment, become traditional due to success and which, because of the same, have been preserved for us in preference to those which they, more or less, reproduce. The date of their editing has, therefore, only secondary importance; it is not valid for marking the epoch of the creation of doctrines contained therein. Therefore, in dating the totality of these doctrines in the epoch of these manuals, as has been done by Abel Rey, is to take an extreme risk. These doctrines are surely much more ancient. One may, however, believe that no other course was open to him. Certainly it would have been still much more risky to put them in an indeterminate antiquity and, most of all, to put all of them there *en bloc*, because the higher they go, with reference to their expression in these manuals, the more chance there is of their being mixed up, during various periods, with more recent notions.

Fortunately, we do not find ourselves faced with the dilemma of either having to rejuvenate, against all evidence, the ancient doctrines or of having to make them old at random. The special classical manuals of Indians constitute only a part of the immense literature of ancient India. It is therefore, legitimate for us to see if we can find out, in more ancient literary strata, the appearance of doctrines, which they have systematised for teaching. In this way we have the chance to locate them nearer their origin and sometimes to find even the stages of their constitution.

This is what we have tried to do for the medical doctrines. It is only after having put them in their place in the current of Indian thought, where they arose, and after having determined their antecedents that we could proceed to compare them with similar Greek doctrines. We will strive chiefly to seize their first manifestation or the formative elements in the oldest texts, so that we can go as far as possible in the historical past of ideas. We will be led to observe that a number of ideas, which had been believed to be borrowed by India from the Hellenic science, as long as they had been studied only in classical manuals more recent than the great Greek works, have, in fact, in India more ancient bases than these great works and that the two medical traditions, Indian and Greek, have had a parallel development. We will have, therefore, to envisage their eventual exchanges in the light of those historical conditions which have made them possible.

The problem of the existence of these exchanges does not have an interest only for the history of ancient sciences; it constitutes a part of the more general history of relations between the Orient and Occident, too often discussed on the basis of *rapprochements* of general ideas which are much less characteristic than those of special doctrines.

On the other hand, the study of special doctrines of sciences is called for, even outside the sphere of comparative researches, even inside each civilisation, because these doctrines are not limited to the savants. They are all known to all the thinkers, at least in their main lines. They determine a part of their ideas and often they constitute a fund of notions on which they agree with one another more easily than on all the problems of Metaphysics or of Religion. This fund is more closely common than any other and to all those belonging to the same culture. The historians of occidental thought are devoting themselves more and more to a consideration of the influence of scientific ideas on the Occidental philosophers. Here we must note, however, that in India speculation concerning nature and physiology has, in parallel, commanded many concepts of the thinkers and of men of all types. We have, therefore, while undertaking this study, to try to call attention at least to the interesting doctrines and which by their large diffusion, characterise, on certain points, Indianism in its entirety, while at the same time they are important for the history of sciences and of the ancient currents of thought, no matter how modest elements they may be in themselves.

J. FILLIOZAT

CHAPTER ONE

CLASSICAL INDIAN MEDICINE : THE ĀYURVEDA

THE PRINCIPAL and oldest texts of the classical Indian medicine are the *Saṁhitās,* the "corpus" said to be of Bhela, Caraka and Suśruta. The first has reached us in one single and incomplete manuscript. The other two are not available in their original form because we know that they have been revised by more recent authors. None of these three texts represents a first effort at systematic description of medical science; on the contrary, all the three suppose an already established tradition, to whose foundation they have not contributed. They limit themselves merely to collecting the facts of the above-mentioned tradition and to teaching it. This tradition claims to have links with the Veda; it is that of the *Āyurveda,* of the "science of longevity", which is considered sometimes as a "secondary part" *(upāṅga)* of the *Atharvaveda*[1] and sometimes as a "secondary Veda" *(upa-veda)* of the *Ṛg-veda.*[2] Theoretically the Āyurveda consists of eight "parts" or "articles" which are so well-known as its characteristic members that the expression "eight parts" *(aṣṭāṅga)* is currently used to denote the science of medicine. The texts of Bhela, Caraka and Suśruta, though not observing it, are aware of

---

1 Suśr., *Sūtr.,* 1, 3 *(...āyurveda nāma yad upāṅgam atharvavedasya...),* cf. also Caraka, *Sūtr.,* XXX, 20, where it is said that "the doctor should show respect to the *Atharva-veda,* which among the four Vedas, belongs properly to him." *(bhiṣajā...vedānām ātmano' tharva-vede bhaktir ādeśyā).* In Suśr., *Sūtr.,* XXXIV, 6, it is said that the "Brahman has given the name of *āyurveda* to that part of the Veda which has eight parts." *(Brahmā vedāṅgam aṣṭāṅgam āyurvedam abhāṣata)* and the same passage, in verse 4, says that "the *Atharva-veda* announces hundred and one deaths" *(ekottaram mṛtyuśatam atharvāṇaḥ pracakṣate);* This is an allusion to *AV,* VIII, 2, 28 which, in effect, refers to "a hundred and one deaths."

2 *Caraṇavyūha,* 38; *Prasthānabheda,* IV.

this division. This division has been popular chiefly with more recent authors.

The Legends about the Origins of the Āyurveda :—According to Suśruta, medicine was created by the Being who exists by Himself (Svayambhū), that is to say Brahman, in 100,000 *ślokas*. In view of the inability of human beings to learn it in this form, Svayambhū is said to have re-composed it in eight parts and taught it to Prajāpati, who is said to have passed it on to the Aśvins, the Aśvins to Indra, Indra to Dhanvantari appearing in the form of Divodāsa, the king of Kāśi. At last Dhanvantari, on the prayer of a group consisting of Aupadhenava, Vaitaraṇa, Aurabhra, Pauṣkalāvata, Karavīrya, Gopurarakṣita and Suśruta, taught it to men. Suśruta is, therefore, supposed to have recorded the very words of Dhanvantari himself.

Caraka has the same thing to say concerning the origin of medicine and its transmission upto Indra (*Sūtra*, I, 4,5). Indra is said to have revealed it to Ṛṣi Bharadvāja, who was sent to him by all the well-known ṛṣis desirous of knowing the means of combatting diseases. Bharadvāja is said to have immediately communicated his knowledge to other ṛṣis. One of them, Ātreya Punarvasu is said to have subsequently trained six disciples: Agniveśa, Bhela, Jatūkarṇa, Parāśara, Hārīta and Kṣārapāṇi (ib., 29-30). Of these, Agniveśa is supposed to have been the first to compose a book for teaching (ib., 31). The *Caraka-saṁhitā* represents itself to be the manual "composed by Agniveśa and reconstituted by Caraka"[1] and it claims to reproduce the actual words of Ātreya Punarvasu himself.

The legend of the origin of the Āyurveda is inseparable from the legends concerning the origin of many other sciences. Almost upto our times, it has been an Indian practice to take back the first teaching of sciences and letters to superior gods. The script is supposed to have been invented by Brahman, Astronomy to have been revealed by Sūrya, the grammar of Pāṇini to have been elaborated by Śiva, in whose mouth besides the Tantras place the teaching of all sorts of things. Indra also, though less frequently, is a god of teaching; tradition

[1] As is indicated by the colophons of chapters which start with the words *ityagniveśa-kṛte tantre caraka-pratisaṁskṛte*.

ascribes him another grammar and Barth (*Oeuvres*, III, 223) has identified the source of this last association with a passage of the *Taittirīya-saṁhitā* where it is said that Indra made speech distinguishable (VI, 47, end).

The sources of the legend concerning the origin of the Āyurveda are more complex. It is evident that the Aśvins, because of their reputation as divine doctors, had already been, in good time, designated, as we will see, to play a role in the transmission of the medical science. Because of other legends and because of his relations with the Aśvins, Indra, for his part, was already a suitable character for their transmission. In the *Chāndogya-upaniṣad* (VIII, 15) it is said that the supreme science was given by Brahman to Prajāpati, by Prajāpati to Manu and by Manu to human beings, but a little earlier, the same text (VIII, 7-12) has given all the details of the teaching by Prajāpati to Indra On the other hand, according to the *Ṛg-veda,* Indra has been aided by the Aśvins "as a son by fathers" (X, 131, 4-5). In his commentary on a repetition of the same passage in the *Vājasaneyas* (X, 33-34), Mahīdhara tells us how the asura Namuci having drunk all the vigour of Indra, the Aśvins and Sarasvatī have, even then, furnished him with the means of killing this asura. This was not the teaching of medicine but this did put him under obligation to the Aśvins. It is, therefore, understandable that Indra easily came to be regarded as having received instruction in medical science from the Aśvins and propagated it in his turn, although there are different traditions some calling Indra the master and some the pupil of the Aśvins. Moreover the *Sautrāmaṇi* ritual associates Indra with the Aśvins; this ritual is even thought to represent the curing of Indra by the Aśvins when the former had fallen ill by drinking too much of soma; here again Indra is indebted to the Aśvins. Clearly, this sum-total of mythological facts contains all the elements which have served to constitute the legend of the origin of the Āyurveda upto its teaching by Indra.

At the same time, in the light of the indications furnished by the *Chāndogya-upaniṣad,* we can observe that from the period of this text, legends regarding the origin of the science, similar to those of the classical period, had already been current. The two traditions differ as to the pupil of Indra; Dhanvantari, mentioned by Suśruta being a post-Vedic god and Bharadvāja, who is mentioned by Caraka, being a Vedic ṛṣi. But this divergence is only apparent because the two personages are, from antiquity itself, closely interconnected. In effect, the Dhanvantari mentioned by Suśruta is also Divodāsa, and Divodāsa is Vedic and is mentioned in association with Bharadvāja in three passages of the *Ṛg-veda*: "While protecting, you have made the route circular for Divodāsa, for Bharadvāja, O Aśvins"[1]; In hymn VI, 16, Bharadvāja himself invokes Agni: "O thou, pressing these plentiful goods for Divodāsa and serving for Bharadvāja"[2]; thirdly Indra is told: "Thou hast given by power, O powerful one, treasures to Divodāsa pressing, O very fast one, to singing Bharadvāja."[3] This should suffice to show that these two personalities were closely related to each other, and could easily become the substitutes of each other and that the traditions of Suśruta and Caraka regarding the pupil of Indra, reach back to the same group of ancient data.[4]

This conclusion is in accordance with the fact that the doctrinal contents of the two texts are the same. Moreover, this conclusion does not allow us to believe that the names of Divodāsa and Bharadvāja can be linked with historical character. Of course persons with these names have existed, but the two mentioned by medical manuals are surely mythical.

The introduction of the personage of Dhanvantari seems to constitute the real divergence of the tradition of the *Suśruta-*

---

1 *yád áyātam dívodāsāya vartír bharádvājāyāśvinā háyantā*. *RV.*, 1, 116, 18.

2 *tvám imā vāryā purū dívodāsāya sunvaté, bharádvājāya dāśúṣe*. *RV.*, VI, 16, 5.

3 *aśikṣo yatra śacyā śacīvo divodāsāya sunvaté, sutakre bharádvājāya gṛṇaté vásūni*. *RV.*, VI, 31, 4.

4 Besides, the *Śāṅkhāyanagṛhyasūtras* (II, 14, 4) directly associate the name of Bharadvāja with that of Dhanvantari. The *Pañcaviṁśa-brāhmaṇa*, XV, 3, 7, makes Bharadvāja to be the purohita of Divodāsa. The *Jaiminīyabr.* [I, 222, (W. Caland), *Das Jaim. in Auswahl*, Amsterdam, 1919, No. 82, p. 86] presents Divodāsa as a king desirous of becoming a ṛṣi.

saṁhitā from that of the *Caraka-saṁhitā.* In India every eminent being can be presented as a god become man. Although he is only a fictive personage, Divodāsa has not escaped this rule. The god whom he incarnates is more recent than himself. Dhanvantari is not mentioned in the Vedic literature, except in its latest stratum, that of the *Sūtras;* generally speaking, though not always, he is a god in the epic and in the Purānas and quite often he is a *parvenu* among the gods. At the time of the churning of the ocean by the devas and the asuras, he emerged out of the waves carrying amṛta or the liquid of immortality. (*Mahābh., Ādip.* 1140; *Rāmāyaṇa,* Bombay, I, XLV, 32; Gorresio, I, XLVI, 30). The *Bhāgavatapurāṇa* sees in him "a part of Viṣṇu" (*Viṣṇor aṁśa,* VIII, VIII, 34) or, what amounts to the same thing, "part of Vāsudeva" (*Vāsudevāṁśa,* IX, XVII, 4).[1] In the first passage, he is called the "observer of the Āyurveda" (*āyurvedadṛś*) and in both of them it is specified that he has a share in the sacrifice (*ijyābhāj, yajñabhuj*). It is also said that Dhanvantari "has obtained as his part in the sacrifice the immortal life to which a stop had been put."[2] This insistence of the Purāṇa can be easily explained if it is considered that the participation of Dhanvantari in the sacrifice could not be secured on its own. The *Gṛhya-sūtras* had admitted this participation (*Āśvalayanagṛ,* I, 3, 6; 12, 7), but it has been contested for a long time. This is evident from texts such as the *Viṣṇupurāṇa* and the *Harivaṁśa.* According to the former, Dhanvantari was a prince, born as a grandson of Kāśirāja, in the family of Āyus. In an earlier life, he had been born at the churning of the ocean and had obtained the right of being reborn in the family of Kāśirāja to be able to divide the Āyurveda in eight branches and become a participant in the sacrifice (*yajñabhāj,* IV, VIII, 4). The *Harivaṁśa* describes how after his birth from the ocean, he immediately demanded from Viṣṇu his part and place in the

---

[1] It makes him the twelfth incarnation of Bhagavanta in this world and calls him Dhanvantara (I, III, 17). cf., in general Louis H. Gray, *The Indian God Dhanvantari* in J.A.O.S., 1922, pp. 323-337.

[2] *Yajñe ca bhāgam amṛtāyur avāpa ruddham...* II, VII, 21. Burnouf understands it to mean that he has recovered that part of the *amṛta* which had been taken away by the *asuras* but another reading is *ruddhe;* in this case it is the sacrifice to which a stop had been put.

sacrifice; this request was not granted as the shares in the sacrifice had been fixed a long time earlier. As a compensation, he was promised divine status and cult in a second birth. He was, then, born as the son of a king of Kāśi (Kāśirāja) who had honoured him and he received the Āyurveda from Bharadvāja.[1] The texts further agree in making Divodāsa the great-grandson of Dhanvantari.[2] Under this form, the tradition offers us three personages where the *Suśruta-saṁhitā* knows of only one. Moreover, the fact that the oldest ancestor of the master of Āyurveda, Dhanvantari is known as Āyus, can lead us to think that the legend of Dhanvantari has been forged at leisure. It is, in any case, probable that some king of Kāśi had, in antiquity, acquired a reputation in medicine and that the legends, now preserved, might have been the result of the efforts to reconstitute from the Indian point of view, the life and the geneology of that prince who was accepted as a divine incarnation. If one were to view things from this angle, it will have, at least, to be accepted that extremely ancient mythical personages such as Divodāsa and Bharadvāja have, in various ways, been introduced into these legends. We have already seen that these two last-mentioned ones, sometimes seem to mingle into one. In the *Harivaṁśa,* a distinction is made between the two, as one of the two is the master of Dhanvantari and the other his great-grandson. But even here at least the notion of a relationship between Dhanvantari and Bharadvāja is present and this relationship goes back at least to the *Śāṅkhāyana-gṛhyasūtra* (ii, 14) which unites the two names of Bharadvāja and Dhanvantari, just as the *Ṛg-veda* had made a *rapprochement* between those of Bharadvāja and Divodāsa. Therefore, it does not go as far away from the tradition as one would have thought at first view, keeping in view the tradition adopted by the *Caraka-saṁhitā.*

The name of Suśruta on the one hand and that of Ātreya on the other do not let us escape the legend. Suśruta, which signifies "one who has listened well", may be studied in relation

---

1 Calcutta edition, 1523-1539, Ch. XXIX. The translation (in French) by Langlois (Vol. I, p. 129) is based on the manuscripts (Biblio. Nat., Sanskrit 369 and 382). The text of these two is often better than that of the Calcutta edition.

2 Similarly *Bhāgavata,* IX, XVII, 5.

to the epithet *bahuśruta,* "one who has listened to a lot (of things)", "an extremely learned person". As the proper name of a person, this word appears only in the classical texts and in the *Suśruta-saṁhitā* itself. Ātreya denotes "a descendant of Atri" and Atri is a Vedic personage protected by the Aśvins and Indra.[1] He is one of those "Ancients" by whom human beings trace their link with the gods. In effect, hymn I, 139 of the *Ṛg-veda* says: "Dadhyañca, Aṅgiras the elder, Priyameda, Kaṇva, Atri, Manu have known my birth; these, the Ancients[and] Manu have known it. Their line goes back to the gods and our navels are in them."[2] The legend of the transmission of the Āyurveda from the gods to human beings could find in the Vedic tradition no one more suitable than a personage who was not only the intermediary between the gods and men but also the special ward of medical gods and of the instructor god. Being too divine as he represented Agni[3], he could not as well pass for the first human being who learnt medicine from the gods, as did his descendant.

The majority of the hymns of the fifth maṇḍala of the *Ṛg-veda* is attributed to Atri and to the Ātreyas, each of whom has a personal name in addition to his surname. Among these personal names, that of Punarvasu, the Ātreya of the *Caraka-saṁhitā* is not found, but one comes across those of *Vasūyu, Vasuśruta* and *Śrutavid* which make the reader think of Punarvasu and Suśruta at the same time. *Śrutavid* signifies "one who knows what he has heard"; this is, therefore, a name quite near to that of Suśruta. *Vasūyu* can denote, "desirous of riches". For *Vasuśruta,* Monier Williams has proposed the probable rendering of "a person renowned for wealth", a sense which can be brought near to that of the epithet *vasuśravas*. *Punarvasu* is simply the name of the constellation of Gemini[4] and the names of the

---

1 Bergaigne, *Rel. Véd.*, II, p. 468.

2 *Dadhyáṅ ha me anúṣam pūrvo áṅgirāḥ priyámedhaḥ káṇvo átrir mánur vidus, té me pūrve mánur viduḥ. teṣām devèṣu āyatir asmākaṁ tèṣu nābhayaḥ. RV.*, 1, 139, 9.

3 Bergaigne, *Rel. Véd.*

4 One could here state that the Gemini are the Dioscuri who, according to the Indo-European pre-history, are related to the Aśvins. In this way, the name of Punarvasu could be the equivalent of that of the Aśvins and could have been applied to a mythical doctor, boru

constellations normally form the personal names with the sense of "born under such and such a constellation" (Pāṇini, IV, 3, 34). In any case, the frequent use of giving a name to the descendants of Atri, where *Vasu* enters as an element, goes back at least to the period when the traditional list of the descendants of Atri, who were authors of the Vedic hymns, was fixed. Moreover, *Vasu* can denote "good" and *Vasuśruta* "one who has listened to good things", that is to say, "learned in good things"; in this case *Suśruta* can be a variant of the same. The doctor Suśruta, pupil of Divodāsa could be, in this case, definitely another name of Punarvasu Ātreya, pupil of Bharadvāja. The traditions of the *Suśruta-saṁhitā* and the *Caraka-saṁhitā* agreed here although this accord was not apparent at first view and both of them had probably borrowed from a single source the names of the legendary masters of the medical science. To put it differently, they probably constituted a unique tradition, but with two different series of proper names. Otherwise, one has to attribute to chance all the resemblances and equivalences observed between the names furnished on the two sides. One can ask as to why, if the two traditions are in fact only one, they should present themselves under different forms, but this is something quite natural in India.

Quite frequently the sects or schools imitate one another and resort to plagiarism, by changing the proper names of personages whom they quote. A large number of Buddhist and Jaina legends, or Hindu and Jaina ones, attribute the same facts and gestures to their respective heroes. Naturally the two medical schools, which inherited a common tradition, had to adopt, each of them, a different way of describing the same thing. In any case, both in the *gṛhyasūtras* and in the grammatical tradition, Atri is quite often mentioned along with Bharadvāja[1] and even with Ātreya.[2] In presenting Bharadvāja and

---

under the astral influence of stars representing the Aśvins, the medical gods. But in ancient India, the Aśvins do not appear to have been identified with *Punarvasu;* the constellation bearing their name (Aśvayuj, later Aśvins) and to whom they correspond as divinities (*Taitt. S.*, IV, 4, 10) is that of the Ram.

1 For example, *Aśvalāyanagṛhyasūtra*, III, 4, 2; Pāṇini, IV, 1, 117.

2 *Gaṇapāṭha* on Pāṇini, XV, 61 and 62. The *Mahābhārata* (*Bhīṣmap.*, 376) includes "the Ātreyas associated with the Bharadvājas" in an

Ātreya[1] as teachers of medicine, the *Caraka-saṁhitā* has once again made a *rapprochement* between these two names. Of course, here one could ask if this was not there as a souvenir of the fact that at one time a real Bharadvāja had taught Ātreya, but the personage of Bharadvāja is decidedly too mythical and it will be too daring to accord a historical status to his pupil while refusing it to him himself. Most probably the author who has created the legend of the transmission of Āyurveda, as found in the *Caraka-saṁhitā*, has found it proper to suppose that the pupil of Bharadvāja had been the same personage who had been described by tradition.[2]

In any case it is possible that in antiquity a veritable Ātreya was famous as a doctor. In effect several Buddhist texts know of a doctor Ātreya and the sources of these texts appear to be quite independent of the Brahmanic texts and of the *Caraka-saṁhitā*. He is mentioned in the story of Jīvaka, doctor to the king Bimbisāra and to the Buddha, this story not being found in these texts or in this *Saṁhitā*.

Therefore it is an old story preserved in the Buddhist texts, because, except for certain variations of detail, it is the same in the texts of both the North and the South.[3] Ātreya is

---

enumeration of peoples (*ātreyaḥ sabharadvājāḥ*).

1 *Ātreya Punarvasu* and one can observe secondarily, that a supposed author of Vedic hymns (IX, 80-82) is known as Vasu Bharadvāja, that is to say, Vasu descendant of Bharadvāja.

2 The *Bṛhadar.-up.*, II, 6, 1-3, in a long list of pupils and masters, whose knowledge goes back to Brahman, there are found successively between Brahman and the most recent masters, the Aśvins, an Ātreya, master of a Bharadvāja, two other Bharadvājas and Agniveśyas. But a large number of other names separate the names of this last series and the relations between Ātreya and Bharadvāja are reversed.

3 Translations collected together by G. N. Mukhopadhyaya in *History of Indian Medicine*, Vol. III, Calcutta, 1929, pp. 681-744. To be completed with E. Chavannes, *Cinq cents contes et apologues extraits du Tripiṭaka chinois*, Paris, 1911, Vol. II, pp. 55-56(No. 189) and Vol. III, pp. 325-61 (No. 499) with the bibliography of parallel texts, Vol. IV, Paris, 1934, p. 246 (The current title, *Fa kia pi yu king*, read:- various sūtras). See also Mme. Liacre de Saint Firmin, *Médecine et légendes bouddhiques de l'Inde*, Paris, 1916, pp. 24-45. cf. also P. Cordier, *L'enseignement médical dans l'Inde ancienne*, in *Bull. de la soc. franc. d'hist. de la méd.*, 1902, p. 5 of the reprint.

described here as a renowned doctor of Takṣaśilā (Taxila), in the North-west of India. Jīvaka goes to him to study medicine and it does not take him long to surpass his master.[1] It is true that this renowned doctor is not named in Pali sources but in all these sources as also in others it is said that he resided at Takṣaśilā. Jīvaka and this Ātreya are given to be the contemporaries of the Buddha; they could, therefore, have belonged to the end of the fourth and the beginning of the fifth century B.C. Evidently it is perfectly possible that a doctor, descendant of Atri, could have won renown at Taxila during this period. But it does not follow that this person could be really the same who is referred to in the *Caraka-saṁhitā*. Hoernle has not hesitated in identifying the two persons[2], but he has not noticed that his identification raised serious difficulties. Firstly, the surname Ātreya is ascribed in the *Caraka-saṁhitā* not only to Punarvasu but also to a bhikṣu Ātreya[3], (*Sūtr.*, I, 9; XXV, 24).[4] Secondly, the personal name of the Ātreya who was the master of Jīvaka is given in the Chinese transcription in the *Sūtra on the Avadāna of Āmrapālī* and has nothing in common with Punarvasu; It is *Pin-kia-lo*, i.e., Piṅgala.[5] In the last place, the *Caraka-saṁhitā* does not give either Takṣaśilā as the residence of Ātreya Punarvasu or any other place in the North-west. It shows him teach-

1 At the time of the surgical treatment of an insect or a reptile lodged in the skull of a patient. This incident forms the subject matter of popular Indian folklore. According to the Tamil sources the master is Agattiyar (Agastya) and the pupil lives at Teraiyar (cf., M. S. Purnalingam Pillai, *Tamil Literature*, Mannirpalam, 1930, p. 29 and *Bull. de la soc. franc. d'hist. de la méd.*, janv.-fev., 1934, p. 39). For a similar story in modern Hindustani: Garcin de Tassy, *Bagh o Bahar*, Paris, 1878, p. 44.

2 *Studies in the Medicine of Ancient India*, Part I, *Osteology*, Oxford, 1907, p. 8.

3 One could be led to believe that this bhikṣu Ātreya could have more chances of being identified with the Ātreya of the Buddhist sources than Punarvasu. But, besides the fact that this *bhikṣu* is not necessarily a Buddhist, the title of *bhikṣu* does not belong exclusively to the Buddhist monks.

4 In this last passage the bhikṣu Ātreya is one of the interlocutors of Punarvasu; there can, in consequence, be no question of mixing them together.

5 Chavannes, *Cinq cents contes*, Vol. III, p. 334.

ing at Kāmpilya on the Ganges, situated in the kingdom of the Pañcālas (*Vim.*, III, 3).[1]

One can, therefore, believe that one or more Ātreyas, traditionally known as eminent doctors, have existed, but one cannot admit with Hoernle that the Ātreya Punarvasu who is said to have received the medical science from the mythical Bharadvāja was the Ātreya, who in the Buddhist sources is made a contemporary of the Buddha. The legends of the origins of the Āyurveda, as found in the two medical *saṁhitās*, do not seem to be based on any historical souvenir. They appear to have been built out of conjectures, based on the data of the Vedic tradition relating to doctor-gods, to their wards and to Brahmanical masters.

The Tradition of the Text of the Suśruta-saṁhitā:—The personage of Suśruta not being historical[2], the *Suśruta-saṁhitā* shows itself to be, not as the personal work of a certain Suśruta, but as the anonymously edited manual of a school

[1] In those parts of the *Caraka-saṁhitā* which have been revised or re-edited by the latter-day continuator of the book, Dṛḍhabala, and who, because of this fact, has lesser authority, he is shown to be on the Kailāsa (*Cik.*, XIII, 1; XXI, 1) or on the Himavant (*Cik.*, XIX, 1; XXX, 1) but this is a special story-effect.

[2] Hoernle accepts him as historical (*Osteology*, p. 8). From the fact that the tradition presents him as a pupil of the king of Kāśi and makes him teach specially surgery, he has inferred that he belonged to the "University of Kāśi" (Kāśi is mentioned as a centre of sciences in the Jātakas). In comparing the nomenclatures of bones in the *Suśruta-saṁhitā*, the *Caraka-saṁhitā* and the *Śatapathabrāhmaṇa*, he had convinced himself that Suśruta had known Ātreya, an author who was a contemporary of the Buddha (VI-V Century B.C.), and that the *Śatapatha*, whose composition he dated in the VI Century B.C., had followed the Osteological teaching of Suśruta. Ātreya and Suśruta had, therefore, both of them, belonged to the VI century B.C., the former holding school at Taxila, the latter, somewhat younger, teaching at Benares. But where Hoernle sees a reference of Suśruta to Ātreya, the latter is not mentioned in the text; nor is Suśruta mentioned in the *Śatapathabrāhmaṇa*. The tradition of the *Suśruta-saṁhitā* has possibly followed the *Brāhmaṇa* as much as it has been followed by the latter. Both of them may have borrowed from a common source. A. B. Keith has already made a number of reservations on the inferences drawn by Hoernle on this subject (*Z.D.M.G.*, 1908, p. 136). In fact these inferences arbitrarily introduced certain fallacious precisions in the history of the Āyurveda.

which had selected a Suśruta for patron. We know, by the very tradition of this school, that this manual has reached us after having been retouched at least once. The commentator Dalhaṇa (XI-XII century A.D.) affirms in effect that Nāgārjuna has been the "reconstructor" (*pratisaṁskartṛ*) of the *Suśruta-saṁhitā*.[1] Cordier has put forward the hypothesis that he has also completed the earlier text by adding thereto the last section which now forms part of the *Saṁhitā* and which is known as *Uttaratantra*, "Last section (of the book)".

The name Nāgārjuna is that of a Buddhist savant, on whose date the traditions do not agree but who is generally made to be the contemporary of the Indo-Scythian king Kaniṣka and of a Sātavāhana king. Now Kaniṣka seems to have reigned from A.D. 144[2], the Sātavāhana dynasty also being concurrently in power. The Chinese pilgrim Hiuen-tsang, who visited India between 629 and 645, also places Nāgārjuna under a Sātavāhana and describes him as a master in the science of preparing elixirs for long life and as a Buddhist savant. In this he was following a widespread tradition which associated the name of Nāgārjuna with Indian alchemy.[3] Several texts of alchemy, many therapeutic formulas, a résumé of medicine, considerably condensed but of great authority, the *Yogaśataka*, and a text of black magic, the *Kacchapuṭa* are all ascribed to him.

---

1 *Nibandhasaṅgraha, Sūtrasthāna*, I, 1. This fact has, first of all, been pointed out by Umesacandra Gupta, *Vaidyakaśabdasindhu*, Calcutta, 1894, p. 18 of the Sanskrit preface and 36 of the English preface. This has been placed in proper perspective by P. Cordier, *Nāgārjuna et l'Uttaratantra de la Suśrutasaṁhitā*, Anatanavarivo, 1896, and *Quelques données nouvelles a propos des traités médicaux sanscrits antérieurs au XII s.*, Calcutta, 1899, pp. 1 & 8.

2 R. Ghirshman, *Begram*, Cairo, 1946, p. 105.

3 cf., P. C. Ray, *History of Hindu Chemistry*, 2nd edn., 1911, Vol. II; S. Lévi, *Kaniṣka et Śātavāhana*, in J.A., Jan.-March, 1936, p. 104, and ff. Hiuen-tsang (S. Julien, *Mémoires sur les contrées occidentales*, Vol. II, p. 98) says that Nāgārjuna was well-versed in the science of medicinal herbs, used to take big tablets for maintaining his life and had attained the age of several centuries. This is to make of him a master of the *rasāyana*, the science of elixirs of youth, which is one of the eight articles of the Āyurveda and is related simultaneously to medicine and alchemy and, in the *Suśruta-saṁhitā*, more to medicine because the preparations described therein have chiefly plants for their base.

It is difficult to accept the attribution of all these texts to the Buddhist savant. The majority of these have nothing Buddhistic about them and some are ascribed to other authors, if we are to trust the colophons of certain manuscripts containing these texts. This is how the *Yogaśataka* eventually passes as a work of Vararuci while the *Kacchapuṭa* and the *Rasaratnākara* (sometimes their titles are interchanged) are ascribed to one Siddha Nityanatha.[1] The alchemical *Rasaratnākara* could really go back to the period of the Buddhist Nāgārjuna (IInd century A.D.) if it has really been imitated, as thought by L. Wieger, by the Chinese Taoist alchemist of the IIIrd century A.D., Ko-Hong, surnamed Pao-p' on-tseu.[2] The *Yogaśataka* is of a later date if the Chinese pilgrim Yi-tsing, writing in the VIIth century A.D., wrote about this text, as being an abridged text of medicine very popular and recently composed. He, however, does not give the name of this manual.[3] But as Yi-tsing has not mentioned the name of the author, we do not know if this work was at first ascribed to a Nāgārjuna, who, in this case, would be a more recent homonym of the Buddhist savant, or if the real author has been later dispossessed of his work to the benefit of Nāgārjuna. That is why we do not know if we can identify the "reconstructor" of the *Suśruta-saṁhitā* mentioned by Dalhaṇa, with the author of the *Yogaśataka* belonging to the VIIth century, or that it should be believed that the assigning of the name of Nāgārjuna is only an echo of the legend describing the great Nāgārjuna as a master of medicine and alchemy.

Happily we have elsewhere some indices of calculating the

---

1 cf., J. Filliozat, "Nāgārjuna et Agastya, médecins, chimistes, et sorciers", *Acts of XXth Inter. Congress of Orient.*, 1938, Brussells, 1940, p. 228.

2 cf., L. Wieger, *Histoire des croyances religieuses et des opinions philosophiques en Chine,* 3rd edn., Hien-hien, 1927, p. 395. The Arab writer Al-Beroni, of the XIth century, places a hundred years before his own time, an alchemist Nāgārjuna (E. Sachau, *Alberuni's India,* London, 1910, Vol. I, p. 189). It is to him that a part of the alchemical texts, attributed to the Buddhist savant of the IInd century, should be attributed, but the tradition describing the latter as an alchemist is of a very ancient date, as it was already in usage at the time of Hiuen-tsang.

3 J. Filliozat, *Fragments des textes koutchéens de médecine et magie,* Paris, 1948, p. 32.

date when the text of the *Suśruta-saṁhitā* was finally fixed. The medical manuscript found by Bower in Central Asia, at Koutcha, and published by Hoernle[1], mentions Suśruta, as also Ātreya, Bhela and other authors. Hoernle has determined the date of this manuscript with a somewhat illusory precision, but which, from the point of view of palaeography, belongs to the period of the IV to the VIth centuries; its script is clearly older than that of the script of Koutcha, of which we have examples dating from approximately A.D. 640.[2] Therefore, the *Suśruta-saṁhitā,* in its totality, goes back at least to the first centuries of our era. Elsewhere, the texts attributed to Vāgbhaṭa, the *Aṣṭāṅgasaṅgraha* and the *Aṣṭāṅgahṛdayasaṁhitā* follow and eventually reproduce the *Suśruta-saṁhitā* as it has reached us. They also reproduce the verses of the *Yogaśataka,* slightly anterior to Yi-tsing (VIIth century). The *Aṣṭāṅgahṛdaya* is quoted in the *Kitab-al Fihrist* in Arabic, in 988, under the name of *Asankar* or *Astankar*. These two texts, therefore, belong to the period between VII to Xth centuries. The *Yogaśataka* itself supposes the existence of the *Uttaratantra,* the last section of the *Suśruta-saṁhitā,* as it terminates with a similarly named section and, to all appearances, is conceived as the pendant of the whole work. One can, therefore, admit that in the VIIth century at the latest, the *Suśruta-saṁhitā* had been fixed in its present form, having already been re-adapted by the "reconstructor". Only interpolations of detail or variations have crept into the body of the text from that time up to the period of the commentaries which have reached us. The first constitution of the *Suśruta-saṁhitā* goes back much higher. Although it appears to have adopted the same legend concerning the origin of the Āyurveda as the *Caraka-saṁhitā,* as both of them designate the same legendary masters by other names and although it teaches the same doctrine, the *Suśruta-saṁhitā* is not a plagiarism of the *Caraka-saṁhitā*. The school of *Suśruta* has specialised in surgical treatment or in the application of cautery and the *Caraka-saṁhitā* in

---

1 *The Bower Manuscript,* in *Archaeological Survey of India,* Vol. XXII, Calcutta, 1893-1912.

2 Passport on wood, cf., S. Lévi, *Le tokharien B., langue de Koutcha,* in J. A., Sept.-Oct., 1913, pp. 321-22; cf., Filliozat, *Fragments,* p. 8, 23 and ff & plates, concerning the script of Koutcha in question.

such cases refers back to the specialists called "Dhānvantarīyas", that is to say, to the school of Suśruta[1], which was already constituted along with its original teaching at the time of the *Caraka-saṁhitā*. The language of the *Caraka-saṁhitā* is classical and does not correspond to a definite epoch. Certain parts of the text are in prose combined with mnemonic verses or in alternating verse and prose; other parts are entirely in verse. This manner of presentation brings this text near certain parts, in prose and verse, of the *Mahābhārata* and also of the *Arthaśāstra* assigned to Kauṭilya and which would belong to approximately 300 B.C. if the attribution were correct. Provisionally we can consider the *Suśruta-saṁhitā* as a work of the last centuries before our era, which has reached us during the first centuries of the Christian Era in an already well-defined form.

The Tradition of the Text of the Caraka-saṁhitā:—In the *Suśruta-saṁhitā*, the teaching of Divodāsa-Dhanvantari is said to have been transmitted by his direct pupil, Suśruta. In the *Caraka-saṁhitā*, on the contrary, the words of Bharadvāja, the substitute of Divodāsa, are not repeated; it is those of his pupil Ātreya, the opposite number of Suśruta, which are quoted by a pupil of the latter, Agniveśa. From this it appears that the work should be called the *Agniveśa-saṁhitā* rather than *Caraka-saṁhitā;* besides, as we have seen, the colophons make of it the *Agniveśatantra* "reconstructed" by Caraka. Caraka is not, therefore, of the rank of Suśruta but belongs rather to that of Nāgārjuna and there is no one corresponding to Agniveśa in the tradition of the *Suśruta-saṁhitā*. The following table summarises the entire legendary history of the origin and of the transmission of both of the texts and shows the theoretical position of Bhela.[2]

---

1 *tatra dhanvantariyāṇām adhikāraḥ kriyāvidhau, vaidyānām kṛtayogānām vyadhaśodhanaropaṇe*: "in this case (when the phlegm is ripe), the technique to be employed is the affair of the Dhānvantarīya doctors, who have made themselves experts in cicatrisation by piercing and by detersion."—Caraka, *Cikit.*, V, 42. *dāhe dhānvantarīyāṇām atrāpi bhiṣajam balam*: "as regards cauterisation, it is the Dhānvantarīyas who are strong."—Caraka, *Cikit.*, V, 61.

2 We leave aside the co-disciples of Agniveśa and Bhela such as Hārīta, to whom are attributed *saṁhitās* of questioned authenticity and which, because of this, we will not utilise here. On the *Hārīta-*

Agniveśa is again a mythical figure. The *Mahābhārata* knows of an Agniveśa or Agniveśya as receiving the secret of the arms (*Dhanurveda*) from Bharadvāja; this was a magic arm of Agni. He communicated this secret to the son of Bharadvāja, Droṇa. Hence, here, Agniveśa receives lessons from Bharadvāja just as he does in the *Caraka-saṁhitā;* the only difference lies in the fact that in the medical treatise he receives it by intermediaries and not directly. The *rapprochement* of the two stories shows that, on both the sides, it is a legend; there is no reason to believe that the Agniveśa, first a pupil, then master of Āyurveda, is a personage more historical than the Agniveśa, at first a pupil, then master of Dhanurveda. It is, even then, possible that a medical author had received the name or surname of a mythical master, as it seems to have happened in the case of Ātreya.

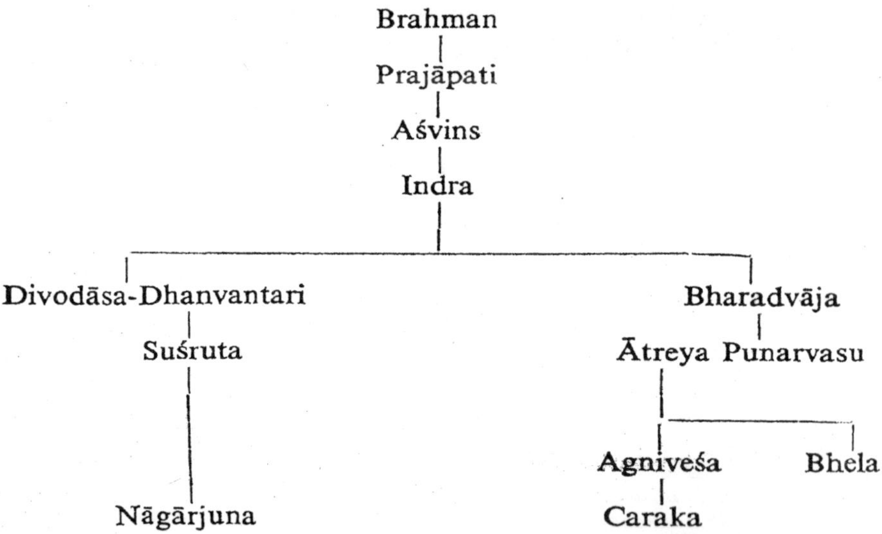

Caraka, who is not a pupil of Agniveśa but who revised the work wrongly or rightly ascribed to Agniveśa, has more chances of having been a historical personage. Certain Buddhist

saṁhitā, cf., J.A., 1934, p. 127 & ff. However we should also point out that several Hārītas and Agniveśas have, besides Carakas and the school of Ātreya, constituted various branches of the school of the *Black Yajurveda,* cf., L. Renou, *Les écoles védiques,* in *Cahiers de la soc. as.,* Paris, 1947, p. 134. We will discuss later on the eventual relations between the Carakas and Ātreyas of the Vedic schools and those of the medical ones.

texts in Chinese talk of a certain *Tche lo kia* or *Tche le*, i.e., Caraka or Cara, who was the doctor of the king Kaniṣka. This fact has been simultaneously recognised by Sylvain Lévi[1] and by Takakusu.[2] The first source, the *Tsa pao tsang king*[3], (which, in Sanskrit reads *Saṁyuktaratnapiṭakasūtra*) is an anthology of tales translated in Chinese, in 472 or a little later, by Ki Kia ye and T'an Yao. It refers only to the friendship of Kaniṣka for his doctor who by his advice keeps him protected from all diseases. The second source, the *Fou fa tsang yin yuan tchouan*[4], is said to have been translated by Ki Kia ye and T'an Yao; but H. Maspero has shown that the work in its present form is a forgery, composed in China on the lines of other works, towards the middle or the end of the VIth century.[5] One cannot, therefore, give any credit to the details given in this work, concerning the relations of Caraka and Kaniṣka, the former himself offering

---

1 *Agniveśam (Agniveśyam) mahābhāgam Bharadvājaḥ pratāpavān, pratyapādayad āgneyam astram astravidām (dharmabhṛtām) varaḥ. agnes tu (agniṣṭuj) jātaḥ sa munis tato bharatasattama, bharadvājam tad āgneyam mahāstram pratyapādayat:* "The ascetic Bharadvāja communicated to the eminent Agniveśa (°sya) the weapon of Agni; the excellent one among the experts of weapons (among the supporters of the Law), the sage born of Agni (the bard of Agni) then communicated, O the best of Bharatas, this mighty weapon of Agni to the son of Bharadvāja."—*Ādip.*, 5107-5108. In brackets the variants of the Poona edn., 1,121, 6-7. The same facts are summarised still further, *Ādip.*, 6465. Reference is made by Droṇa to his studies under Agniveśa, *Ādip.*, 5172 (Sukthankar reads this time Agniveśa, yet the same reading should be kept in the three passages). And again *Ādip.*, 5524-5525, gives Agastya and not Bharadvāja as the teacher of Agniveśa. Last of all, Agniveśya is described by Droṇa (*Droṇap.*, 3476) as having received the magical protection of Bṛhaspati; he is not, therefore, the pupil of only Bharadvāja but this detail is of no importance to our subject.

---

1 *Notes sur les Indo-scythes*, in *J. A.*, Nov.-Dec., 1896, pp. 451, 473 480 & ff.

2 *A Record of the Buddhist Religion* by I-tsing, Oxford, p. lix.

3 Catalogue by Nanjio, 1329, Taisho Issaikyō, 203, translated by Chavannes, *Cinq cents contes. . .* Vol. III, p. 1-145 (which summarises, without giving them in full, the tales already translated by S. Lévi).

4 Nanjio, 1340, Taisho, 2058.

5 About the date and the authenticity of the *Fou fa ysang yin yuan tchouan*, in *Mélanges d'indianisme. . . .*, Sylvain Lévi, Paris, 1911 pp. 129-149.

his services as a doctor to the king, and by means of clever obstetrical moves, twice saving the queen on her death-bed while in the throes of delivery[1], leaving the king who did not pay much attention to his advice and retiring from the world. It is necessary at least that these details be confirmed by a reliable source. In any case, the fact of the presence of Caraka in the court of Kaniṣka could be true, as it is also attested elsewhere and for the moment, this is all that matters here for fixing the date of the revision by Caraka of the text attributed to Agniveśa. But we cannot be sure that the legend of Kaniṣka has not placed in the court of this prince a celebrity of another epoch, either older, or more recent. It is true that the *Tsa pao tsang king,* translated in Chinese only about three hundred years after the reign of Kaniṣka, existed in Sanskrit before and had, therefore, been composed at a date quite near to that of Kaniṣka. The memory of the real contemporaries of this prince could have been faithfully preserved till then and, in any case if it were the question of a more recent author, the Caraka in question could not have lived a long time after the IInd century.

On the other hand, even if the doctor of Kaniṣka was effectively called Caraka, we are not certain that he was the same Caraka, who has revised the *Agniveśa-tantra.* Several doctors have possibly had the name of Caraka. The name of Nāgārjuna was that of an alchemist of the Xth century, mentioned by

---

1 Dr. Liétard in his "Le médecin Caraka", in *Bull. de l'Acad. de médicine,* session of 11 May 1897, p. 3 of the reprint, thought that the operation referred to was the extraction of a still-born child with its feet downwards and that Caraka considered as normal only a delivery with the head downwards, thus following the doctrine of Hippocrates (which could have easily reached him in N. W. India where ruled Kaniṣka) and ignored at that time the more advanced doctrine of Soranus of Ephesus (beginning of the IInd century). But there is nothing in the text which leads one to believe that the child was coming out with feet first or, and that is more important, that Caraka considered a delivery as abnormal if it was not with the head first. It was a case of dystocia and Caraka put his hand in the womb, brought out the child from its envelope, succeeded in extracting it and gave as prognostic the recurrence of the same trouble in case of a new delivery. These vague indications are an honour to his obstetrical cleverness, but they do not reveal anything concerning his theories. Similarly it was not necessary to know the teachings of Hippocrates for knowing that in a case of delivery, the normal presentation is that of the head first.

al-Beroni, while in the VIth century it was, for Hiuen-tsang, the name of a great master of alchemy and medicine. It is therefore not excluded *a priori* that our medical author might have been anterior to the epoch of Kaniṣka. The name of Caraka is an old one. It is that of a school of the *Black Yajurveda,* the *Caraka-śākhā,* which consists of, besides other sub-divisions, those whose *saṁhitās* have reached us in a more or less complete form under the names of *Kāṭhaka, Kapiṣṭhala-kaṭhasaṁhitā* and *Maitrāyaṇī-saṁhitā.*[1] This school is opposed to that of the *Taittirīyas,* which has given us the *Taittirīya-saṁhitā* and for stronger reasons to the schools of the *White Yajurveda,* represented by the *Vājasaneyī-saṁhitās.* The scholars of the *White Yajurveda* and the *Taittirīyas* often blame the *Carakas.* A passage of the *Taittirīya-saṁhitā* (VI, 4, 9) could be interpreted as covering under the same reprobation the Carakas and the doctors:

"The head of the sacrifice had been cut. The gods said to the Aśvins: "You are doctors, put back the head of the sacrifice." They replied: "Let us select a boon that the libation be drawn by us right here!" They drew for them the libation of the Aśvins. Then they put back the head so that the (libation) of the Aśvins is drawn for re-establishing the sacrifice. The gods said of them: "They are impure, they are the doctors roving among men." Thus a Brahmin must not take to medicine, because the doctor is impure and unworthy of the sacrifice. After having purified them by the *bahiṣpavamānas,* they (the gods) drew for them the (libation) of the Aśvins. Thus it is that after *bahiṣpavamāna* has been recited, that the (libation) for the Aśvins is drawn..."[2]

The saṁhitās of the *Caraka-śākhā* explain the same incident somewhat differently:

Kāṭhaka, XXVII, 4:

"The head of the sacrifice has been cut. The Aśvins who did not drink soma were the doctors of the gods. The gods said to them: "You are doctors, put back the head of the sacrifice." They replied: "Let us demand a boon: that we may drink the soma among the gods, that the

1 cf., L. Renou, *Ecoles vėdiques,* pp. 129, 144, 150 & ff., p. 203 & ff.

2 *Yajñasya śiro'chidayata, té devā aśvínāv abruvan, bhiṣájau vaí stha, idám yajñásya śiraḥ práti dhattam íti. tāv abrūtām, váram vṛṇavāvahai gráha evá nāv átrāpi gṛhyatām íti. tābhyām etám āsvinám agṛhṇan. tato vaí taú yajñásya śiraḥ prátyadhattām, yád āśvinó gṛhyáte, yajñásya niṣkṛtyai taú devā ábruvann ápūtau vā imaú manuṣyacaraú bhiṣájāv íti. tásmād brāhmaṇéna bhesajám ná kāryam, apūto hy eṣo'medhyó yó bhiṣák, bahiṣpavamāṇéna pavayitvā tābhyām etám āśvinám agṛhṇan tasmād bahiṣpavamānė stutā āśvinó gṛhyate. . not,.*—*Taitt. S.* VI, 4,9.

libation be drawn for us." The gods, having purified them by means of the *bahiṣpavamāna,* drew the libation for them, the pure ones, the ones worthy of the sacrifice. Thus it is that (only) after the *bahiṣpavamāna* has been recited, that the (libation) for the Aśvins is drawn..."[1]

Maitr., VI, 6, 2:

".....The created head of the sacrifice had been cut. For him the gods searched an expiation. Then, the Aśvins, who did not partake of the soma, were the doctors of the gods. They ran to these two as one rushes to a doctor: "Put back the head of the sacrifice." They replied: "That we should also have a share in the same." "Select!" said (the gods). They said: "That the libation be drawn for us, that we may have access to soma-drinking." The Aśvins then put back the head. (The gods) having purified them by the *bahiṣpavamāna,* drew the libation for them, who had become pure, worthy of the sacrifice. Thus it is that after the *bahiṣpavamāna* has been recited that the (libations) for the Aśvins are drawn..."[2]

The different *saṁhitās* are thus unanimous in admitting the impurity of the *Aśvins* who are not soma-drinkers originally although, as says the *Ṛg-veda,* the "drinkers of nectar" (*madhupa,* I, 180, 2).[3] But the *Taittirīya-saṁhitā* goes a step farther than the rest, it vilifies the doctor and says that the Aśvins are impure like "doctors roving among men." Certainly, the promiscuity with human beings places them below the gods, but the term employed to say that they are "roving," *cara*, is a

1 *....Yajñasya vai'siro'cchidyata, atha tarhy aśvinā asomapau bhiṣajau devānām āstām, tau devā abruvan, bhiṣajau vai stha, idam yajñasya śirah paridhattam iti tā abruvatām, vāryam vṛṇāvahai, somapītho nau deveṣu astu, Graho nau gṛhyatām iti, tau devā bahiṣpavamāṇena pāvayitvā tābhyām śucibhyām medhyābhyāṃ bhūtābhyāṃ graham agṛhṇaṁs, tasmāt, stute bahiṣpavamane āśvino gṛhyate..* (ed., Schroeder., Leipzig., 1909. Vol. II, p. 143). The *Kapiṣṭhalakaṭha-saṁhitā* gives, with small variations about the same text (XLII, 4, ed., Raghuvira, Lahore, 1932, p. 251).

2 *Yajñásya vai sṛṣṭásya 'siro'cchidyata, tásmai devāḥ prāyáścittam aicchann, átha vā etaú tárhi devānām bhiṣájā āstām aśvínā ásomapau, tā úpādhāvan, yáthā bhiṣájam upadhāvanty evám, idám yajñásya śíraḥ prátidhattam íti. tā abrútām, bhāgó nā astu, vṛṇāthām íti, abruvaṁs, tā abrūtāṃ gráhaṁ nau gṛhṇantu somapīthám áśnavāvahā íti, tád vā aśvinau prátyadhattām, tásmād āśvínibhi abhiṣṭuvanti, aśvínau hi pratyádhattām, taú vai bahiṣpavamāṇénaiva pāvayitvā tābhyām pūtábhyām yajñíyābhyām bhūtābhyām gráham agṛhṇaṁs, tásmād bahiṣpavamāné stutā aśvinaú gṛhyete* (ed., Schroeder, Leipzig, Vol. IV, 1886, pp. 79-80).

3 This is explained by Indo-European facts, cf. G. Dumézil, *Jupiter Mars Quirinus,* Paris, 1941, pp. 124 & ff., where the parallel legends of the *Śatapathabrāhmaṇa* & the *Mahābhārata* are given together. The notion of the impurity of doctors has remained a classic thing, cf. *Manu,* III, 180, IV, 212, although the prohibition ordained by the *Taitt, S.* to the Brahmin against his practising medicine, has not had the force of Law. The *Bhāgavatapurāṇa,* IX, III, 26, reminds the reader that the Aśvins had been at first excluded from the offering of soma because they were called "doctors".

syńonym of the name of the Carakas and one may believe that the *Taittirīyas* have fired a passing shot at the rival school of the Carakas, who have not inserted anything similar in their *saṁhitā*. This will be all the more effective if medicine had a place of honour among them. In that case this will also explain their silence about it. Besides, as regards the *sautrāmaṇi,* the rite of offering liquor (*surā*) to the Aśvins, to Sarasvatī and to Indra, Hillebrandt has supposed a relationship between the fact that there is a *caraka-sautrāmaṇi* and the fact that the medical *Caraka-saṁhitā* makes out a case for liquor.[1] This *rapprochement*, in itself, is not very characteristic because it is quite natural that liquor be praised as medicine in a book of medicine. But, in all cases, the Carakas are not animated against the "*cara* doctors", as are the Taittirīyas and the doctor Caraka could have been one of them.

This does not at all signify that the author of the revised version of the *Agniveśatantra* lived at the time when the Vedic *saṁhitās* of the Carakas were elaborated but it can indicate that he belonged to their school, already favourable to medicine at a time when its rival used to attack the "*cara* doctors". In fact, the extremely brahmanic contents of the *Caraka-saṁhitā* evoke the idea that its editor was rather a Brahmin of a Vedic school than a doctor practising at the court of an Indo-Scythian prince. Moreover, if it is considered that another school of the *Yajurveda* was the Ātreya[2] school, one will be led to think that it was not because of mere chance that the chief masters of one of the great medical traditions are precisely an Ātreya and a Caraka. It is at least probable that the association of the medical tradition in question with the circles close to the Vedic schools was desired, as it could plausibly have been derived from the latter. If, therefore, Kaniṣka has had a Caraka for his doctor, it is nevertheless possible that a Caraka still older might have been the veritable editor of our actual *Caraka-saṁhitā*.

---

1 *Ritual-Litteratur* (Grundriss), Strasbourg, 1897, p. 159. A. B. Keith, *The Veda of the Black Yajus School*, Harvard Or. S., XVIII, p. cxxii, contests the *rapprochement* without any decisive reasons and prefers to see in the *Caraka-sautrāmaṇi* that of the school of Carakas. But the two points of view are not contradictory if the doctor Caraka has some relation with the school of the Carakas.

2 L. Renou, *Ecoles védiques*, p. 134.

One cannot, in any case, rate this text very high. Its style is not Vedic; it resembles that of the *Suśruta-saṁhitā* and of the *Arthaśāstra*. The work can be anterior to the Christian era but not by a long period of time.

According to a tradition, which should now be examined, Caraka was the incarnation of the mythical serpent Śeṣa, who became a human being, in order to write under the name of Patañjali, the *Mahābhāṣya* and the *Yogasūtras*. This is apparent from one of the preliminary invocations of the *Āyurveda-dīpikā*, a commentary by Cakrapāṇidatta or Cakradatta (XIth century), on the *Caraka-saṁhitā*: "Adoration to the Lord of the serpents, the destroyer of the troubles of the mind, of speech and of body by *Pātañjala*[1], the *Mahābhāṣya* and the work reconstituted by Caraka."[2] A later author, Śivarāma, the commentator of the *Vāsavadattā*, describes Patañjali as a grammarian, a master of yoga and a doctor.[3] The invocation of Cakradatta, however, does not signify that the three works are of one and the same author; the three authors could also have been considered as the three successive incarnations of Śeṣa. The tradition, which finds its echo in the invocation, does not, therefore, imply that the *Caraka-saṁhitā* was, at an earlier date, regarded as having been revised by the grammarian Patañjali himself or as belonging to the same period. One can, however, as we have seen, place Caraka in the IInd or in the Ist century B.C., which was the period of Patañjali."[4]

1 *Pātañjalamahābhāṣyacarakapratisaṁskṛtaiḥ, manovākkāyadoṣāṇāṃ hartre'dhipataye namaḥ*, verse 4. This verse has been reproduced with the variant *hantre* in the *Patañjalicaritra* of Ramabhadra Diksita, an author who cannot be dated beyond the XVIII century, cf., S. N. Dasgupta, *Yoga Philosophy*, Calcutta, 1930, p. 54.

2 That is to say, the *Yogasūtras*.

3 cf., G. N. Mukhopadhyaya, *History of Indian Medicine*, Vol. III, p. 799.

4 Ordinarily it is admitted that Patañjali belongs to the middle of the IInd century B.C., partly as he talks, in the present tense, of a sacrifice which is being held on the orders of the king Puṣyamitra. But since this is only an ordinary example of grammar, it is naive to believe that he was composing his work during the sacrifice itself. On the other hand, he mentions the Śakas who were, in that period, still far from India but who invaded the country in the beginning of the Ist century B.C. (cf., La Vallée de la Poussin, *L'Inde au temps des Maurya*, Paris, 1930, p. 201) However, his place in the line of grammarians puts him at least in the Ist century B. C.

But the problem is complicated by the fact that still other texts are ascribed to Patañjali. There has been, for a long time, a discussion on the possibility of joining together the Patañjali of the *Mahābhāṣya* and that of the *Yogasūtras*.[1] Moreover, al-Bēroni frequently quotes and summarises *Pātañjala*.[2] This is a work on mysticism apparently quite close to the *Yogasūtras* but differing from them, notably by the fact that it contains a section on alchemy. Now Śivadāsasena in his commentary on the *Cakradatta-saṅgraha* (a work of the commentator of Caraka)[3] also invokes several times as an authority on alchemy Patañjali or his *Pātañjala*. One can admit the existence of several Patañjalis but it is to be feared that we find ourselves once again in the presence of legendary attributions. In effect these attributions remind one of those which are ascribed to Nāgārjuna, which include an ensemble of philosophy, alchemy and medicine; now the name of Nāgārjuna signifies "The White one among the serpents"[4] and the legend says that Patañjali, the incarnation of the serpent Śeṣa, was born while falling (*pat*) in the shape of a serpent, in the hands of the grammarian Pāṇini at the moment when the latter was making an *añjali*.[5] Of course this etymology has no linguistic value but it explains all that which the legend has made of the grammarian Patañjali, who was not probably a historic personage. This being so, one may ask if Patañjali, claimed as a doctor and an alchemist like Nāgārjuna, is not a double of the Buddhist Nāgārjuna[6] as we have seen that Divodāsa and Bharadvāja on the one hand, and Suśruta and Ātreya Punarvasu on the other, were the doubles of the same

---

1 cf., Mircea Eliade, *Yoga*, Paris, 1936 pp. 27 & ff.

2 E. Sachau, *Alberuni's India*, Vol. I, pp. 68 ff & *passim*.

3 cf., G.N. Mukhopadhyaya, *op. cit.*, pp. 771 & 783-785 (references to pages of an unspecified edition), the quotations in question are to be found in the Chapter LXVI (*Rasāyanādhikāra*) of the edition of Jīvānanda Vidyasagara, 3rd edn., Calcutta, 1897, pp. 706 & ff.

4 The Tibetan translation of the name, *kluí sgrub*, signifies "Perfect among the serpents".

5 cf., H. H. Wilson, *A Dictionary of Sanskrit & English*, see Patañjali. Moreover the *Mahābhāśya* of Patañjali is sometimes called *Phaṇibhāṣya*, "the commentary of the hooded serpent".

6 Śivadasasena invokes at the same time, as authorities in alchemy, Nāgārjuna and Patañjali and as a consequence makes a distinction between the two, but this only proves that in his times, different works were attributed to them.

mythical personages. In that case, Caraka confused with Patañjali by virtue of their being the incarnation of the same serpent, or even simply identified with Patañjali, could have been confused with Nāgārjuna. The reviser of the *Caraka-saṁhitā* and that of the *Suśruta-saṁhitā* will then be one.

In that case one would be tempted to suppose that historically it has been so and that the two big medical *saṁhitās* have been revised by one and the same author, who has been given two different names by the traditions of the two schools. But this conclusion is too hazardous. It is quite possible that the grammarian Patañjali, the doctor Caraka and the Buddhist savant Nāgārjuna have existed independently and that the stories which identify them or which make them identical, have come into being secondarily. In effect these names are attested much before we have proof of the existence of these legends. The origins of these can be linked with the name of Nāgārjuna or with ideas which have given him this name. In India it is a common usage to demolish the claims of others, not by denying them, but by appropriating them. Senart has shown that the serpent has often played the same role in the Buddhist and Vaiṣṇava stories.[1] Nāgārjuna is said to have seized the doctrines of the Mahāyāna from the Nagas, who had been keeping them hidden in the depths of the *Pātāla* and Viṣṇu is said to have brought out from the same depths the Vedas, which had been stolen by the Asuras or by the Nagas."[2] It was natural that a Buddhist savant and a Brahmanic savant or a group of Brahmanic savants, both parties having relation with the serpents, made a pair. If once the revision of the *Suśruta-saṁhitā* had been attributed to Nāgārjuna, if it were really the work of a savant of that name, it was necessary that the reviser of the *Caraka-saṁhitā* also became the incarnation of the mythical *Nāga*, as his school would not have liked to have been left behind. It does not follow in the least therefrom that the two personages must have been the same historic personage. From this we can only conclude that the stories told about the classical redaction of the two *saṁhitāṣ* have a common source;

---

[1] cf., notably regarding the serpent *Śeṣa: Essai sur la légende du Buddha*, 2nd edn., Paris, 1882, p. 218, notes in general, Chap. V.

[2] Senart, *ibid*, p. 389.

this is all the more understandable since the texts manifestly belong to the same epoch.

As regards the connection of the legend of Caraka with that of the grammarian Patañjali, this forms part of an ensemble of concordances between the legends of the transmission of grammar and that of the transmission of medical science. We have already seen that a tradition attributes the teaching of grammar to Indra. Pāṇini (VII, 2, 63) quotes the opinion of a Bharadvāja who could have been a real personage and whose name only signifies "descendant of *Bharadvāja*". But chiefly Kātyāyana, the predecessor of Patañjali-Caraka, is sometimes, as the exegetist of Pāṇini, called Punarvasu[1], just as in the medical traditions the teacher of Caraka passes for having been Punarvasu. The late character of the attribution of this name to Kātyāyana indicates that probably this is only a secondary adaptation of the story of the doctors to that of the grammarians, but this attribution gives an example of the way in which the Indians have readapted the history of their sciences.[2] This is then another sign that the stories of the origins and of the transmission of the Āyurveda are not at all altered history but are the ideal reconstitutions of a history that had been lost or neglected and the names given to the authors of the big medical *saṁhitās* are not, undoubtedly, those which they really had, unless they had precisely selected these names or had received them as surnames. The medical *saṁhitās* cannot therefore be dated surely according to the possible epochs of their supposed authors. It is only their intrinsic composition, the state of their language and their place in relation to the texts of known date which allow the assigning to approximate period for their composition.

Essential Doctrines of the Ayurvedic texts:—The large *saṁhitās* are didactic texts in prose and verse of varied metres. The prose passages generally contain mnemonic verses which summarise them. The chapters entirely in verse are specially those that contain the enumeration of symptoms or therapeutic prescriptions. They are, therefore, the ones which it is most

---

1 In the latter-day dictionaries, cf. Bohtlingk & Roth, see the word.

2 We may also remind here that the *Yogaśataka* is sometimes attributed to Vararuci instead of Nāgārjuna and that the name of Vararuci is often given to Kātyāyana.

useful to know by heart for practising, whereas the passages in prose generally deal with the theoretical principles. The choice of prose or verse seems, therefore, to have been dictated chiefly by a pedagogic desire. Their alternation is not the sign of the intervention of several authors in the composition of the *saṁhitās*. The prose-parts, chiefly in the *Caraka-saṁhitā*, remind one of the theoretical accounts of the *Brāhmaṇas* and the *Upaniṣads*. In a certain number of cases they have the same dialogue-form as in these later texts, but the language has the characteristic of being more recent.

The *Suśruta-* and the *Caraka-saṁhitās* have, as a whole, the same contents. Their divisions are identical or analogous. The same is the case for their theoretical and practical data, but the *Suśruta-saṁhitā* is much more rich in the field of surgery than the *Caraka-saṁhitā*. Both of them generally present their teaching in an extremely condensed form. But because of the abundance of matter, they are, nevertheless, voluminous. They profess a rational system which excludes magic and mysticism. They invoke the intervention of demons only in special cases: delirium of possession and the diseases of children. Ordinarily they explain the state of health and of disease by the interplay of constitutive elements of the organism, of the alimentary and general regimes and by the influences of time and season. It is only in the case of certain therapeutic prescriptions, or in the case of ceremonies connected with birth that religion and magic are brought in.

Experience has manifestly played an important role, as is always the case in medicine, in the establishment of therapeutics. But we are still far from the state where we could say that medical practice as taught by the Āyurveda is empirical. The data of experience are organised according to a general theory of physio-pathology. This is a complex theory. In the texts can be found the traces of the different currents of thought which have simultaneously exerted an influence on its formation. The general theory of the Sāṁkhya, which enumerates the formative elements of the universe, is added on to particularly medical conceptions. These latter see in the body a composition of chief elements which forms the material content of all things in the universe: Space or emptiness—(*ākāśa* or *antarikṣa*), wind or air (*vāyu*), fire (*tejas*), water (*ap*) and earth (*pṛthvī*), to which various texts add thought (*cetanā*) which sits inside this body[1] as is frequently done by the Buddhist texts which call this thought, *Vijñāna*.

These chief elements form the differentiated substances of the organism which, in their turn, are the "elements" (*dhātu*) of this organism and are seven in number: the organic juice (*rasa*) which is the chyle, the blood (*rakta*) which is the chyle coloured in red, the flesh (*māṁsa*), fat (*medas*), bones (*asthi*), the marrow (*majjā*) and the sperm (*śukra*), all of which, starting from *rasa* derive one from the other[2]. The *rasa* is therefore the primordial substance of the organism and certain authors took it to be the essence of water which generates everything.[3] Besides, in all things there is a *rasa*, a "taste", the liquid element which constitutes simultaneously the substratum and the sign of the properties, of the virtues of this thing.[4]

The substances contain a liquid of principle effulgence (*tejas*) which makes them alive and which is known as *ojas*, that is to say, "force."[5] It is the material of vitality and it may be

---

1 Caraka, *Śār,* I. 14; Suśr., V, 1, In the sperm, Caraka recognises only four of them, because he does not take into account space (*Śār*., II, 4); the same is the case with the embryo (*Śār*., II, 35). An opinion attributed specially to Bharadvāja also does not consider space (Caraka, *Sūtra,* XXV, 21). This does not contradict the theory of five elements as, in the passages under consideration, space can be considered as omitted simply because there was no need to mention it in the context of the particular topic under discussion. On the other hand, the allusions to general doctrines found in the Buddhist texts generally refer to four elements, the same as those of the Greeks, cf., *Mahāvastu*, ed. Senart, Vol. III, p. 65; P. Demiéville in *Hôbôgobirin*, fasc. III, p. 264.

2 Suśruta, *Sūtr.*, XIV, 6.

3 Such is the opinion ascribed to Vāryovida in Caraka, *Sūtr*, XXV, 13: "Things and diseases of various types are born of the *rasa,* because the waters are rich with the *rasas*, waters about which it is said that they are the cause of creation" *(rasajāni tu bhūtāni vyādhayaśca pṛthagvidhāḥ, āpo hi rasavatyas tāḥ smṛtāḥ nirvṛtti-hetavaḥ).* This opinion has antecedents from the *Ṛg-Veda* onwards, X,129, 1 & 3, where water is described as the origin of things. The waters are also the primordial element according to a classic passage of Manu (I, 8 & 10). But the theory of Manu is a creationism, which is not the case with the one ascribed to Vāryovida.

4 On the *rasas*: Caraka., *Sūtr*., XXVI, an important discussion of theories.

5 Suśr., *Sūtr*., XV, 13-14.

called "vital juice". It stays in the heart; the breath (*prāṇa*), which is going to be discussed shortly hereafter is based on it and it is distributed in the body along with *prāṇa*, by the blood-vessels.[1]

Such is the substance of the body. The interplay of the three chief elements, which enter into its composition, namely, wind, fire and water, gives it life and movement. But when they are excited or when on the contrary, their action stops, disease comes in. They are, therefore, simultaneously the three elements, *tridhātus* and the three troubles, *tridoṣas* of the organism. The wind *vāta* or *vāyu*, introduces itself into the body in its own form just as in nature, that of a breath, *prāṇa*; the fire in the form of bile, *pitta*, and water in that of phlegm, *kapha* or *śleṣman*. Each of them has many special forms.

The *prāṇa* is divided into *prāṇa* proper, "breath of the front", which stays in the mouth and ensures respiration and deglutition; *udāna*, "breath which goes upwards", which produces speech; *samāna*, "concentrated breath", which provides the necessary amount of air to the internal fire for cooking, that is to say, for the process of digestion of the aliments; *apāna*, "breath which goes downwards", ensuring the functions of excretion and delivery; finally *vyāna*, "diffused breath", which circulates in all the limbs and explains their movement.[2] In effect, all the movements of the body are related to the action of the wind; this is by analogy with what passes in the Universe where the wind is the motor *par excellence*.

Fire, represented by bile in five forms, is the *pācaka*, the cooker of aliments; the *rañjaka*, the colouring agent, which turns the *rasa* red for making it into blood; the *sādhaka*, the "realiser", by means of which desires are excited; the *ālocaka*, the "observer", which shines in the eye and allows the sight to function and the *bhrājaka*, the "illuminator" which shines in the skin.[3]

Water for its part, under the various forms of *śleṣman*, is that element of the organism which is humid, cold and is the connector of all the elements together. It stays chiefly in the

---

1 Caraka, *Sūtr.*, XXX, 6-11
Suśr., *Nid.*, I, 11 & ff.
ibid., *Sūtr.*, XXI, 7

stomach, which is the centre of its functions. In the chest, it maintains the junction of the head and arms and supports the heart. In the throat and the tongue, it ensures gustation. In the head, it favours the sensorial faculties. In the articulations, it brings about coaptation.[1]

The seasons, the habitat, the type of life and the various types of nourishment help or hinder the action of wind, fire and water according as they affect the activity, the over-heating or the cooling (of the body).

Nosology studies the symptoms of diseases and thereby is related to observation, but it tries to interpret these symptoms as a function of the system of the physiology of the three elements. Its principal aim is to determine the etiology or, as it is known in the Ayurvedic texts, the *nidāna*, the occasion when troubles arise. This occasion, determined by the time, the regimen, the behaviour or such other cause, consists in the excitation or the slowing down of the one or several of these elements. Diagnosing does not consist of only recognising a disease but also of a judgement concerning the rôle exercised by the mind, the bile or the phlegm. A haemorragic fever will come from *rakta-pitta,* from "blood and bile"; from the bile because it is hot and from the blood because it appears and it overflows. Descriptions are given concerning all the supposed manifestations of the excess or the absence of each of the three *doṣas,* or of the combinations of any two among these when excited or of the concourse (*sannipāta*) of the three.

Therapeutics is dominated by the ideas that have been conceived about the soothing or exciting action of drugs, of aliments, of diet, of the place of habitation, on the mind, the bile or phlegm. In the presence of the patient, once the symptoms have been recognised, once the rôle of such and such a *doṣa* has been determined, the Indian doctor must prescribe a medicine having the antagonistic effect on the *doṣas* concerned. A treatment based on a theory which is false could have been singularly hazardous; yet the theory is sufficiently supple and vague for adjusting itself to the data of pure experience, although all the time it appears to excel the latter. In fact, the action of the remedies had been known by the usage, and, if a

[1] ibid., *Sūtr.*, XXI, 11.

particular drug had a soothing effect on the certain morbid manifestation believed to be caused by the wind, this drug was ranged among the drugs antagonistic to the wind, an explanation of this fact being invented later. It was therefore definitely the experience which guided the choice of the medicines and the general theory was only a later effort to explain simultaneously the mechanism of the normal functioning of the body, that of the pathological accidents and that of the action of the treatment. Thus the system of the Āyurveda is a dogmatism which interprets experience.

This system is comparable to some of the medical systems of Greek antiquity, which were also elaborated in the centuries preceding the Christian era. The collection of Hippocrates contains the elements of the doctrine which was fixed later with a rigour comparable to that of the Ayurvedic theory and which relates to four humours: blood, bile, atrabile and phlegm, corresponding to four chief elements and to their properties, hot, dry, cold and humid. The existence, with regard to the humoral doctrine of the Greek world, of the Ayurvedic system of the three *doṣas* should evidently be recognised as one of the facts dominating the general history of ancient medicine. Both of them have been simultaneously recognised as authoritative since antiquity, one in the Indian world and the other in the Western world. Both of them are still followed. The Greek doctrine survives in the countries of Islam. The Indian system not only continues in India, but at present it is even undergoing a vigorous renaissance. It has been adopted since an early date, in all those countries which have been under the influence of India, as far as Mongolia, from which it has come, towards the end of the last century and the beginning of the present one, to provoke in Russia an infatuation for the medical system called the "Tibetan", because it had reached the Mongols through the Tibetans.

Both of them being based on the representation, which the "physiologists" made of the Universe, the medical theories of Greece and India make a pair, not only because historically speaking, they have had an equal diffusion in two comparable worlds, but also because they are related to analogous speculations, because their organic constitution is similar and they are scientific in the same sense, inasmuch as they are efforts at a purely natural explanation of vital, normal and pathological phenomena.

We should, therefore, look for the birth of a scientific Āyurveda in the texts which have preceded it. The mythical character of the stories, of its origin and its transmission, which it itself contains, should not be allowed to convince us that its doctrines are sullied with myths. We have seen that the tradition concerning the masters of the Āyurveda was full of Vedic reminiscences as the supposed Vedic authors have Vedic names. We will also see that the antecedents of the classical doctrines of the *Āyurveda* are equally Vedic. There is, however, a contrast between the value of the expositions concerning the history of the Āyurveda which is nil and that of the meritorious efforts made to explain rationally health and disease. But the legend of the origin and the transmission of the Āyurveda is only pseudo-historical with a veneer of the scientific doctrine. This doctrine is derived from Brahmanic speculations, if not valid by themselves, at least by the tendency of the spirit that animated them; moreover, it is partly based on the observation of normal and pathological facts, thus giving it a connection with reality. The legends of the origins, on the contrary, although they utilise the data from the Veda and refer to the names of authors of yore, do not seem to be based on a tradition with a historical basis, ancient and solid. In studying the relations of the Veda and the Āyurveda, we will, however, examine the extent to which it may be described as accurate.

CHAPTER TWO

PRE-ARYAN AND INDO-ARYAN DATA ON MEDICINE

1. The First Data

It is only since 1922 that the excavations carried out by R. D. Banerji and the Archaeological Survey of India, have brought to light, at Mohen-jo-Daro in Sindh, the remains of the civilization known as the Indus Valley Civilization. These remains are related to the ones revealed by the excavations at Harappa in the Panjab. Despite the absence of any real decipherment of the inscriptions found there and despite the incomplete state of excavatory work of great depth, this discovery has already given rise to a multitude of fantastic theories. However many facts are already accepted; at least everybody agrees on points of major importance. The old age of the ruins is attested to by the thickness of the alluvial stratum which had covered them and also by the discoveries made outside India, at Kish, at Ur, at Tello and at Susa in the strata going to 3rd millennium B.C. of seals manifestly coming from the Indus or belonging to the same type of those of the Indus.

Evidently we can know nothing positive concerning the position of medicine in the Indus civilization. But the ruins of the extremely large town excavated at Mohen-jo-daro are particularly remarkable in view of the uncovered remains of the large-scale works of public sanitation. All the houses have a place for washing. In poorer houses this consists of an ordinary room with a water-proof floor sloping towards a drain. In bigger houses, there are proper bath-rooms. The drains of the houses end in a system of street-drains which is spread over all the streets. The biggest building contains a bath of 55 meters by 33 meters, with a tank of 13 meters by 7 meters, having a depth of 2.5 meters and with many subsidiary constructions manifestly used for the purpose of baths.

It is asked if the big bath could be compared to the thermal baths of the Romans, used for hygiene, hydrotherapy and sports or was it meant for religious purposes. Of these two the former hypothesis is much more probable as the importance of the individual installations shows very well the liking of the habitants for ablutions and bath.

But did the water used in the big bath have any medicinal properties ? Nothing allows us to suppose so. If the big bath were the only hydrotherapic installation favoured in the town, one could think so. But the individual installations could not have been uniquely destined for cures ; they were put up for daily use. We can, therefore, conclude that in all likelihood, the ruins of Mohen-jo-daro attest, from the 3rd millennium B.C., to the existence of personal and urban hygiene in India.

Much later, hygiene and hydrotherapy come to have a great importance in the eyes of the doctors of the classical periods and they become very popular in the convents as also in private life.[1] Therein one can observe a persistence of the tastes and usages going back to the Indus civilisation. But it should not be forgotten that such tastes and such usages are born naturally in a tropical country. In any case, the well-developed ideas of hygiene, apparent from the monuments of the Indus, was neither necessarily scientific nor even medical. A system of hygiene can be medical and scientific only if it is based on the conceptions of prophylaxy and therapeutics. Otherwise, it remains only commonplace cleanliness or luxury. The hydrotheraphy of Suśruta[2] and Caraka[3] provides for treatments by *svedas*, the "sudations" achieved by extremely varied methods, generally much more complex than baths and shower-baths. The choice of these methods is dictated by the properties of soothing or exciting the various vital elements of the organism, which are ascribed to these methods. Drugs are incorporated in the water to be used. Nothing can indicate if, at Mohen-jo-daro, hydrotherapy already had assumed forms comparable to those described by the doctors of the classical period.

1 cf., J. L. Doreau, *Les bains dans l'Inde antique, monuments et textes médicaux*, Paris, 1936.

2 *Cikitsāsthāna*, XXXII, Baths (*Snānas*) are specially discussed in *Cikit.*, 56-64.

3 *Sūtrasthāna*, XIV.

The discoveries of the Valley of the Indus, moreover, consist of several products which could have been used as remedies. The horns of a cervidae, the *sambar* (or *sābar* in Hindi, SKT. *Śambara, Rusa aristotelis Jerdon*) have been found without any other remains of the animal and consequently should have been collected for their own sake. Precisely similar horns are even now utilised in popular Indian medicine. Bitumen has also been found and this substance is included in scientific pharmacopoeia of Sanskrit, under the name of *Śilājatu.* Lastly cuttle-bones, which could also have had a medical use, were contained in pottery unearthed by Majumdar at Othwan-jo-Buthi.[1] The use of similar products in therapeutics unfortunately does not have any characteristic significance. It proves nothing concerning the medical knowledge of the people of the Indus Valley civilization. We cannot therefore form any idea of the same. The material remains of this civilization would suggest that this knowledge could have been in a sufficiently advanced stage, especially so because the discovery of the Indus seals in Mesopotamia shows the relations they had with the region where the Sumerians or the Babylonians had developed an important medical tradition from an early age. From the period of Mohen-jo-daro scientific exchanges have possibly taken place between Mesopotamia and the Indus Valley. This is all that we can say for the time being and as a consequence, when the Vedic Aryans entered India in the 2nd millenium B.C., they may have found there already developed medical notions, which were probably related to those of the Sumerians. At this moment it is impossible for us either to confirm or deny this theory, but we will be able to show that at the time of their arrival the Indo-Aryans carried with them, if not an elaborate science of medicine, at least ideas which have entered as elements in the formation of Āyurveda.

THE INDO-IRANIAN DATA

The comparison of passages concerning medicine in the oldest texts of India and Iran, that is in the Vedas and in the *Avesta*, is likely to indicate some of the notions which had been formed during the period of the Indo-Iranian community and

1 E. Mackay, *La Civilisation de l'Indus*, French Edn., Paris, 1936, pp. 181, 185, 186.

have been preserved both by the Iranians and the Aryans who entered India. These notions are not very numerous and are quite vague. But nevertheless it is worthwhile taking them into consideration. It is necessary to take stock of these ideas so that it may be possible to see which elements of classical Indian medicine can be traced to the period of the old Indo-Aryan community and which have been acquired at a later date. But this stock-taking is quite a delicate affair because all that is common to Indians and Iranians of the historical period does not necessarily go back to the Indo-Iranian community. The two peoples could have separately borrowed the same notions from a third people or better still, either of the two could have communicated its own acquisitions in the subject to the other.

In fact, the relations between India and Iran have been permanent since antiquity. Darius had established two satrapies in the basin of the Indus from the end of the 6th century B.C. and the annexation of a part of the Indian territory of the West could have taken place even in Cyrus' time. After the destruction of the Persian empire by Alexander and the short occupation of these satrapies by the latter, India won them back. Yet the relations between India and the Iranian regions continued to be unbroken. The Iranian people of Upper Asia and of Iran itself, the Śakas, the Parthians and the Kuśānas conqured vast territories of India several times and stayed there as rulers for long periods. The Sassanids also penetrated into the country or maintained regular relations with its sovereigns. From a very early date a continuous traffic with Iran and, across Iran, with the Western countries had been established which passed through regions now in Afghanistan and across the Iranian territory. We will refer back to this traffic when we discuss the eventual relations between the savants of India and those of the Hellenic world. In the intellectual sphere, the existence of Buddhism in Bactriana and in Sogdiana, on the routes which bypassed the Pamirs to the west and led to Central Asia and to China, is the clearest trace of the Indian contribution to the Iranian territories. Reciprocal proofs are available to show the Iranian influence on India from the epoch of Aśoka, in the middle of the IIIrd century B.C. and even from the Achaemenid period. One can, therefore, conclude that a part of the common heritage of India and Iran, especially in the domain of scientific ideas, in whose formation emulation, always and everywhere, plays a big rôle and which could not have been developed to such an extent in the prehistorical period, can be dated back to the period of the exchanges rather than to that of the original community.

The relatively later dates of our Iranian sources (texts) make it likely that they contain borrowings from India and they developed certain indigenous ideas under the influence of India, either as an example or as a reaction against her. We should be very cautious in ascribing to the hoary past of the Indo-Iranians those concordances of ideas which may be due to latter-day communications or, on the contrary, in considering as cases of recent borrowing those ideas which may have emerged in the original community.

The *Avesta*, called "recent", is our oldest source for the knowledge of medicine in Iran, as the Gāthās do not contain any reference to medicine. It is not *a priori* impossible that an element under Indian influence has been able to react, directly or not, on the redaction of some of its passages. According to Parsi tradition, the Achaemenid *Avesta* had been burnt by Alexander, except for the passages dealing with astronomy and medicine, which had been translated into Greek. Later on, in the 3rd century A.D., after the Chief Priest Tansar had undertaken, on the order of Ardaser I, the restitution of the *Avesta* already begun under the Arsacidian Parthians, Sahpuhr I, the son and successor of Aradaser (241-272), caused to be inserted therein certain passages relating to medicine, astronomy and cosmogony which had been "scattered in India, Greece and elsewhere".[1] Ordinarily, it is not thought necessary to believe in this traditional account.[2] But of course there is no decisive argument against it. In any case, the Avesta of the Sassanian period, which is today partly lost, did really contain, notably in the *Huspāram-nask*, certain passages relating to medicine, as can be seen from the résumé included in the

[1] cf., J. Darmesteter, *Le Zend-Avesta*, Vol. III, Paris, 1893 (*Ann. Mus. Guimet*, Vol. XXIV, p. xxi-xxii).

[2] A. Christensen, *L'Iran sous les sassanides*, Copenhagen, 1936, pp. 136-7.

Pehlavi *Denkart* (of the IXth century).[1] The same *Denkart* has kept the tenor of a medical text but the technical passages which would be the most important for judging about its doctrines are unfortunately vague.[2] This text seems to attest a Hellenistic influence, notably when it allows a big rôle to the cold, to the dry and to the hot which are *phukhron, eiron, ugron* and *thermon* in Greek. The points of resemblance with Indian medicine which have been pointed out, do not have much significance.[3] For the rest, it takes up the data of the Avesta which are thus mixed up with foreign notions.

Elsewhere, an Indian influence appears to be quite manifest. The biography, or better still, undoubtedly the autobiography of the doctor of Khusro I (king from 531 to 579), Barzoe, who had brought from a journey in India the Book of Kalilagh and Damnagh, that is, a version of the *Pañcatantra,* contains a summary of embryology, which has, it seems, justly been recognised by Hertel, as containing typical Indian notions.[4] This is how, according to Barzoe, delivery is caused by a wind and this is precisely the teaching of classical Indian medicine. But even in this case, where the reality of a contact with India of the VIth century is beyond any doubt, as it had brought the Pehlavi imitation of the *Pañcatantra,* it will not be possible to assert that the notion of the rôle ascribed to wind in delivery was known in Iran before Barzoe. He was more likely to have found this notion again in India instead of having brought it from there. Actually, this notion could have had its origin either in Indo-Iranian pre-history or could have been borrowed from India before the 6th century B.C. The first eventuality cannot be rejected because, as we will see, the concept of the physiological rôle of the wind is very old. The second one is made possible by what is known of the Indian contribution to the famous school of medicine established in the 5th century

---

1 cf., A. Christensen, ibid, pp. 414 & ff.

2 *Denkart,* ed. Peshotan senjana, Bombay, 1874-1928, Vol. IV, pp. 181 & ff.; & transl., pp. 220 & ff. A study & transl. in L. C. Casartelli, *Un traité pehlevi sur la médicine,* in *Muséon,* Nov., 1886, pp. 532 & ff.

3 Casartelli, *op. cit.,* Ist article, pp. 314 & ff.

4 cf., Christensen, *op. cit.*; pp. 418 & ff. The autobiography of Barzoe has been edited & translated by Th. Noeldeke, *Barzoes Einleitung Zu dem Buche Kalila wa Dimna...* Strasbourg, 1912.

at Gundesapuhr, in Susiana, by the Nestorians expelled from the Byzantine Empire.[1]

On the other hand, several Indian texts on medicine, starting from the *Caraka-saṁhitā* show that for a long time before (these texts), Iranian doctors had been in contact with India and had been able to learn precisely the Indian theory regarding the physiological rôle of the wind. Several times and exactly in the chapter which deals with the functions of the wind,[2] the *Caraka-saṁhitā* brings in, in an assembly of savants assembled round the master Ātreya, a certain Kāṅkāyana Bahlikabhiṣaja "K. the doctor from Bactria". The title of "Bactria" shows clearly his Iranian origin and even his name signifies that it is "Sogdian". This is, at least, what appears to be most probable when it is seen that his name denotes a patronymic signifying "a descendant of Kaṅka" and that *K'ang* or *K'ang-kiu* in Chinese is a transcription of the name of Sogdiana.[3] It is true that Sogdiana and Bactria are separated by the course of the river Oxus but there is no contradiction in a man coming from Sogdiana, in practising medicine in Bactria. Kāṅkāyana plays only a secondary rôle in Indian medicine but it is significant that this Iranian is presented in one of the fundamental texts of the Āyurveda as having been admitted into a circle of Indian doctors. By this example it can be seen that in the absence of direct historical evidence, it can be sometimes quite delicate to

[1] cf. Reinaud, *Mémoire sur l'Inde*, in *Mém. de l'Acad. des Inscr. et Belles-Lettres*, Vol. XVIII, 2nd part, Paris, 1849, p. 309 on the continuity of Indian scientific contribution to Iran even after the invasion of Islam, cf., following pages, specially those concerning medicine, p. 316 et ff.

[2] *Sūtra*, XII. Kāṅkāyana also appears in Caraka, *Sūtr*, I. 12; XXV, 22; XXVI, 8&*śār.*, VI,21; MS Bower, ed., Hoernle, 935. Vāgbhaṭa; *Aṣṭāṅgasaṅgraha, cik.*, X (ed. Gaṇeśaśarman, Vol. II, p. 64); Cakradatta, *Cikitsāsaṁgraha*, V, 19 (*Kāṅkāyanaguṭikā*); XXX, 35, (*Kāṅkāyanamodaka*); Nityanatha, *Rasaratn ākara*, ed. of Bombay, 1897, p. 490 (*Kaṅkāyanaguṭikā*); *Śārṅgadharasaṁhitā*, 2, VII, p. 50 et ff. (*Kāṅkāyanaguṭikā*). He is mentioned in the commentary of Daḷhaṇa on Suśruta, *Sūtr*, I, 2. The preparations ascribed to him include besides the *guṭikā* (pill) and the *modaka* (cake), or *vaṭaka* (fried cake) whose récipé is given by G. Mukhopadhyaya, *Hist. of Ind. Medicine*, (Vol. II, Calcutta, 1926, pp. 464 & 466). The proposed identification, in this book, of Kāṅkāyana with the Kankah mentioned by Reinaud, *Mémoire sur l' Inde*, p. 314, is impossible, as the personage discussed by Reinaud belongs to the Muslim period. In the *Kauśikasūtra*, a Kāṅkāyana is twice mentioned, without, however, being designated as a Bactrian or as a doctor.

[3] cf., Chavannes, *Documents sur les Ton-kiae occidentaux*, index.

interpret recognised concordances between Indian and Iranian medical data.

The medical data of the Avesta,[1] as it has reached us, are mostly contained in the *Videvdāt* (*Vendidād*) which appears to belong, in its totality, to the beginning of the Arsacidian period[2] (250 B.C.—A.D. 224), although the materials are older. This work gives us information concerning doctors and fixes their fees (VIII. 36) but, of course, it does not contain any account which could be really called medical. It distinguishes three types of doctors practising with the aid of knife, of plants or of the holy word (*manthra spenta*) the last being the most esteemed (VII. 44, cf., also *Yast*, III, 6).

This classification has been commented upon several times. Christensen[3] has made a *rapprochement* between this passage and another which is given in the *Aphorisms* of Hippocrates (VII. 87) and according to which, all that can not be cured by medicines, is cured by fire and that which cannot be cured by fire is incurable. He thinks that this Greek classification has been able to exert some influence on the Iranian one and observes that the latter is completed in the *Denkart* by the mention of fire (and also of the "burning" which he interprets as denoting the fumigation by means of aromatic herbs and which most probably is cauterisation by means of caustics). But the Greek classification and that of the *Videvdāt* agree only in the total number of their elements because the holy word is not mentioned in the *Aphorisms* and the fire is missing in the *Videvdāt*. Hence there is no significant trace of influence. Much more important, however, is a remark of Darmesteter, taken up and emphasised recently by Mr. Benveniste. According to this remark the Avestan classification of doctors corresponds to that of Pindarus regarding curative processes (*Pyth.*, III. 91).[4] The concordance being, in this case, complete, it follows that, in all probability, the tradition of a deliberate division of medicines

1 Noted many times, notably by H. Fichtner, *Die Medizin in Avesta untersucht auf Grund der von Fr. Wolff besorgten Ubersetzung der heligen Bücher der Persen*, 1924.

2 Christensen, *op. cit.*, pp. 33 & 415.

3 ib., p. 415.

4 Darmesteter, *Ormazd et Ahriman*, Paris, 1877, p. 293, No. 2; E. Benveniste, *La doctrine médicale des Indo-Européens*, *Rév. Hist. Rel.*, July-Dec., 1945, pp. 5 & ff.

in three classes, drugs, surgical means and charms, is Indo-European. But this does not reveal anything concerning the eventual existence of the already determined processes and of already established doctrinal concepts, dating from the Indo-Iranian period and which could have been in vigour in the period of the *Videvdāt*.

The holy word referred to in the *Videvdāt* is the formula *Airyemā isyo* (*Yasna*, LIV).[1] This formula is personified in the Avesta and Ahura-Mazda himself invokes it against the 99,999 diseases created by Aṅra Mainyu, offering in return thousands of heads of cattle and a benediction (*Vid.*, XXII). The word *manthra*, designating the "word" and more precisely the magic formula corresponds exactly to the Vedic word *mantra*. The rôle ascribed to it, which is quite an important one because it is the recourse of Ahura Mazda against the Evil Spirit is, upto a certain extent, comparable to the power imputed in India to the *mantras* and chiefly to the similar and important rôle which, in the Vedic texts, is assigned to the "Voice" (*vāc*) or of the sacrificial formula (*bráhman*), which has also become a personified god. The *bráhman* is often for the Vedic gods that which a *manthra spenta* is for Ahura Mazda in his struggle againt Aṅra Mainyu. This *bráhman*, who "gives victory in the combat" (*pṛtanāsu sahyāḥ, RV.*, I. 152,7) is useful to the gods in their combat against the enemies. It is by him that Agni expels the demon of abortion (*RV.*, 162. 1 & 2) or kills the Yātudhānas (*AV.*, 1, 8, 4). It is by means of the *bráhman* of his singer or by that of the Soma that Indra has exalted his courage or his force (*RV.*, II. 17, 3).[2] Again it is with his aid that Bráhmaṇaspáti, the "Master of the *bráhman*", made sovereign (*RV.*, II. 24, 15),

---

1 Regarding this formula, G. Dumézil, *Le troisième souverain*, Paris, 1949, p. 47 & ff. Regarding the curative role of the Avestan Airyaman/the Vedic *Aryaman:* ib., p. 81 & ff.

2 *asya ... bráhmaṇā śuṣman airayah*. *Sāyaṇa* explains *asya* as designating the *stotṛ*; Geldner asks if it is not the *soma*, which has been under discussion, under this hypothesis; he translates *bráhman* as "magic force". In fact it is conceivable that in lieu of a formula, a "virtue" is ascribed to the soma. This example could be invoked to support the theory of Hubert and Mauss who see a *rapprochement* between the Indian *bráhman* and the Melanesian *mana* which is the magic force and sometimes simultaneously the formula possessing that force. (*Esquisse d'une théorie générale de la magie*, in *Année soc.*, 1902-1903 (1904), pp. 111, 117 & ff). But in spite of this example the *bráhman* is, probably even in this example, essentially the formula having a magical virtue whereas the *mana* is only secondarily a formula.

has "torn" *Vala* (ib., 3). These are some of the examples to which can be added others where the *bráhman* is replaced by the "voice" (*vāc*) or the "voices", by the "hymn" (*arká*) or even by the *mantra*. It is specially said about *Bráhmaṇaspáti* that he "enunciates the elogious mantras in which the gods Indra, Varuṇa, Mitra and Aryaman have pleased themselves",[1] now the last-named of these is the Vedic counterpart of the Avestan Airyaman.[2] It seems, therefore, that the concepts relating to the formula of curative magic are, generally speaking, Indo-Iranian, but the contents of the invocation *Airyemā isyo* is trivial and does not have in India its special counterpart capable of making us think that from the Indo-Iranian period itself a precise formula of magical therapeutics had come into being. Similarly the words denoting "remedy", charm, or drugs, *bheṣajá* in Vedic, *baesaja* in Avestan, are the result of one and the same Indo-Iranian form but they, in no manner, suppose that the "remedies" which are respectively designated by them, can be taken back to an Indo-Iranian therapeutics which had already been traditionally contributed.

The origin of plants and probably of the surgical knife is indicated by the *Videvdāt*. Zarathustra asks Ahura Mazda as to who had been the first doctor. Ahura replies that his name was Thrita who obtained from Ksathra Vairya the means to counter various diseases. Ksathra Vairya is the Aməsa spənta who presides over metals, also it is thought that Thrita received the knife from him (*Vid.*, XX. 2-3).[3] At the same time Ahura

---

1 . . . . *bráhmaṇaspátir mántram vadaty ukthyám|yásminn índro váruṇo mitró aryamā devā ókānsi cakriré.* (*RV.*, I, 40, 5).

2 Secondarily one may observe that Mithra plays an important role in the Avesta, that Indra is present there under this name or under that of Andra, a demon. But he responds to Vərəthragna of the camp of Good and that Varuṇa, 'the Asura of the gods' (*AV.* I, 10, 1) corresponds for a considerable part of his mythical personality to Ahura Mazda.

3 On this subject one may also see the remarks of Darmesteter *Haurvatāt & Ameretāt*, Paris, 1875, p. 53, note which shows that Manu, father of men, has also, as described in the Vedas, obtained several remedies. But this is only a vague analogy with the personage of Thrita (Moreover Darmesteter does not insist on this point) and the details on either side do not agree. The same author (p. 55, n. 2), makes a just *rapprochement* between the epithet *vispobis* 'of all the remedies', applied to the tree of Vourukasa (*Yast*, XII, 17) and the Vedic epithet having the same sense, *viśvábheṣaja*. In the *Ṛg-veda*, it does not qualify a tree but the wind (X, 137, 3) or the waters (I, 23 20 & cf & X 137, 6 where the same idea is expressed in a different manner) once even the hand of a singer (X, 60, 12), but in the *Atharvaveda* it is applied most of the time to

Mazda has given innumerable medicinal plants which encircle the mythical tree Gaokərəna (ib., 4). These plants are associated with waters and with the liquid of immortality, the *haoma*. This *haoma* has a terrestrial form of golden yellow which is made use of in liturgy, but the Gaokərəna grows in the waters of the lake Vourukasa and produces a white *haoma* which, one day, will give the good persons immortality whereas a sea of molten metal will submerge the evil-doers. Besides, the waters and the plants are related to the Aməsa spənta, Hauravatāt and Amərətat, the arch-angels of health and immortality.[1]

Many of these notions and particularities are found in Vedic India. The *soma*, which corresponds to the *haoma*, is both the sacrificial liquor and the king of plants. Among other hymns, the *oṣadhīstuti*, the "praise of plants" (*RV.*, X. 97) is addressed to him, this hymn being ascribed to *Bhiṣaja*, the "cure-man". The quality of the sovereign remedy of the *soma* has been proclaimed on many occasions.[2] It is specially said (*RV.*, I, 23, 19) and repeated in other forms that : "In the water is the liquor of immortality (*amṛta*), in the waters is the remedy (*bheṣaja*)".[3]

The mythical hero of the Avesta has for its counterpart the Vedic Tritá, but the two personages are not equivalent. Thrita is the third of four mortals who first of all extracted the

---

plants, the *jangiḍa* (II, 4, 3,; X, 35, 5), the plant of Kaṇva (*Kaṇvasya vīrudh*, VI, 52, 3); the nitatni (VI, 136, 3) the totality of plants (VIII, 7, 26) and the *kuṣṭha* (XIX, 39, 5).

1 cf., Darmesteter, *op. cit.*, *Rapprochement* with the Nāsatyas: G. Dumézil, *Naissance d' archanges*, Paris, 1945, pp. 157-170.

2 Numerous references in Bergaigne, *Rel. Véd.*, I, 152 & ff: 192. The soma-plant has most frequently been identified with an asclepiade. It seems that several species have been employed at different times and in different places, cf., Aurel Stein, *On the Ephedra, the Hūm Plant & the Soma*, in B.S.O.S., 1931, Vol. VI, p. 501-514. For the *rapprochements* between the *soma* and the *haoma*, cf V. Henry *Sóma & Homa* in *Ann. Mus. Guimet*, Bibl. Vulg., Vol. XX, Paris, 1906, pp. 51-80; G. Dumézil *Le Festin d' Immortalité*, Paris, 1924 (numerous references in the index). Jogeshchandera Ray, *The Soma Plant*, in *Ind. Hist. Quart.*, XV, 1939, p. 197, makes the identification of the *soma* plant with the Indian hemp extremely probable. According to a decisive remark of this author, it is in any case out of the question that this plant supplied an alcoholic drink as the effects of this drink are immediate when it is prepared extemporaneously by pressing and with the addition of water. The alcoholic fermentation required a long interval between preparation and consumption. (This will bring it very near *bhang*.-trsltr).

3 cf., *infra*, p. 46.

haoma (*Yasna*, IX. 4-13). The second is Āthwya, father of Thraetaona. Sometimes, the name Āthwya has been identified with the epithet āptya, "of the waters", which joins itself to the name of Trita, but it is extremely doubtful if the supposed correlation is exact, Āthwya and Thrita constitute two distinct personages and chiefly the phonetic correspondence in very much open to question.[1] "Trita" signifies "the third"[2] and he is one of those who prepare the soma,[3] just as Thrita is that of the haoma. Thraetaona would have for his counterpart the Vedic Traitana, an insignificant personage (*RV.*, I. 158, 5) whereas in the Avesta he is a hero of premier rank, who put to death the demon Azi Dahāha. In effect, the exploits of Thraetaona correspond more with those of Trita, the enemy of demon Viśvarūpa. In any case, only Thrita in the Avesta and Trita in the Veda have roles related to medicine, but whereas Thrita is the first doctor, Trita, on the contrary, is the first transmitter of evil.

According to the *Atharvaveda* (VI. 113, 1): "On Tṛtá (-Tritá) the gods have wiped off their sins. Tṛtá has wiped them off on men; if, later, the seizer (grāhi) has taken hold of you, that the gods destroy it for you by means of the incantation".[4] The ritual usage of the hymn, one found at a sufficiently late date,[5] without the possibility of affirming or denying its ancient origin, is that of exorcising the sin due to the marriage of the younger brother before that of the elder one and one could be led to think that the "seizing one" is the seizure of moral guilt having no relation with the disease. Yet the hymn, X. 161 of the *Ṛg-veda* makes a close *rapprochement* between the *grāhis* of the two afflictions, whose relations with the sin we will precisely see and which are nevertheless diseases: "I deliver you by means of the oblation so that you may live free from the

---

1 On the entire question, cf., K. Ronnow, *Trita Āptya, eine vedische Gottheit*. Uppsala, 1927, p. XXIII & ff.

2 This interpretation is more or less certain but it is not excluded that the name has not been originally used in another sense.

3 Bergaigne, *Rel. Véd.*, II, 328, thinks that it has acquired this sacerdotal role by means of a secondary transformation; yet the quality of Thrita, the third preparer of the *haoma*, seems to show that this role is Indo-Iranian.

4 *tṛté devā amṛjataitád ènas tṛtá enaṃ manuṣyéṣu mamṛje/áto yádi tvā grāhir ānaśé, tām te devā bráhmṇā naśayantu.*

5 *Kauśikasūtra*, 46, 26.

unknown evil and from the royal evil; if the seizing one has taken hold thereof, of it, O Indra and Agni, deliver it."[1]

Tṛtá or Tritá is hence an intermediary like Thrita, a "third" person if one so wishes to call him between the gods and men, but whereas Thrita passes on to human beings the remedies of Ahura Mazda, Tritá communicates to them a morbific defilement of the gods. Hence between these two mythical personages, there is a similarity and a contrast at the same time but the contrast is less strong than the similarly, as Tritá is far from having, in the Veda, an entirely malefic rôle, as he has prepared the soma, a liquor like the *amṛta*.[2]

Often enough his fatal rôle has not been correctly recognised. In order to identify Tritá completely with the Avestan Thrita, Haug has covered this rôle by means of tendencious translations.[3] He has understood the passage, which we have just quoted as signifying that Tritá extinguished diseases in the human beings just as the gods had extinguished it in him, but *mṛj* can not denote "extinguish" and Bloomfield has quite justly recognised in Tritá the "scapegoat" of the gods.[4] Haug has equally claimed that in the *Ṛg-veda* (VIII. 47, 13) disease was sent to him for being "pacified" and he has added that reference is made in the Avesta to this circumstance "by the surname *Sāma*, which signifies pacifier". But this assertion is false because there is no question of pacifying in the *Ṛg-veda* (VIII. 47, 13) which says: "That which openly, that which secretly, O gods, is badly done, on Trita Āptya, all that place far from us; your help be benign, your help is good help".[5] This passage, when compared with the preceding one, provides good evidence that Tṛtá or Tritá is the divine scapegoat but the men on whom he

---

1 *muñcāmi tvā haviṣā jīvanāya kam, ajñātayakṣmād uta rājayakṣmát, grāhir jagrāha yádi vaitád enam, tásyā indrāgni prá mumuktam enam.*

2 cf.. Ronnow, *op. cit.*, chap. II; *Das Lebenswasser*, p. 64 & ff.

3 Martin Haug, *Essays on the Sacred Language, Writings & Religion of the Parsis*, ed. by E. W. West, London, no date (1878?), p. 277 & ff.

4 *Trita, the Scapegoat of the Gods* in J.A.O.S., 1894, p. CXIX & ff.

5 *yád āvir yád apīcyám dévāso asti duṣkṛtám, tṛté tád víśvam āptyá āré asmád dadhātanānehásо va ūtávaḥ suūtávo va ūtávoḥ.* Elsewhere (*AV.*, VI, 84, 3) the favourable epithet *anehas*, 'benign', which designates the absence of "(hostile) designs" (cf., L. Renou, J. A., 1939, p. 211) applies to *Nirṛti*, in order to turn away her fatal influence and when she does not rage, this epithet suits her quite well. *Nirṛti* can, therefore, have a relatively favourable aspect, cf., *infra*, concerning the double character of gods and demons.

tries, in his turn, to discharge a disease, request the gods to take it back and send it back to him with their own affliction, so that this personage, though indirectly and in return, is also the scape-goat of human beings. There is thus quite a distance between this rôle and that of a cure-giver and it is surprising that Pischel has tried to make Tritá a doctor.[1]

Beneficent when he presses the soma, maleficent when he wipes off on human beings the impurity which the gods have wiped off on him, useful when one can, thanks to the gods, throw on him this impurity, Tritá in so far as he has a relationship with the diseases or with the soma, the liquid of immortality, does not possess a unequivocal character, whereas the Avestan Thrita appears as only a beneficent character. But there is here nothing surprising in a Vedic personage and it does not prevent him from going back to the same mythical Indo-Iranian figure, to whom goes his Avestan counterpart. Moreover, it is probable that he responds better than the other one to the image which can be conceived of their common mythical ancestor.

The equivocal character of gods and demons becomes a commonplace thing in India from the time of the Veda. This can be linked with the general and very important fact that in the Veda many notions have two opposite values, one favourable and the other unfavourable, as it is well attested by the Vedic vocabulary, which is extremely ambivalent.[2] This causes astonishment to our minds, used, by a long Christian tradition, to the classification of beings and of notions as good and bad ones. In reality, the mixing of contrary tendencies is quite constant. It

---

1 Basing himself on an indeterminate passage (*RV*.. II, 34. 10) and disregarding the precedents, cf., *Gotting. gel. Amzeigen*, Gottingen, 1894, p. 426, & ff., *Résumé* by Ronnow pp. IX & 39. See ibid., pp. V to XX, the principal theories on the subject of Tritá. Besides that of Haug, referred to above, to add among others, the identification, summarily but cleverly presented, of Trita Āptya on the one hand with Thrita and Athvya on the other in V. Henry, *Le Parsisme*, Paris, 1909, p. 220.

2 cf., L. Renou, *L' ambiguité du vocabulaire du Ṛgveda*, in J. A., 1939, p. 161-235; see particularly on the character of the gods, p. 220 & ff. Bergaigne, *Rel. Véd.*, Vol. III, p. 3 has already studied the turn-by-turn beneficent and redoubtable character of 'sovereign gods', but they are not the only ones to play a double role *vis-á-vis* human beings. cf. also J. Filliozzat, *Etude de démonologie indienne. La Kumāratantra de Rāvaṇa et les textes paralleles*, in *Cahiers soc. As.*, IV, Paris, 1937, on the favourable role of *Rāvaṇa*, p. 136 & ff.; on the maleficent role (rare, but cf., L. Renou, J. A., 1939, p. 224) of *Viṣṇu*, p. 72, on that of *Gaṇeśa* p. 78.

is by means of an idealistic systemisation to which we are accustomed, that we separate them and then divide them among completely conceived superhuman figures. But since such a systemisation was not thought necessary everywhere, it has not been created everywhere. Greek mythology, as that of India, admits, though to a lesser degree, the ambiguity of the character of gods ; this permits us to believe that this ambiguity is Indo-European. The Iranian dualism, on the contrary, opposes radically and mechanically, the Good and the Evil. It is not possible to accept that, under this absolute form, it is primitive. It is more likely that the mythical Indo-Iranian personalities, such as Thrita-Trita had been, in their origin, equivocal and have remained the same in the Veda whereas in the Iranian texts they have been secondarily made to specialise into the Good and the Evil ones. Moreover even in the Avesta, there are traces of the ambiguity of action of divine personalities and these traces can be interpreted as the survivals of concepts anterior to the dualist systemisation. This is an important question for the chronology of ideas and we will come to that on the subject of Vāyu.

The Iranian systemisation necessarily takes the origin of all the diseases back to the spirit of the Evil, Aṅra Mainyu (*Vid.*, XXV. 2) or to various other beings connected with him. Chief among them are, on the one hand, the *yātus*, the *pairikās* and the *jainis*, exorcised conjointly at the end of the *fargards*, XX, XXI, XXII of the *Videvdāt* and on the other hand and with less surety, the *drugs* (*druj*) *Nasu* and *Jahi*.

The Avestan *yātus* are the demon-sorcerers, indeed human sorcerers (*Yast*, II. 11 and VIII. 44). Similarly in the *Ṛg-veda*, *yātu* denotes sometimes sorcery, sometimes the demon-sorcerer. The latter one is specially the *yātudhāna* ("one who carries [in himself] sorcery" and the man can be yātudhāna) because the singer of *Ṛg-veda* (VII. 104) utters imprecations against one who calls him *yātudhāna*.[1] The *pairikās* and the *jainis* are the

1 cf., already De Harlez, *Avesta*, Paris, 1881, p. CXXXII. *RV.*, VII, 104, 16 puts as parallel ones the person who has called a singer a *yātudhāna* and the person who has declared himself to be pure, although being a *rakṣāsa*, this seems to assimilate the *yātudhānas* and the *rakṣās*. In the classical Sanskrit literature, these two types of beings are closely related; for example the *Rāmāyaṇa* (Bomb., VII, 59, 15) makes them descend simultaneously of the *Yadus* and the *rakṣasa* (or *rākṣasas*); they can play a role in the production of diseases to which we will allude later.

female demons who do not have their counterparts in the Veda unless it be that these two names are related to that of the evil *jāyānya* or Jāyenya (cf., *infra*), but this cannot be admitted as valid.[1] The *drugs* are the demons of "untruth",[2] ordinarily female ones and have for counterparts the Vedic *drunhs* (cf., *infra*). But here only the corresponding general concept is Indo-Iranian as the various *drugs* known in the Avesta, are not found in the Veda. In the Avesta, Jahi is the *drug* of luxury ; she is mentioned beside a list of diseases (*Vid.*, XXI, 17), but she is in this neighbourhood only because of her evil character and not necessarily as a morbid cause. The same holds for *daevi* and other impure beings mentioned with her.

More important is the *drug* Nasu for whom Hertel and Reinhold Müller have desired to find a Vedic counterpart and in whom they have desired to see the witness of the Indo-Iranian concept of the igneous nature of disease.[3] The hymn X. 163 of the *Ṛg-veda* consists of a charm for chasing the *yákṣma* from all the parts of from body which are successively named. In the *Videvdāt* (VIII. 35-72), the purification of corpses by means of water is discussed and the limbs from which water chases away, turn by turn, the *drug* Nasu, are enumerated. There is perforce a resemblance between the two enumerations without their having a common Indo-Iranian origin. However Hertel and Müller had thought that the *rapprochement* of the two texts revealed the existence of a worry among the Indo-Iranians, which we will call a prophylactic one, and he had proposed that the Avestan *drug* was regarded as a demoniacal fire. Earlier, he had suggested that the *yákṣma* drew its name "from the high temperature of those who are caught by it",[4] but he had not noticed that there is no proof to show that the *yákṣma* was necessarily feverish. His conviction was essentially based

1 For *pairikās*, Darmesteter had once suggested an entirely forced etymology, tending to relate this name to the vedic *apsaras* or *apsarā* (*Ormazd et Ahr.*, p. 177, note 2) because he had by means of an equally forced comparison, identified the *pairikās*, ancestors of the *perīs*, the fairies of Iran with the *apsaras* of India.

2 cf., Nyberg, *Die Rel. des alten Iran*, p. 133.

3 Reinhold, F. G. Muller. *Die Medizin im Ṛg-veda*, in *Asia Major*, Vol. VI, 1930, p. 315-387, including Johannes Hertel, *Nachtrag zu Ṛg-veda* X, 163; *Vendidad*, VIII, 35-72, p. 377-385.

4 cf. also *Vid.*, IX, 15 & ff., which deals with the purification of the man made impure by the contact of a corpse.

on the equivalence which he had proposed yákṣati = yájati[1] and on the sense of "changing into fire" which he claimed as the original sense for *yaj*=to sacrifice.[2] From all this, it resulted that the disease had been a malignant fire for the Indo-Iranians.

This theory is a tissue of hypotheses which cannot stand at all. It has been conceived chiefly by virtue of an already conceived Vedic interpretation. Hertel has not been the first who tried to see everywhere in the Veda, only one essential theme. The old mythologists found everywhere in it the storm, Regnaud the soma, Hertel always the fire[3]. The mere fact that each of these systems has been defended is sufficient to demolish all of them together, because it proves that the storm, the soma and the fire, all three play a considerable role and in consequence it will not be possible to accord exclusive importance to any of them. In any case, to a reader not informed about the Avesta, the *drug* Nasu does not appear, to be of igneous nature. It is variously qualified but it is under the hideous form of an insect that it is shown by the *Videvdāt* (VII. 2 & 5; VIII. 16 & IX. 26) and this form particularly suits it because this is the form of the flies of corpses, because it is precisely the *drug* of the corpses.[4] Moreover, as we will see, it is not a disease but an eventual cause of disease. The fact that the *yákṣma* and the *drug* are successively expelled from all the limbs of the body, cannot establish their community of origin; this is the usage in all cases of evil impregnation and it is not found solely in India and Iran.

It is, however, possible to establish a *rapprochement* between the *yákṣma* and the *drugs,* not as going back to the

---

1 *Die arische Feuerlehre,* I, Leipzig, 1925, p. 24, approved in the last resort by R.F.G. Müller, *Grundlagen altindischen Medizin in Nova Acta Leopoldina neue Folge,* 11, No. 74, Halle, 1942, p. 12.

2 *Die arische Feuerlehre,* p. 20. In any case an Avestan *yaska* does correspond to the Vedic *Yákṣma* (we will discuss it once again), the former having the general sense of disease.

3 ibid., p. 119.

4 In his alread accepted interpretatien of the Avestan data, cf. H.S. Nyberg, *Die Religionen des alten Iran,* deutch von H. H. Schaeder, Leipzig, 1938, p. 20.

5 *nasu* is manifestly related to the Latin *nec-are,* Greek *nexus.* 'corpse'. Hertel translates *drug* as 'destruction' (vernichtung) and *nasu* as putrefaction (Vernesung) but cf. *infra.*

Indo-Iranian concept of an igneous physical impurity, but because of the relations existing between the physical evil or the material impurity on the one hand and the sin on the other. The Avestan *drugs* are chiefly the demons of sin and impurities. The *drug*, *par excellence*, is covered and fertilised by the sinners, voluntary or involuntary ones: the one who refuses to give a piece of cloth to the faithful indigent, one who urinatès near one's foot, one who has a nocturnal pollution and one who, at the age of fifteen, has intercourse with a prostitute *(Vid.*, XVII, 34-5). This clearly shows that physical impurities and moral defects can he assimilated. The *drug* represents therefore all the evil elements attached to human beings in their bodies and in their spiritual personalities. In so far as it is attached to the bodies, it can give rise to diseases (*Vid.*, IX, 48). It had been probably observed that the contact of corpses was not only repugnant but also dangerous and that the disease which had led to death stays attached to the body, because it is said that various afflictions are found in those depots where corpses are exposed, in the *dakhmas (Vid.*, VII, 58). The dog, chiefly certain dogs having special characteristics, were considered as being capable of putting the *drug* Nasu on the run (VIII, 16-18) and it is not, undoubtedly, because the dog is a creature of Ahura Mazda (*Vid.*, XIII, 39), highly valued for his utility in keeping watch over the herds and men. The dog keeps his tongue and his teeth surprisingly clean even when he nourishes himself on carrion; he could, therefore, appear to possess a virtue which destroyed putrefaction. Similarly it is probable that other beings who nourish themselves on corpses in stages of decay—birds, wolves, flies—were thought to have a quality of purification because it was agreed that they did not pass on the impurity with which they were in contact (*Vid.*, V, 3-7).[1] It is clear that these ideas have hardly anything to do with medicine; they are, in the first place, the result of instinctive repulsions and then that of a unitary concept of evil. Lastly they are the observations leading us to the belief that the dead spread a morbific power to which is opposed an anti-morbid

[1] The text observes that otherwise the impurity will extend itself everywhere because of the multitude of corpses. The wind figures in the list of beings who do not pass on the impurity.

magical virtue found among beings who can expose themselves to contagion with impurity.

If the Vedic *yákṣma* is not, like the *drug*, a cause of disease, it has at least some relationship, like the *drug*, with sin or bad disposition (*infra*, p. 80). It even seems that one must consider it as the physical evil produced by a sort of *drug*. Actually the word *druh* is used in expressions characterising the disposition of the man who contracts *yákṣma* because of an act of impiety towards Mitra and Varuṇa: "the man who, O Mitra and Varuṇa, the impure (*abhidruḥ*) man, who does not press for you the waters (the juice of the soma), the artful (*akṣṇayādruḥ*) himself deposits the *yákṣma* in his heart . . ."[1] Accordingly, one may observe that the *yákṣma* is exercised conjointly with the *druh* in the *Atharvaveda* (II, 10, 6). The root *druh*, in the classical language, signifies "to cause harm, being hostile", but in the Vedic, this hostility consists of all that twists the normal order, the *ṛta;* it is the heresy, the impiety, indeed it is the error or the falsehood. The Vedic *druhs* are originally related to the Avestan *drugs*, which are the antagonists of the *asas*, the Avestan counterpart of the *ṛta*. The sense of the Avestan *drug* is justly "falsehood" or "disorder".[2]

But as usual, the role of the Vedic *druhs* is equivocal, whereas that of the Avestan *drugs* is solely bad.[3] A Vedic *druh* can be of service if one can make use of it against the evildoer or can send the evildoer to break himself against it: "The person, O Maruts, who having a bad desire in his thoughts, O Vasus, wishes to strike against us, let him loosen

---

1 *Jánoyó mitrāvarunāv abhidhrúg apó ná vām sunóty akṣṇayādhrúk/ svayám sá yákṣmaṃ hṛdaye ní dhatte...(RV.*, I, 122, 9).

2 cf. in the last place, Nyberg, *Die Rel. des alten Iran*, p. 133.

3 It is the *drug* itself which in *Vid.*, XVIII, 13 & ff. explains all that is favourable and all that is harmful to her, thus giving the means to combat her. One can here make a *rapprochement* between this fact and the one that in India the discussion of an anti-demon ritual is ascribed to Rāvaṇa, chief of the Rakṣasas who in the Veda are specially known as the demons who cause abortion, and that this Rāvaṇa had, even from before the time of Galien (IInd century *A.D.*), become known as a doctor (cf., Filliozat, *La Kumaratantra*, pp. 170 & ff.). One could therefore conclude that the personage of the Avestan *drug* has, like Rāvaṇa, been subjected to a favourable evolution. According to Nyberg, op. cit., p. 67, it is with pleasure that she talks to Sraosa who has put aside his formidable mace. But probably it should be understood that she talks because of the fear that he may not seize her again.

himself against the toils of the *druh*! Beat him with the most burning beetle!"[1] Elsewhere the *druhs* which pursue the departures from the *ṛta* belong to Mitra and Varuṇa: "All these, O male ones (Mitra and Varuṇa), are infallible, they are yours, in them one has seen neither marvel nor prodigy, the *druhs* pursue the monstrosities of human beings . . ."[2] In other words, the *druhs* pursue, without miracle, naturally, the shortcomings in the natural order and they punish these as a revenge, acting in the capacity of the guardians of *ṛta*, Mitra and Varuṇa.

In any case it appears to be certain that the concepts of the Vedic *druh* and the Avestan *drug* go back to a general Indo-Iranian idea about the wrong done to the normal order, to anamoly in all its forms, of which the diseases are a part, but correctly speaking, they are not medical concepts. One cannot, on its basis, talk of an Indo-Iranian medicine.

The diseases mentioned by the Avesta are probably the demons of diseases.[3] Their names are extremely obscure[4] and were already so under the Sassanians, because some of them have been left without a translation in the Pehlavi version of the *Videvdāt*.[5] Moreover, they are very rarely related to the Vedic names of diseases. The Avestan word *gada*, "ruin, evil", is currently found in classical Sanskrit under the form *gada*, "disease", and appears in the Vedic in *agadá*, "doing well". The name of the disease *pāman* is common to the Avesta and the Vedas (*AV*., V, 22, 12). Neither in the *Avesta* nor in the *Atharvaveda* is its sense made clear by the context. However, in the *Atharva*, the *pāman* is said to be the cousin "of the fever"; it is, therefore, probable that it is inflammatory. Moreover, the *Chāndogya-upaniṣad* brings in a personage, Raikva, who "scratches himself" for a *pāman*, from which he suffers (*pāmānam kaṣamānam*, IV, 1, 8); it is also, therefore, a

---

1 *yó no maruto abhí durhṛṇāyúś tirás cittāni vasavo jighāṅsati/druháḥ pāśān práti sá mucīṣṭa tápiṣṭhena hánmanā hantanā tám* (*RV*., VII, 59, 8).

2 *ámūrā víśvā vṛṣaṇav imā vām ná yāsu citráṃ dádṛśe ná yakṣám/drúhaḥ ṣacante ánṛtā jánānām*...(VII, 61, 5),

3 The chief passages where its enumerations are found are *Vid*., VII, 53 XX, 3; XXXI, 18.

4 cf., Nyberg, op. cit., p. 340.

5 cf., Haug, *Essays*...., p. 363, note 3.

pruriginous affection, generally believed to be itch. But it can also be any type of pruriginous dermatose and it is not wise to admit without any proof that the itch, properly speaking, was clearly distinguished since the Vedic period itself, especially as in the classical Indian medicine, the *pāmā* corresponding to the Vedic *pāman*, corresponds to eczema rather than to itch. Suśruta says: "The diagnosis of the *pāmā* is done according to the tiny vesicles accompanied by discharge, according to the pruritus and the peripheric inflammation" and he continues this time in characterising the veritable itch which he calls *kacchū*: "By the pustules accompanied by a great deal of inflammation, appearing on the buttocks, on the hands and on feet, this is how itch is represented".[1] Moreover, the Avesta has the name of a disease corresponding to *kacchū*: *kasvī(s)*, as has been kindly indicated to me by Mr. Benveniste, who has also informed me that *pām* denotes in Afghan the itch. One may, therefore, admit that *pāman* denotes from the Indo-Iranian epoch an "itch" in the general sense and not in the medical sense properly speaking.[2]

There is yet another contrast between the Avestan and Indian nomenclatures of skin-diseases. In effect, the Avestan

---

1 *sāsrāvakaṇḍūparidāhakābhiḥ pāmāṇukābhiḥ piḍakābhir ūhyā/sphoṭaiḥ sadāhair ati salva kacchūḥ sphikpāṇipādaprabhavair nirūpyā.—Suśr, Nid.*, V, 11 12. The eruptions of the vesicles at the places of the choice of the itch, which are the very ones indicated by Suśruta, are actually the very important symptoms of the itch, but unlike the groove and the swell of the epiderm above the parasite not described by Suśruta and whose importance has been definitely established among us only in the 19th century, they are not pathognomonic. It is true that the *pāmā* and the *kacchū* sometimes appear to be mixed up. The Tibetan version of Vāgbhaṭa's *Aṣṭāṅgahṛdaya* (*Nid.*, XIV, 9) renders *pāmā* as *gyan pa* which, according to Jaeschke (*Dict.*, see the word), denotes a skin-disease, hereditary and non-contageous, therefore, something else than the itch. But in the Sanskrit-Tibetan dictionary of *Tse-ring-oung-gyal* (published by J. Bacot, Paris, 1930) *gyan pa* is rendered both as *pāmā* and as *kacchū* (variant of *kacchū*). The Tibetan version of Vāgbhaṭa, ib , *Cik.*, XIX, 84, again employs *gyan pa* for explaining *kacchū*, although the *Mahāvvutapatti* (Sakaki edn.) gives *pāmā—gyan pa* and *kacchuḥ—khyi rño.*, 'itch of dog'.

2 Because of semantic evolution the sense of linguistically related terms can differ from one language to another. The equivalent of Skr. *kacchū, AV. kasvī (s)* is found in the Koutchéen language in the form of *kasvo* but corresponds in sense not to the Sanskrit *kacchū* but to the Sanskrit *kuṣṭha*, denoting the totality of dermatoses including leprosy, cf., J. Filliozat, *Fragments de textes koutchéens de médecine et de magie*, Paris, 1948, see the word in the index.

druka has been identified with the Sanskrit *dadruka.*[1] In the two words—*ka* represents a suffix and *dadruka* is more usually found in the form of *dadru.* In Vedic neither *dadru* nor *dadruka* is found, but beginning from *Suśruta*, *dadru* is referred to in medical texts. This author describes it conjointly with the *pauṇḍarīka:* "The *pauṇḍarīkas* have the aspect of the leaves of blue lotus, the dermatose *dadrus* have the colour of the flower of flax or are of copper colour; they are serpiginous and pustulous. The traits common to both are the elevation, the circularity, the pruritus and the slow rate of evolution.[2] These indications do not allow to identify the diseases in question, these can be those of several different dermatoses.[3]

One could think of a *rapprochement* between the Avestan *azivāka* (varient *azavaka*, of *Vid.*, XX, 12, 18 & 23) and Vedic *ajakāvá* (*RV.*, VII, 50, 1). But even if the equation was phonetically speaking, incontestable, it will remain uncertain. The sense of *azivāka* is unknown; only that it is a disease is clear. The sense of *ajakāvá* identified by Bergaigne[4] with *ajakā*, the name of an eye-disease in classical Sanskrit, is problematical. It has been proposed to translate it as 'scorpion', though without much reason.

It should therefore be admitted that there is no common nosological nomenclature pertaining to the Veda and the Avesta, except in so far as it concerns a few skin-diseases and this leads us to think that in the Indo-Iranian period there was no fixed nosology which the Aryans could have brought with them into India. The anatomical terms common to the Vedic and the Avestan are the names of the organs or of various parts of the body related to ordinary general knowledge.

---

1 cf., W. Krogmann, *Zeit. für vergl. sprach*, Vol. LXV, 1938, p. 141.

2 *puṇḍarīkapattraprakāśāni pauṇḍarīkāṇi/atosipuṣpavarṇāni tāmrāṇi vā visarpiṇi pīḍakāvanti ca dadrukuṣṭhāni/tayor dvayor apy utsannatā parimaṇḍalatā cirotthānātvam ceti sāmānyarūpāṇi* (*Nid.*, V, 5).

3 This is, what is, actually indicated by the translation 'ringworm' (dartre), adopted by K.L. Bhiṣagratna in his version of the *Suśruta* and by the majority of authors, as the term does not possess a precise medical value. It follows therefore that the two ailments were considered as having extremely similar aspects and that they were willingly mixed up by the Tibetans. Śāyaṇa in his commentary on the *Chāndogya Upan.* gloses *pāman* by *kharju*, a relatively popular term, little used in the Sanskrit nosology and which includes the itch and all types of pruritus.

4 *Etude sur le lexique de R.V.*, see the word.

Therefore nothing proves the existence of an Indo-Iranian medicine, already fixed as the outline of a science. The therapeutics by means of magical imprecations itself, which is the only one whose examples are found in the Avesta, does not have any significant concordance with the ones which are known to us by an infinite number of the Vedic passages. The Avestan formulae are simple and have very little by way of characteristics. Parallels can be easily found for them in the Veda but, long ago, de Harlez has also been able to compare them with the 'Accadian' incantations.[1]

It does not follow that Indian medicine owes to Indo-Iranian ideas nothing other than the notions recorded by us, such as the relationship of the physical evil with the twists to general good order or those of the curative virtues of the waters, the plants and the holy formulae; all these notions, despite their relationship with medicine, are not at all scientific. On the contrary, some of the fundamental concepts of the theoretical system of classical Indian medicine appear to have been inherited from the Indo-Iranian concepts, non-scientific at the time of its origin, but utilised for the dogmatic construction of the Āyurveda.

The Āyurvedic theory of three essential principles, which are of the human or animal organism and at the same time of the cosmos, i.e., water, fire and wind, is not given in outline in the Avesta, but a part of the notions which has remained classical for each of these principles is common to the Avesta and the Veda and goes back, in all probability, to the Indo-Iranian period.

The Waters:—In the *Veda*, the waters play a cosmic role to a considerable extent. They constitute the condition for the march of the universe and of the life of beings; they are also the Mothers *(ambí) par excellence (RV.*, I, 23, 16); the immortality is in them *(amṛta,* ib., 19). Celestial or terrestrial, they correspond from one world to another, the rivers of this lower world having a replica in the sky. In the beginning, all was only "water without form".[2] Being the essential principle of

[1] *Avesta*[2], pp. cciii & 207, No. 6 ('Accadian' of his time answers ordinarily to what we call 'Sumerian').

[2] *ágre' praketáṃ salilám sárvam ā idám* (*RV.*, X. 129, 3).

the world, they must have been later on naturally considered not only as a vivifying liquid but again as one of the primordial elements of microcosmic organism.

In the Avesta, the waters which cure and purify (*Yasna*, LXIV, 1-5), are not only the source of health but also and chiefly as in the Veda, one of the primordial elements of the universe and of the living bodies. A part of *Yasna*, XXXVIII is devoted to them. They are invoked here under the names given them by Ahura Mazda, such as *azi*, *mātar*, *agənya*, *darəgudâyaṅh*. These names are variously explained. Neryosengh, in his Sanskrit translation of the *Yasna*, explains *azi* in relation to water, in the form of phlegm (*kapha*)[1], *mātar* 'mother' in relation to the waters which are in the semen of the man and the woman at the time of the sexual union[2]; the *agənya* will be the 'bloods[3]' and lastly the *darəgudāyaṅho*, whose name he translates by *durbalakapālakāḥ*, 'cups of the weak', would be waters which are inside the matrix[4], they being, therefore, those with which the embryo is saturated (hence the designation of 'cups of the weak'). In the same text other designations follow where Neryosengh sees the waters of the plants and of the grains, those which are 'in the body' of the Earth and lastly 'the milks'.[5] This interpretation, if it were correct, would peremptorily prove that in ancient Iran there used to be some speculation on the physiological rôle of the waters, just as has been the case with the Indian doctors. But Neryosengh, the Parsi priest, could have been suspected of interpreting the passage too much in the Indian way and to have himself introduced therein, without any right, the traits which remind us of the ideas of the Āyurveda. However, Neryosengh did not translate the Avestan text directly and according to his personal conjectures, he rendered the Pehlavi version in Sanskrit, which had already explained the various

[1] *ajiśnāmni kapharūpiṇī*, 33, 13, Fr. Spiegel, edn., *Neriosengh's Sanskrit-Übersetzung des Yasna*, Leipzig, 1861 p. 163.

[2] *āpo yāḥ antaḥ sambandhe naranārībijayoḥ.* (ib).

[3] *ageniaonāmnyaḥ/rudhirāṇi* (ib.).

[4] *durbalakapālakā nāmnyaḥ/āpo yāḥ autargarbhasthāne* (ib.).

[5] *āpo yaḥ antaḥ jagatigātre mātaro jītaio ceti nāmnyaḥ kṣīrāṇi* (15); the term of *jagatigātra* is a little equivocal. It can signify the body of the earth or the body of the totality of living beings.

[6] *Die Rel. des alten Īran*, p. 284.

denominations of the waters as the designations of different liquids, organic and others. The Pehlavi translation can, in its turn, be suspected of having, by virtue of the cosmological and physiological ideas prevalent under the Sassanians which could have been subjected to Indian influences, lent to the Avestan text a significance which it did not have in view. In fact, the Pehlavi version and Neryosengh differ a little in detail, which leads one to think that they did not follow a tradition which had been rigórously fixed from the time of the origin of the text, and lastly in the names of the waters in our passage, Nyberg sees only the epithets of the waters, respectively invoked as full-grown cows, as cows who are calving and as cows with milk, which give the nourishment of *drigu*, that is to say, undoubtedly of the 'poor' in the scheme of sacred things.[1]

It will, therefore, be imprudent to base ourselves definitely with too much of confidence on the data of the Sassanian tradition and on those of Neryosengh to claim that the ancient Iranians had already felt the ideas of the Indian doctors concerning the rôle of the waters in the economy of the human body. It remains, nevertheless, true that the Avestan notions regarding the waters are related to those of the Veda. In the Avesta, according to the text which has just been discussed, the waters are the Mothers, as in the Veda and, if they are compared to the cows, the same comparison is found quite ordinarily in the Veda.[2] Elsewhere, as we have seen, the waters have, in the two texts, the same relationships with the plants and with the *haoma* and the *soma* respectively. Speculations concerning them, therefore, manifestly go back for their essential part to the Indo-Iranian period and right from that period, they held, in the explanation of Nature, a first place, which predestined them to receive later on a similar one in the system of physiology.

The Fire:—The same is true of the fire. Under the principal name of *atar* in the Avesta and of Agni in the Veda, it plays an essential rôle, specially in the cult. The Veda recognises it everywhere in the universe under multiple forms; it is the lightning, the Sun, the terrestrial fire and shows itself in many other idden or manifest forms. In one of them some-

1 cf., ib., p. 194.
2 cf., Bergaigne, *Rel. véd.*, I, p. 259.

times hidden, sometimes manifest, it is specially in relation with human beings or better still with the beings of five races, those of the cardinal points and of the sky.[1] He is at that time the *vaiśvānará*, the 'pan-human'. In this capacity he has been conceived, at the end of the Vedic period and may be earlier still, as a physiological element with a precise function. The *Bṛhadāraṇyaka-upaniṣad* situates it in man and ascribes to it the rôle of the digestive fire: "This Agni, the pan-human one, who is man, it is by him that all edible food is cooked".[2] The hymn of the *Ṛgveda* to the Puruṣa, to the cosmic Man, had already caused to be created by His mouth, the fire accompanied by Indra (*RV*., X, 90, 13), but it is possible that there is only a reference to the warmth of the breath therein. Another hymn, a charm of the *Atharvaveda* seems to have already implied the idea of a relationship between digestion and the *vaiśvānará* fire because it constitutes a benediction of the nourishment partaken and not only does it demand that Agni render this nourishment as 'well presented in oblations' (*suhuta*) but also desires that nourishment eaten when not due (*ánṛtena*) and of doubtful character, be made 'of honey' (*mádhumant*) 'by the greatness of the great Agni, the vaiśvānará' (VI, 71, 3). It is possible that at first this hymn had been conceived for a purely ritual use and solely destined to render offerings of nourishment or a *dakṣiṇā* given to a Brahmin in conformity with the *ṛta*. But, if followed to the letter, it was well-made at least for preparing the notion, found in the *Bṛhadāraṇyaka-upaniṣad* of the rôle of the fire in the digestive functions[4].

[1] Bergaigne, *Rel. véd.*, II, p. 156.

[2] *ayam agnir vaiśvanāro yo'yam antaḥ puruṣe yenedam annam pacyate yad idam adyate* (V, 8, 1,). In the *Chāndogya-up*, it is the light of sky (*divojyotis*), equivalent to the fire, which is ahead of man (III, 13, 8).

[3] Similarly according to the *Bṛh-up*., (I, 1.1) the situation of the vaiśvānara fire has taken place in the open (*vyātta*) mouth of the Cosmic Horse.

[4] In the *RV*., X, 5, 1, Bergaigne saw a reference to the internal fire. This passage, he wrote, in "giving to the fire the epithet *bhūri-janmā*," 'one who has many births', adds that he 'radiates from our heart, (*Rel. véd*, I, p. 34). The text is: *ékaḥ samūdró dharúṇo rayīṇām' asmád dhṛdó bhūrijanmā vi caśṭe*...The interpretation of Sāyaṇa is altogether different. He takes *hṛdó* for an accusative plural and renders *ví caṣṭe* as *vi paśyati*, 'sees', and by *jānāti* 'knows', quoting in support of his interpretation a traditional phrase, '*mano vai devā manuṣyasya jānanti*', 'the gods, in sooth, know the thoughts of men (Actually the *manas* is frequently localised in the heart). He invokes'

Besides, in the *Ṛgveda*, the fire is considered as a power of development hidden inside everything, because it is called the one who is the embryo of the waters, of the woods, the embryo of the immobile things and that of the mobile things.[1]

In the Avesta, besides the fact that *Atar* presents the general traits which relate him to Agni and go back, in all probability, to the Indo-Iranian period, some of his special forms appear to be related to the special forms of Agni. *Yasna* (XII, II) successively invokes the fires, *bərəzisavah*, *vohufrayāna, urvāzista, vāzista* and *spənista*. Neryosengh translates the first name as *udagrajyotiṣ*, "eminent light", and explains that this is the ever-luminous fire found near Ahura Mazda, but the Pehlavi version renders it as 'of great utility'. The fire *vohufrayāna* literally 'who aims the good', is according to Neryosengh who agrees with the tradition, the 'excellent friend', one who finding itself permanently in the body, eats and drinks. The fire *urvāzista* becomes *vanaspatiṣṭha* in Sanskrit meaning 'one who lives in the trees', 'one who always drinks but never masticates'.[2] The fourth is the fire in the form of lightning (*vidyudrūpa*) which neither drinks nor eats and the last one is the fire found in milk (*payahṣṭha*). The existence of the fire in plants, specially in wood, from where it is drawn out by friction, is a notion quite common in the Veda. But it is chiefly the fire *vohufrayāna* whose rôle of the element of body presiding at nutrition is important for observation as that aids us to reconstitute the physiological ideas of the Indo-Iranians, because it corresponds exactly, by means of this rôle, to an aspect of the Vedic fire, *Vaiśvānara*. Perhaps one could say that the functions ascribed by the Iranian Sassanian tradition to this fire do not really go back to the epoch when the Avestan text was conceived and we have seen that the similar function

---

besides the rule of Pāṇini. VII, 1, 39, to justify his interpretation of the ablative *asmat* by the genitive *asmākam*. But one can also translate as follows: The unique (Agni), the ocean carrying riches, from us, from the heart, he who has many births, sees on all sides". This implies the belief in an organic central fire identical to the universal fire and conceived as a principle of knowledge.

1 *gárbho yó apām gárbho vánānām gárbhaś ca sthātām gárbhaś carāthām* (1, 70, 3).

2 Edn. of Spiegel, XVII, 64, 65: *agnim uttamasakhāyam ā/ yaḥ sadaiva dehastho bhakṣati pibati ca/agniṃ vanaspatiṣṭham ā/ yaḥ sadaiva pibaty eva na khādati.*

of Agni *Vaiśvānara* is not formally described in the most ancient stratum of the Veda. However, the agreement of the two traditions, Iranian and Vedic, leads one to think that these notions of this function must be Indo-Iranian. Otherwise, it will be necessary to suppose, and without there being much basis for the same, a borrowing by Iran from India or reciprocally, or it will be necessary to admit that the Indo-Iranian concept of fire was such that it has, in the two countries, separately given rise to a similar application in physiology. But the last hypothesis will amount to saying that the Indian and Iranian notions of the rôle of fire in the organism do possess, in any case, a remote but common Indo-Iranian origin.

The Association of the Fire and the Waters:—Not only are the general ideas concerning the cosmic and physiological functions of the waters and of the fire, common to ancient India and ancient Iran, the Veda and the Avesta share certain more special concepts such as that of the association of the fire with the waters. This association is mythically manifested in the name of a personage whose name is found in the two texts in the form of Apām Nápāt, 'grandson (or descendant) of the waters', in the Veda[1] and under that of Apam Napāt in the Avesta. Originally it was certainly the fire of the clouds which shows itself in lightning and falls on earth in the form of the thunderbolt with the rain; the same also enters the plants with the waters that they absorb and which reappears in the combustion of wood ignited by means of friction.[2] In the Veda, as fire, as Agni, it is essentially made,

[1] cf., Bergaigne, *Rel. Véd.*, I, p. 17 a ff; II, p. 16 & ff.

[2] Mr. E. Herzfeld has suggested an altogether different interpretation (*The Aryan Myth of naphta*, II, World Congress of Petrol, Paris, 1937. Vol. IV, *Hist. & Arch. of Petrol*, session of 14 June 1937, p. 21-23). In his opinion, even the name of naphtha comes from *napāt*. Moreover and chiefly, in the *Yaśt*, XIX, the fire and *Azi Dahaka* wish to seize the *akhrata khvarnah* but it is Apam Napāt who succeeds in getting hold of him. From this Mr. Herzfeld concludes that his *akharta khvarnah* is the very essence of Apam Napāt; here he understands *akharta khvarnah* as signifying "flame which does not require nourishment" and he thinks that this designation applies to naphtha. In this way the myth of Apam Napāt becomes a myth of naphtha. It is difficult to agree with this thesis. Even by admitting that the *akharta khvarnah* is the "flame which requires no nourishment", it is not possible to recognise therein the naphtha which is simply a combustible liquid.

in contrast with the waters of the females, in whom he engenders an embryo (*RV.*, II, 35, 13), although he is himself their son or their embryo. Husband or son of the waters, he is also their father, because Agni, whom he represents, has engendered the waters (*RV.*, I, 96, 2). In the Avesta, similar comparisons of the relations of natural elements with family relationships are not found, but Apam Napāt is also the male spirit of the waters and he distributes them (*Yast.*, VIII, 33). The two texts ascribe him detailed traits which are almost identical. In the Veda, 'he has engendered all the beings' (*viśvāny...bhuvanā*, *RV.*, II, 35, 2) and he is described as 'pushing forward the rapid ones [horses]' (*āśuheman*, *RV.*, II, 31, 6; 35, 1; VII, 47, 2).[1] In the *Avesta*, he has formed human beings (*Yast.*, XIX, 53) and is said to be *aurvat-aspa*, 'having rapid horses' (*Yasna*, VI, 4; LXIV, 6; *Yast.*, II, 9; XIX, 52, 53). Moreover because of the jumbling together, in the Veda, of the myths of Agni with whom he is mixed up, of Soma, who also often shows himself as a liquid fire[2] and of the waters linked up both with Agni and Soma, Apām Napāt is placed in relation with the storm clouds, celestial mountains. At least Agni, merely in its aquatic form, is called 'son of the mountain' (*ádreḥ sūnuḥ*, *RV.*, X, 20,7), whereas Soma is both the mountain-plant and celestial liquid 'milked from the mountain'[3], that-is-to-say in the celestial mountain, in the clouds. On his side, the Apam Napāt of the Avesta is described as the 'eminent master' (*ahura bərəzat*) and this designation is found

It is rather a case of pure glory of a fire without hearth; lightning is a fire of this type. Moreover, the word naphtha does not appear to go back to the name of Apām Napāt but to the Accadian *napṭu* (cf., A. Boissier, *Choix de texts relatifs á la divination assyro-babylonienne*, Vol. II, pp. 37-8; Ch. Virolleaud in *Babyloniaca*, III, 240).

1 It is not specified that they are horses. Elsewhere (I, 186, 5) it is a case of male *(vṛṣan)* fast ones of Apām Napāt: Bergaigne has, without hesitation, admitted that horses are meant (*Rel. véd.* II, p. 18); Geldner has translated it as "bulls" although he has suggested in a note the word "stallion" with a question mark and has referred to VI, 29, 2, where *vṛṣan* is juxtaposed with *aśva*. 'horse'. The *rapprochement* with the Avesta seems to settle the question.

2 Bergaigne, *ib.*, I, p. 168; II, 30 & ff. Cf. I, p. 33, on fire passing in the plants and therefrom in the body of man by means of the rain which moves him. Regarding the fire placed in the waters by *Varuṇa*, cf., *RV.*, V, 85, 2.

3 *duduhānó ádraū*, *RV.*, IX, 96, 10; cf., Bergaigne, *e. véd.*, II, pp. 31-32.

later in the name of the cosmic mountain, al-Borj.[1] Although the same may not be the case with this last detail elsewhere, it is clear that the concordance between the Vedic and the Avestan ideas regarding the association of the waters and of fire in nature, supposes the existence, from the Indo-Iranian period itself, of concepts which were absolutely apt to have served as the starting points for the later speculation of Indian physiologists concerning the presence of the organism of the fire in the form of a liquid.

The Wind:—According to the Āyurvedic doctrine, the last and the most active of the elements of the body, the wind, seems to have, like the water and the fire, already been regarded by the Indo-Iranians as the motor *par excellence.*

The Vedic wind is called *Vāyu* or *Vāta*, the former being specially that of the wind-god, the latter that of the element-wind, although this specialisation of sense is not absolute.[2] The Avestan wind is also *Vāyu* (alias *Vaya*) or *Vāta*, with a tendency to the same distribution of sense as in the Vedic. This tendency has been kept intact till the Pehlavi where *Vāi* derived from Vāyu is rather the god or the spirit and *Vāt* (from *Vāta*) is the wind or the air.[3]

The hymns of the *Ṛgveda* are far from giving to the wind as much of importance, as they give to the fire or even to the waters. They, however, invite him to the sacrifice and sometimes even before all other gods as in the *Ṛgveda*, I, 134, 6 (where it is called *ápūrvya*, 'without precedent'), but herein we should see nothing more than an example among thousands of the constant habit of the Vedic *ṛṣis* to invoke each god turn by

---

[1] Name drawn from the Avestan bərəzat 'raising himself high,' 'big' *Nafədro apam (Yasna,* I, 6) genitive of *Naptar (Napāt*) *apam* is translated by Neryosengh as the "navel of the waters" (*nābhim* [accus] *apām*, Spiegel Edn., 1, 15). That-is-to-say, undoubtedly their generator and their centre of radiation as in classical India, the navel is considered as the point of departure of the vessels, nourishing the body. The Parsi priest among other things, adds that the sovereign Burja (al-Borj) is the spirit of women and that it is made of water (burjasvāmī strīṇām iajdo (=Av. *Yazata)* jalamayaḥ).

[2] Bergaigne, *Rel. véd.*, I, p. 25.

[3] Stig Wikander, *Vayu, Texte and Untersuchungen zur indo-iranischen Religions geschichte,* Teil, I, Uppasala, Leipzig, 1941 (*Questiones indo—iranicae,* I), p. 75.

turn as the most eminent, indeed as the unique one.[1] Actually, Indra, for example, with whom Vāyu is conjointly invoked several times (I, 2, 4-6; I, 23, 3, etc.), is quite often placed in the first rank and he also, twice, is called 'without precedent' (VIII, 21, 1; 78, 5) whereas elsewhere it is Agni (III, 13, 5) who receives this epithet. It remains nevertheless true that his cosmic importance, although rarely celebrated, is clearly recognised and highly proclaimed. The hymn X, 168 of *Ṛgveda* describes Vāta as the 'king of the entire universe' (*viśvasya bhuvanasya rājā*, verse 2), 'the first-born taking part in the order' (*prathamajā ṛtāvā*, verse 3), 'the soul (or breath) of the gods, the embryo of the universe' (*ātmā devānām bhuvanasya gárbho*, verse 4). The last words of the hymn, *tásmai vātāya haviṣā vidhema*, 'to that wind we should render homage by means of an oblation', are like an answer to the question of the

---

1 Max Müller, in his famous theory of the Vedic religion, has seen in this habit, the expression of a religious form intermediary between polytheism and monotheism, the henotheism or the kathenothelsm (cf., for instance F. Max Müller, *Origine et developpement de la religion...* French translation by J. Darmesteter, Paris, 1879, pp. 236 & ff). But in believing that it implied, in the presence of each god, a forgetting of all the others, he has somewhat exaggerated its importance (cf., *Physical Religion*, London, 1891, p. 181). He has not taken sufficient note of several facts. First of all, the authors of hymns are numerous and are of different ages and each one could have had the divinity of his choice, or better still, each one could follow the fashion of his period and of his milieu; It is one of the characteristic traits of the sects of classical India that each tends to appropriate for his gods or for his heroes, the glory or the exploits of the gods or the heroes of the other sects (cf., the reciprocal borrowings of the Buddhist, Jaina and Hindu legends) and it will not be surprising that the Veda had already become Indian by the same tendency among its authors. Secondly, the simple desire of giving to each god the maximum of praise fatally led to all of them being praised in the same manner. Moreover, the fact of ascribing to several gods successively the first place does not necessarily imply a contradiction; one, for example, who is "without precedent" is not necessarily the only one who should be such a one, because the epithet can be applicable also to each of his counterparts. It is true that the formal contradictions are numerous, that a particular specific exploit is once ascribed to one mythical being and then to another, but these contradictions seem to have been deliberately looked for, in the texts where the paradox is set up as a normal literary procedure and they are logically compensated by the idea that in definitive the gods are a single being under different forms (*RV.*, I, 164, 46), at least beginning from the moment when this idea had come forth. The epithet of *ápūrvya* retains nevertheless, in the case of wind, a special value because the wind is the first among the gods to arrive at a sacrifice and this priority is already Indo-Iranian (cf., G. Dumézil, *Tarpeia*, 1947, pp. 49 & ff). It appears to be due to this reason that the wind has the attribute of velocity in the race.

well-known hymn to the unknown supreme god (8, 121), *kásmai devāya haviṣā videhma*, 'to which god do we render homage by means of an oblation?' Elsewhere Vāta is again the soul (*ātman*) of Varuṇa (VII, 87, 2), the sovereign god of the Order, of *ṛta*. Again Vāyu is elsewhere invoked (VIII, 26, 21) as the master of *ṛta (ṛtaspati)* and protects 'by the *dharman*', an equivalent of *ṛta* (I, 134, 5).

The close relationship, thus affirmed with insistence, of the wind with the normal cosmic Order betokens, from the Veda itself, the rôle of the motor and of the regulator of the Heavenly bodies which will be later on ascribed to the wind by the astronomy of classical India. (*Sūryasiddhānta*, II, 3 & XII, 73). But other features show that the life of the body also was conceived in relation with the wind. In the Veda, the concept of reciprocal relations between the Universe and the body is quite clearly shown. On dying, the human being must dissolve himself in nature: 'that the eye go to the Sun, the soul to the Wind, to the Sky and to the Earth according to the Order. Go to the Waters, if there it is advantageous for you, establish yourself in the Plants as your body'.[1] The eye, i.e., the flash, the fire of the eye, and the soul, the warm breath of the living one, which alone are named here as the elements of the human being had certainly been conceived as of the same nature as the fire and the wind of the universe as they are referred back to them. The sky, the waters and the plants, inhabited by the fire, could also receive them. As regards the earth, it is undoubtedly the residue of the solid organism which the division according to the natural Order ascribed to her. One may also see in this passage, as it has already been pointed out by Anna Moreshwar Kunte[2] a type of the announcement of the concept, later become classical, of the organism as formed of five elements (*pañca-bhautika*), if at least it is admitted that here the sky is a prefiguration of space (*ākāśa*) recognised in the classical doctrine. On the other hand, the world is sometimes represented in the image of a big human body (*pu-*

1 *śūryam cákṣur gachatu vātam ātmā dyām ca gacha pṛthivīm ca dhármaṇā* |*apó vā gacha yádi tátra te hitám óṣadhiṣu práti tiṣṭhā śariraiḥ* (*RV*., X, 16, 3).

āṅgahṛdayam, Bombay, 1880, Vol. I, p. 11 of the English introduction, note 5, (2nd edn., 1891, p. 5, column 1).

ruṣa) standing, whose head is the sky, the navel the atmosphere and the feet the earth (*RV.*, X, 90, 14). Among other cosmic elements, the Sun is born of His eye and the Wind of His breath.[1] According to the *Bṛhadāraṇyaka-upaniṣad* (beginning) it is the body of the horse which is placed limb by limb in comparison with the universe not so much because the world is conceived as the figure of the cosmic Horse but because the horse of the sacrifice must represent the world in miniature. It is the wind again which is the breath of this horse. In the *Atharvaveda* it is said that Tvaṣṭṛ and Vāyu have brought the breath (*ātman*) to a bull (*ṛṣabha*) which is an animal of the sacrifice and at the same time a symbolically celestial bull (IX, 4, 10). Lastly, the *Atharvaveda* affirms, in terms which could not have been more decisive, the identity of the *prāṇa* and of the wind (*vāyu*), "the breath (it is said) is *Mātariśvan:* it is the wind which is

---

[1] The complete text of the passage is as follows: *Candrámā mánaso jātáś cákṣoḥ sūryo ajāyata/múkhād īndraś cāgníś ca prāṇād vāyúr ajāyata* (X, 90, 13). "The Moon is born from his spirit, the Sun from his eye, and from his mouth are born Indra and Agni; the Wind is born from his breath". But this text is taken up again with a noteworthy variant in the 2nd part of the *Vājasaneyī-saṁhitā*, XXXI, 12: śrotrād vāyūś ca prāṇáś ca, mūkhād agnir ajāyata, "from his ears the wind and the breath, from his mouth the fire were born". Here the Wind and the Breath are not drawn one from the other, they are brought together as twins. If their origin is placed in the ear of the Cosmic Man, it is undoubtedly because the Vedic poetry voluntarily emphasises the noise of the Wind (*RV.*, IV, 22; VIII, 91, 5; X, 168, 1) which is heard but which is not seen (X, 168, 4). If the breath (*prāṇa*) is said to have issued from the ear and not from the mouth or the nostrils as one may have expected, it is apparently because it was conceived as the image of the wind, the audible element, rather than as the image of the breath of a man. *Vāc*, the Speech, which is the Cosmic Noise but which, in the form of human voice, comes from the Breath, is besides assimilated to the Wind (X, 125, 8) and the singer pushes forward his praises as the wind the clouds (I, 116, 1, cf., Bergaigne, *Rel. véd.*, I, p. 279) as if the speech and the song drew their power from their participation in the nature of the Cosmic Wind. . . . In an article (*Rév. philos,* Nov.-Dec., 1933, p. 420) I had proposed that in the Vedic comparison of the human body and the Cosmos, efforts had been directed more towards explaining the body by the Cosmos rather than the Cosmos by the body. Mr. Mus has objected (*BEFEO*, 1933, p. 849 and *Barabudur*, Hanoi, 1935, p. 445) that, from the hymn to the Puruṣa saying formally that the wind was born from the breath of the Puruṣa, one should, on the contrary conclude that the world was first conceived anthropomorphically. But the variant of the *Vājasaneyī-saṁhitā* answers this objection. In any case it should be conceded that the assimilation of the Cosmos and of the body is reciprocal and that in particular the wind is the breath of man just as this breath is the wind.

called the breath; it is on the breath that all that was and all that is, all is based".[1] It is true that this hymn, at the same time, identifies the breath with many other forces of nature, but it is to make of it the motor of the universal activity and the entire piece is an amplified counterpart of the hymn X,168 of the *Ṛgveda* where the mind is placed above all.[2]

Tvaṣṭṛ who, associated with Vāyu, animates the mythica bull and Mātariśvan who is identified with Prāṇa-vāta are orignally igneous gods. The first has assumed, at an early date, the rôle of a divine artisan, the second has transformed itself from fire into wind. This is because of the close association of the two elements in the Vedic ideas. This association is not due only to the commonplace idea that the wind is recognised as exciting the fire but because of a notion of the parentage of the nature of the Vāta with Agni and also with the Sun,. Sūrya, who in their company makes a triad (*RV.*, VIII, 18. 9). Moreover the Sun has himself a breath, "he circulates across the brilliant paths, with his breath he breathes down below".[3] Similarly, of the fire which burns, it has been said that it 'breathed' (*prāṇīt*, *RV.*, X, 32, 8), and another time it is said that it became 'at the time of its shooting forth, the flight of the wind'[4] which can be well understood by admitting precisely that it 'breathed'. All this gives evidence

1 *prāṇám āhur mātariśvānam vāto ha prāṇá ucvate/prāṇé ha bhūtám bhávyam ca prāṇe sárvam prátiṣṭhitam* (XI, 4, 15).

One may specially note that in *RV*, X, 168, 2. *vāta* is called. "the king of this entire universe" (*asyá víśvasva bhúvanasya rājā*) whereas in *AV.*, XI, 4. 1, it is the Prāṇa which is said to have "become the lord of all" (*bhūtáḥ sárvasyesvaró).*

antáś carati rocanāsyá prāṇād apānatī RV., X, 189, 2.

vátasya śargo abhavat sárīmaṇi (*RV.*, III, 29, 11). Geldner has understood it as "Der Wind strom enstand, wenn er (the fire) sich in Lauf setzte" and if the current of the wind has been considered as being born at the moment when the fire was starting, that is because at that time the fire was a wind. If, in any case, it could be admitted (but this hypothesis can neither be confirmed nor denied) that here the word *sarga* has one of the senses current in the classical language, i.e., that of 'creature', the translation would be: "it became, at the time of shooting forth, the creature of the wind" and it would then be simply a reference to the fact that the wind sets ablaze the fire which starts. This sense will suit quite naturally because immediately before it is a question of the fire ready to set itself ablaze which, as is said in the text, "has developed within his mother" (and which in that case is Mātariśvan: *mātariśvā yád ánimīta mātári*).

of the already quite complex speculations regarding the wind, the natural force, to whose action is sometimes assimilated that of other natural forces such as the Sun and the fire, the animating power which is found in the bodies in the shape of the breath *(prāṇa)* or of the soul *(ātman)*.

In the Avesta, the speculations regarding the wind are not pushed as far ahead as in the Veda; but it is true nevertheless that the wind is recognised to play a rôle which is quite eminent and that it appears with a number of traits which are similar to those ascribed to it in the Veda.

It is hardly worthwhile to emphasise certain similarities of the two groups of texts on the subject of the wind. These simply show that everywhere the representation of the wind is largely based on the commonplace observation of its action. It is not of much importance whether the *Yast* (VIII, 33) says that the wind brings the rain and that on its side the *Ṛgveda* (VII, 40, 6) wishes that the wind may give the rain. But the importance accorded to the wind on both the sides, as a natural element as also a supernatural being, is more significant. The notion of this importance must go back to the Indo-Iranian community; otherwise it would be necessary to suppose that this notion was formed among the Iranians and among the Indians independently or that it was formed among these people after their separation and that it was then communicated to each other.

But in the absence of all historical data capable of settling the question, these two last hypotheses can be judged only according to their intrinsic probability and which is rather weak. Given the important rôle played by the naturalism both in the Avesta and in the Veda, it would be difficult to suppose that this naturalism did not correspond to the very basis of the Indo-Iranian ideas. It will be still more difficult to conceive that in a largely natural mythology, the wind did not directly have its recognised place. Although one may admit that due to the date of its definitive redaction, the recent Avesta could have borrowed certain data from Brahmanic India, it is probable that the importance accorded to the wind in this Avesta goes back to the Indo-Iranian period as it is similar to the importance given to it in the ancient Veda.

Moreover the Avestan ideas regarding the wind seem to

carry in themselves the mark of their antiquity. In spite of the systematic character of the Iranian dualism, a dualism which rigourously divides, on principle, the beings into good ones and bad ones, the wind appears in the Avesta in an equivocal rôle. Now this exception to the dualistic systemisation can be explained as a case of the survival of an older concept, related to those of the Veda concerning the equivocal character of the divinities.

While examining the passages relative to Vāyu in the Avesta, first of all, it is found that all of them do not proceed from the same spirit. A litany simply proclaims, "we honour the audacious wind created by Mazdā".[1] In the same passage other elements (except the fire) and the chief beings habitually adored in Zoroastrianism are also declared to be worthy of adoration. The *Yasna* again invokes the wind, either under the name of Vāta or under that of Vayu. In XXII, 23, the sacrificer announces his desire to operate for the satisfaction of Ahura Mazda, of Aməsa Spənta, of Mithra, of Rāman (who, as we shall see, is already a personification of the wind) and in the following passage (24), "from Vayu to superior action, who gets the better of other creatures, (and of) that which of you, O Vayu, is of Holy Spirit",[2] wherefrom it results both that the wind is a pre-eminent being and that it is not entirely good. Further on another litany declares: "We honour Vayu which is of the Order, we honour Vayu having the superior action...", etc. (as in the preceding passage).[3] At the end of the *Yasna* comes back another invocation of 'the wind which possesses the Order',[4] but this time it is to the name of Vāta that the epithet *asavan*, 'who possesses the Order', is joined, which proves that Vāta and Vayu are, at least in the *Yasna*, two names of the same wind, simultaneously a mythical element and a mythical personality. Moreover

---

1 *vātəmcā barsīm mazdadātəm yazmaidē* (*Yasna*, Spiegel Edn., XLI, 26, Westgaard and Geldner Edn., XI-III, 3). The phrase is taken up with insignificant variants in the *Vīspered*, VII, 4.

2 *vayaos uparō. kairyehe taradātō anyaīs dāman aetat to vayō yaṭ to asti spentō. mainyaom.*

3 *vaēm asavanəm yazamaide vaēm uparō. kairīm yazamaide.* (*Yasna*, XXV, 5).

4 *vātahe asaono* (*Yasna*, Spiegel Edn., LXIX, 11, Westgaard and Geldner Edn., LXX, 3).

the epithet *asavan* is remarkable as by a characteristic trait it proves the relationship of the Avestan concept of the Wind, Vayu or Vāta with that of the Vedic Vāyu or Vāta, the latter one also, as we have just now seen, places the wind in close relationship with the Order, the *ṛta*, equivalent of the Avestan *asa*.

The *Sīrôza* (I, 21) which indicates the divinities to whom the thirty days of the month are consecrated, makes the 21st that of *Rāman*, of *Vayu* (to whom it gives the same qualifications as are given them by *Yasna*, XXII, 23), of Thwāsa, the atmosphere and of the infinite time, *zrvan akarana*. The 22nd day is consecrated to *Vāta* which comes from the four cardinal points (I, 22). Vayu and Vāta are, therefore, not always assimilated; sometimes the difference in names corresponds to a mythical doubling, so that one of them is sometimes the substitute of another and sometimes his doublet. This trait is an additional resemblance with the Veda where, similarly, the two names are employed one for the other, sometimes figuring together in the same passage, as is the case in the *Atharvaveda*, XIX, 1 & 2.

In the *Videvdât*, the reference to the wind is principally made as a natural element, designated under the name of Vāta. Yima asks Ahura Mazda that his kingdom be free from the hot and cold winds (II, 5). In III, 42, the Law which chases away sins is compared to the wind (Vāta) 'of right'[1] which sweeps the atmosphere (thwāsa). The passages V, 3 to 7 envisage the case of the transport of a dead body by the wind and V, 12 & 13 refer to the wind which dries the earth. In V, 15 & 17, it is a case of the mythical wind but even then, identical to the atmospherical wind, which Ahura Mazda sends out with the waters of the Vouru kasa Sea. Vāta is nevertheless conceived in the same text as personified and doublet of Vayu because both of them are invoked one after the other, Vayu with his qualificative of *uparo kairya*, 'having the superior action', Vāta with those of heroic *(takhma)* and of 'created by

---

dasināt. If in the epoch of the author of the text, the orientation was done by turning the face to the east, as in India. it is the wind of mid-day and precisely, in a comparison of the *Āfrīngān* of Rapithwin. 6, reference is made to the wind of mid-day as a favourable wind. Bartholomae, however (*Altiranisches Wörterbuch*), believes that it is the wind of the east.

Mazda' *(Mazdadāta)*. At the time of their invocation are also invoked once again the supreme entities of Mazdaism (XIX, 13 & 16). Yet the *Videvdāt* knows also of an evil wind the demona, the wind (*Vāta*[1] *daeva*, X, 14) which it exorcises and it sees in Vayu mostly the spirit of death which carries the man fallen in water or in the fire *(Vid.*, V, 8 & 9).[2] On the contrary, a litany of the *Nyāyisn*, (I, 8) invokes the 'Vāta, healthy and of good intentions'.[3]

The *Yast* mention several times Vātạ in the form of a South and North wind *(vāta pourvo apākhtara)*, in that of a bad one (III, 9, 12 & 17) and chiefly refers to his grandiose and propitious figure. Auxiliary of Mithra in his offensives, Vāta is said several times to be one 'which shatters the defences' *(vərəthrajan)*.[4] He shares this epithet with other "victorious" warrior entities of the Avesta and also with the Haoma,[5] which has an important anti-demoniacal function. In the Veda, the parallel epithet *vṛtrahan* is not applied to him directly, but it has a use analogous to that of *vərəthrajan* in the Avesta.; it characterises a group of mythical heroes comparable to those of the Avesta and which includes notably the Soma, but among whom Indra dominates.[6] Now Vāyu-Vāta is frequently associated with Indra in the *Ṛgveda* and this associates him directly with a group of warrior divinities which is the counterpart of the one which includes in the Avesta, its Iranian homonym.[7] Another trait which

---

1 or *vātya*. 'of the wind' (Bartholomae—Wolff).

2 cf., Nyberg, *Questions de Cosmogonie et de cosmologie mazdéennes*. in *JA*., Oct-Dec., 1931, p. 205, where the wind. spirit of death, of the *Videvdāt* is identified with the "pitiless" wind of the *Aogemodaēsā* (77-81).

3 *vātəm spəntəm hudanhəm.*

4 *Yast*, X, 9; XII, 4, 6 & 9; XIII, 47, 48; cf., E. Benveniste & L. Renou, *Vṛtra & Vrthragna; étude de mythologie indo-iranienne* in *Cahiers de la soc. as.*, III, Paris, 1934, p. 20.

5 ibid. 6 ibid., p. 115-116.

7 In the *Atharvaveda*, XIX, 27, 2, the epithet *Vṛtrahan* is even juxtaposed to the name of Vāta but it is related rather to that of Candra which precedes him. In any case, the passage shows once again the wind grouped with the *vṛtrahan* divinities.—B. Geiger, *Aməṣ̌a Spənta's*, p. 79, has recognised an Indo-Iranian trait in the 'conqueror' character of the god of Wind; Mr. Lommel *Die Yasts des Avesta*, Gottingen, 1927, p. 144, has contested the Indo-Iranian character of this trait. For him the Vedic Vāta would have been too late a personification to have been an Indo-Iranian divinity, but in order to

appears in the *Yast* makes a *rapprochement* between the Avestan wind and the Vedic wind. According to the *Yast* (XII, 4, 6 & 9) Vāta along with other entities, accompanied Ahura Mazda at the preparation of the religious service and this reminds us of the invitations given to Vāyu in the Veda.

But the most important passage concerning the Wind is the *Yast*, XV (entire) known as the *Rām Yast*, dedicated to Rāman who is here the same as Vayu[1]; everybody agrees in considering this text as a relatively late one in regard to its redaction. In fact, it presents itself as partly constituted of passages reproduced from other pieces of the Avesta. This is how in paragraph 5 it repeats the passage relative to Vayu of *Yasna* (XXV, 5) and that from 1 to 17 it takes up a legend of *Videvdāt*, (II, 5) in which Yima asks for the prosperity of his kingdom. But as regards Vayu it is richer than the rest of the Avesta.[2] Herein Vayu holds the rank of supreme god. The mythical heroes come in turn by turn to propitiate him, most of them to request for victory and Ahura Mazda himself is the first who invokes him and honours him ritually for obtaining victory over the creation of Añra Mainyu (2 to 4). It is to him and no longer as in the *Videvdāt*, to Ahura Mazda that Yima addresses his prayer. He is mostly asked to confer victory, which reminds one of his warrior aspects found in other *Yasts*, but he also dispenses all sorts of gifts. By his character of *asavan*, of "the possesser of the good Order", he could evidently arrange everything happily. The same was thought about the Vedic Vāyu, to him a similar homage was rendered and to him oblations were made to flow, because he was told: "Thou protectest by the good Order".[3]

---

support this opinion, he simply refers back to a page of Oldenberg, of little consequence on this subject. Moreover, it is not necessary that the wind be personified so that the representation one makes of it be linked with the idea of victory, mainly of an offensive victory consisting in the overthrow of the defence.

1 This *Yast* is edited, translated and profusely commented upon along with the hymn to Vayu of the *Aogemadaecā* in Stig Wikander, *Vayu*, first part of a big study which may be followed by another of Mr. Ronnow on Agni and Vāyu.

2 On the importance of this *Yast*, cf. Nyberg, *Questions*...in *JA.*, Oct. Dec., 1931, pp. 197 & ff.

3 *tvám viśvasmād bhúvanāt pāsi dhármaṇā sūryāt pāsi dhármaṇā* (RV.,

Certain enumerations of the names and the epithets of Vayu are important inasmuch as they specify the representation that is made of him. In these enumerations many traits of details remind one of the Vedic Wind. He is essentially strong and fast (*aurva*, 46, 54, 57), now in the *Ṛgveda*, the speed of the gods or of the mythical horses is several times compared to that of the wind.[1] He has a chariot of gold just as the one possessed by Indra and Vāyu in the *Ṛgveda*, (IV, 46, 4). He is 'blazing' (*saocahi*, 47), 'healer' (*baesazya*, 56), states referred to with pleasure by the Vedic *ṛṣis* while noting on several occasions his action on the fire, while frequently presenting the fire itself as excited by the wind[2] and while desiring, with an oft-repeated word-play 'that the wind may fan the remedy' (*vāta ā vātu bheṣajám*).[3] This last concordance of the Veda and the Avesta is quite significant in so far as it points to an original relationship of concepts, because the idea of making the wind a dispenser of remedy could not have been one of those which suggests itself naturally to anyone who observes his action.[4]

The Vayu of *Rām Yast* as the Vayu or the Vāta of other parts of the Avesta, therefore, very much resembles the Wind of the Veda. There is, however, a distinction to be made between the two in certain aspects. This Vayu is more strongly personified and his character of Cosmic force is extremely vague. He is made to say to himself, "I call myself

---

I, 134, 5). It is quite possible that one may see in *asurya*, as suggested by Sāyaṇa, a reference to the 'demonical' rather than to the 'divine' in view of the extremely equivocal sense of *Asura*.

1 cf., Bergaigne, *Rel. véd.*, I, p. 27.

2 ibid, p. 26.

3 *RV.*, X, 186; cf., also I, 89, 4 & VII, 35,4; cf, Bergaigne, *Rel. véd.* I, p. 34.

Here one could ask if the two names that Vayu gives himself (*Yast*, XV, 45) *fracara*, 'marching forward' and *aipicara*, 'marching back' do not correspond to the two forms of the organic wind, *prāṇa*, 'which breathes forward' and *apāna*, 'which breathes below', the second being specially that of the inferior or posterior part of the body as we will see. Of course linguistically the words differ completely as the Avestan root *car* responds to the Ved. *car* or *cal* which is more recent (cf., Wikander, op. cit., p. 79) and not to *an* but the corresponding ideas are comparable and are undoubtedly related.

Vayu because I pursue (or chase) the two creations, that of Spənta Mainyu and that of Añra Mainyu" (43), but this is for explaining by means of an etymology which is only a play on words, the name of *Vayu* by *Vayemi*, "I pursue". Similarly the following addition is made, "I attain *(apayemi)* the two creations", (43) "I conquer (*vanāmi*) the two creations" and "I operate well *(vohu vərəzyami)*, for the creature, Ahura Mazda and the *Aməsa Spenta*" (44). Here there is no precise idea of any cosmic role ascribed to the wind; there are only the explanations of the qualificatives *apayata*, 'who attains', *vanô-vīspa*, 'who conquers everything' and *vohuvarsta* 'benefactor'.[1] Vayu or Vāta has become a sovereign entity and is no longer a force of nature. It is true that in certain passages of the Avesta the wind is only a metereological phenomenon, but this itself removes it away from the central concept of the wind in the Veda. The Vayu-Vāta of the Avesta do not come in the middle of the material phenomenon and the god, the Vedic Vāyu-Vāta is thus less divine and more of a natural force. The soul of the world, it is the god because of the fulness of its rôle. Being breath, it is a material force and in the unitary explanation which the *ṛṣis* try to give of the world and of the body, he is ready to be conceived as the great cosmo-physiological principle of movement. The form in which he has reached us in the Avesta, does not show that a concept of the wind, simultaneously as a cosmic soul and as a vital breath is as clearly attested as in the Veda. One, therefore, tends to conclude from the comparison of the Avestan and Vedic data on the wind, that a general concept of its eminent rôle in the universe and of its high rank among the powerful entities which co-operate for the maintenance of the Cosmic Good Order is Indo-Iranian, but it is by means of a more recent and exclusively Indian evolution that the wind has been conceived in the Veda as the common motor of the cosmic and individual lives.

This conclusion should, at least, suffice to establish the physiological theory of the Indian doctors of the classical epoch, according to which the wind plays an essential rôle in

1 On these names and their nominatives in—*e* which seem to correspond to an Iranian form of the East, cf., Nyberg, *Questions*...in *J.A.*, Oct. Dec., 1931, p. 201 & note 4.

the organic life, has antecedents which go back right up to the Indo-Iranian epoch where the wind already, like fire and water, the other elements of the physical life, occupied a big place in the speculations. But this is a "minima" conclusion. Many indices show the possibility of the existence in Iran at an early date, of concepts still nearer to those of the Veda than are not those of the actual Avesta and which can eventually go back to the Indo-Iranian period. It is necessary to examine this possibility, which is important not only for a knowledge of the antecedents of the Indian physiology but also for the entire history of the ancient cosmo-physiological doctrines of Iran and the Hellenic world.

The Avesta as it has reached us is not complete, but the analyses of its contents as found in their epoch and given by the Pehlavi books allow us to suspect a part of what has been lost and the cosmological statements of these books seem to reproduce the ideas which were, of yore, really Avestan. In fact, these books sometimes refer to the Avesta and every time we are unable to verify their reference in the actual Avesta, we cannot accuse them of having falsely ascribed to the sacred book the data which were unknown to it. False attributions could not have been accepted in a milieu and at a time when verification was easy. However, the interpretations of the authors could have been sometimes abusive and their indications cannot replace the original texts which have disappeared. We should, therefore, receive the Pehlavi complements of the *Avesta* with circumspection; on another side, it is certain that many of the ideas which were prevalent in ancient Iran were never included in the Avesta. There Pehlavi texts have not created *ex nihilo* all that they contain without having borrowed from the Avesta; a good part of their data can be Iranian and ancient and can even go back to the Indio-Iranian epoch, without ever having been Avestan.

As regards the problem of the Iranian Vayu, the researches of Nyberg have led him to suppose the existence of a veritable religion of Vayu, of a 'vayism', forming the counterpart of a 'zervanism', the religion of the Time and heterodox in comparison to the Avestan Mazdeism, although only traces of its existence be recognisable in the Avesta. A passage of the neo-platonist Damaskios ascribes to Eudemos of Rhodes, an author of the IVth century B.C. and a friend of Aristotle, a piece of information according to which 'the Magis and the entire Aryan race' hold either Topos or Chronos as the World-principle.[1] Nyberg recognises in the Topos the 'thwasa', the atmospere, in chronos, Zrvan, the Time which two are often mentioned side by side in the Avesta and he proposes the identity of *thwāsa* with *Vayu.*[2] In this case this passage will attest the existence of zervanism, of a vayism whose traces he finds precisely in the *Rām Yast*[3] and which could have been more particular in the East of Iran and in the warrior caste. This last hypothesis is based on the fact that in the *Rām Yast* (and generally in the *Yasts*) Vayu has the characteristic of a victorious god and is based on two other facts, namely the presence of the grammatical forms of the East in his adjectives and the frequency of the name of Vāta on the Indo-scythian coins, which are also oriental. It may be objected that there is nothing signiflcant in it, because the Indo-Scythian coins belong to the commencement of the Christian era and the redaction of the *Rām Yast* is also not very old; now if it be necessary to recognise the trace of a vayism in the information ascribed to Eudemos, then this vayism must have been known in the Occident from the IVth century B.C. The coins and the grammatical forms of the East, posterior by many centuries, cannot indicate that the East has been the first home of vayism. It is still more difficult to believe that the Parthians whose domination stated about a century after Eudemos, could have, according to a hypothesis proposed again by Mr.

---

1 Nyberg, *Questions*...in *J.A.*, July-Sept., 1931, p. 103 & ff.

2 ibid, & *Die Rel des alten Ir.*, p. 75. The arguments of Mr. Nyberg are accepted by M. Christensen, *L'Iran sous les sassanides*, p. 149. It can be, however, possible that *thwāsa* corresponds rather to the concept of the aerial space, covering all that has the motive force running around the world. "Topos" indicates a place and not a moving energy. The facts observed by Mr. Nyberg that *thwāsa*, Vata and Vayu are invoked side by side in *Yasna*, LXXII, 10, *Nyāyisn*, I, 8, & *Vid.*, XIX, 16 (also XIX, 13) provokes not so much to assimilating them as to distinguish them, all the more so as in these same passages, other entities which can not be assimilated to them, are also invoked. Examples are those of the *fravasi* of Ahura Mazda and the Mathra Spənta, etc.. It is not, however, doubtful that just as Vāta, Vayu and Rāman are only different aspects of the one and same entity, *thwāsa* can also be considered as the fourth aspect.

3 *Questions*...in *J.A.*, Oct. Dec., 1931, pp. 197, 201 & ff.

Nyberg, played a rôle in the expansion of the cult of Vayu towards the West. But Mr. Nyberg raises the question of the geographical centre of the development of vayism only secondarily. The more important one is to know if it has really existed as an independent religion because that would imply such a big movement of speculations on the wind that it could be the centre of the diffusion of these speculations.

The fact that Vayu appears in the *Rām Yast* as superior to Ahura Mazda seems to support strongly the hypothesis of the existence of vayism as an autonomous religion.[1] One can, however, observe that it is not rare that Ahura Mazda appears in the Avesta below the supreme rank without the necessity of seeing in it each time the traces of the influence of a competing religion. In the *fargard* XXII of the *Videvdāt*, he asks for help against Aṅra Mainyu, from Mathra Spənta and mostly from Airyaman, just as in the *Rām Yaśt*, he honours Vayu by asking him to vanquish the demon. In the Yasts, Ahura Mazda has sacrificed to Ardvī sūrā Anāhitā to ask from him the favour of attaching himself to Zoroaster (V, 17-19) and he honours *Tistrya* (VIII, 25). These cases can be compared to that of *Rām Yast* and if one can invoke the well-attested existence of a special religion of Ardvī sūrā Anāhitā (120), one cannot do the same in the case of Mathra Spənta, of Airyaman, or of Tistrya. The case of the last-named one allows us to understand that basically the homage of Ahura Mazda to any entity does not necessarily place him below the latter. In fact in the *Yast*, VIII, Ahura Mazda says not only: "Myself who is Ahura Mazda, I honour by the expressed name Tistrya, the splendid, the brilliant"[2] (25) but also that he has made him as his equal to enable him to struggle against a *pairikā* (50 & ff). Ahura Mazda, therefore, does

---

1 ibid p. 219 & note.

2 It is true that Mr. Nyberg bases himself chiefly (op. cit., p. 202) on the fact that *Vayu* calls himself in the *Rām Yast*, the vanquisher of the two opposing creations, in support of his opinion that he is, in this text, a superior god to Ahura Mazda. But he could have been the vanquisher of the creation of Ahura Mazda, that is to say, he could have dominated the creatures without dominating the creator himself; it is therefore only the fact that Ahura Mazda has recourse to him which seems to give him a higher rank.

3 On which cf., Nyberg, *Die Rel. des alten Iran*, p. 260 & ff.

4 *azəm yo ahurō mazda tistrim raēvantəm hvarənaṅ uhan təm aokhtō-nāmana yasna yaze.*

not go down in esteem when he honours one of his creatures, because by honouring him he does not accomplish an act of humble piety, but a rite whose efficacy is taught by him, this efficacy being necessary provided that that rite be in conformity with the Order (56). It should not be forgotten that we are dealing here not with Christianity but with a cult where the officiating person who honours the god by his name, does not perform an act of devotion but only magically sets in motion the action of the god. It is, therefore, possible that in the *Rām Yast*, Vayu may not be really superior to Ahura Mazda and it is not indispensable to believe that the veneration of Vayu has been frequent and exclusive for constituting a veritable religion of the wind. Moreover, it is a rule of the Yasts that they exalt without limits the entities to which they are dedicated and place them turn by turn above all. This is how is found in them an echo of the henotheism of the Vedic hymns. In that case, it appears to be possible to admit that the eminent rôle ascribed to the wind in the *Rām Yast*, as also in other parts of the Avesta, comes from the survival and the evolution in Mazdaism of the ancient and the naturalistic Indo-Iranian ideas on the wind. It is not necessary to represent to oneself, the formation of the *Yast* as the result of a syncretism of Mazdaism and of vayism. The hypothesis of survivals explains the concordances noted between the Avestan and the Vedic data. The hypothesis of vayism could equally explain them if it was to be admitted that this religion has precisely preserved the Indo-Iranian notions, but it introduces a superfluous deviation and brings in the risk of finally exaggerating the importance of speculations on the wind in Iranian thought.

Nevertheless, these speculations hold an important place and seem to have been linked with cosmological ideas, much nearer those of the Veda than it can be seen from the actual Avesta. We have seen that the wind and the breath had been assimilated in the Veda, that the breath was regarded as a wind animating the body and that, reciprocally, the wind was conceived as the breath of a Cosmic body. The actual Avesta contains nothing similar to it. It is true that the Vedic myths of the cosmic man, of the cosmic horse, of the cosmic bull must be originally related to the Avestan myths of the primordial bull (gəus) and of the first man, Gayo-marətan. But if one relies only on the Avestan data, then neither man nor bull possesses a body representing the world. It can be that they were originally a celestial man and a celestial bull as was conceived by Darmesteter, but they do not cover the universe. In the *Gāthā Ahunavaiti*, (in *Yasna*, XXIX) the soul of the bull is presented as the spirit of the herds. According to *Yast*, XIII, 87, Ahura Mazda has drawn the Aryan race from Gayo-Marətan. On the other hand, the Pehlavi tradition gives a cosmic significance to the myths of the primitive bull and the primitive man. According to the *Bundahisn*, both are killed by Aṅra Mainyu. From the various parts of the body of the bull are born all sorts of plants, his semen goes to the Moon, whose light purifies it and produces a couple of bovides and then couples of all the animals (Chap. X & XIV).[1] Similarly the semen of Gayo-marətan, gathered on his death, is purified by the light of the Sun and later gives birth to two plants which become the first human couple (XV). All this is presented as having been taken from the Avesta and the *Zādsparam* which takes it up with more details and indicates (IX, 1) that a correspondence of the plants with each limb of the bull is given in the *Dāmdāt nask*.[2] Here it is precisely the case of a *nask* lost from the Avesta, but the assertion can be accepted as the actual Avesta, instead of contradicting these myths, contains several details which corroborate them and most of all because several traits of these myths are Indo-Iranian. The Vedic texts compare with the semen of an animal, the rain which makes the plants grow and which assimilates itself to the celestial Soma, to the Soma whose relations with the Moon are not necessarily of a late origin as is admitted sometimes. In any case, the bull whose semen is in the sky and whose dead body giving birth to plants, represents all the earth and is a cosmic body; He is the world conceived in the image of an animal; He is sometimes conceived by the Vedic texts. This idea has all the chances of going back to the Indo-Iranian epoch.[4]

---

1 cf., translation and study of this *gāthā* in J. Duchesne—Guillemin, *Zoroastre*, Paris, 1948, pp. 193 ff.
Translation, E. W. West, *Pahlavi Texts*, I (*SBE*, V) Oxford, 1880, pp. 30-31, 45 & ff.

3 ibid.. p. 177.

4 It will not be of much use to object that in India the myths of man or

In the Pehlavi texts, one could easily pursue the research for concordances between the cosm-ophysiological doctrines of Iran and India. A passage of the *Bundahisn*, (from the recension usually called the "Big Bundehesh"), published and translated by E. Blochet[1] deals with the human body considered as representing the world. The correspondences established by this text between the elements of the world and the parts of the body are found to a great extent in the Indian texts, but to a lesser extent in those of the Vedic group than those of the classical epoch. The *Bundahisn* compares the movement of the Wind to that of life in the body (VII, 6)[2] and there one may see the parallel of the Vedic conception of the wind and *prāṇa*. The *Denkart* teaches that air circulates as much in the earth as in the human body and produces the earthquakes, an idea which reappears in Caraka.[3] As regards the constitution of the body by the three elements of water, fire and wind, the Pehlavi books sometimes agree with Caraka and other Indian doctors.[4] But in these cases, one should not, however, hurriedly conclude that even the evident concordances between the Iranian and Indian teaching denote the existence of corresponding notions form the Indo-Iranian period. The remarks that we made, in the beginning of this chapter,

---

of the cosmic animals are not found from the most ancient Ṛgvedic hymns (the myth of the Puruṣa is found only in the Xth maṇḍala). Very old ideas can be found in relatively late texts. The concept of the world as a body is frequent among the people of inferior culture, it can therefore perfectly have been a part of the Indo-Iranian ideas. Moreover, the relative age of the hymns is sometimes appreciated without any serious criterion, by reason of sentiment. The older Vedic scholars have introduced in science the prejudice that hymns containing theosophical, philosophical and other speculations were necessarily more recent than those whose contents are more purely naturalistic. To their mind, all that concerned speculation was not sufficiently "primitive" to be able to belong the base itself of the Veda. But one can no longer accept such ideas if it is thought that much before the first Vedic hymn was composed (and this hymn itself supposes a degree of civilisation which admits the usage of speculations) various peoples not far removed from the Vedic Aryans, those of Mesopotamia, had both, speculations and various sciences.

1 *Textes religieux pehlevis,* in *RHR*, Vol. XXXI, Paris, 1895, pp. 3-10 of the litho text,, pp.243-51 & 253 for translation and commentary.

2 Translation, West, op. cit., p.27.

3 *infra.* The theses of *Denkart* are quoted by L. C. Casartelli, *La philosophie religieuse du mazdeisme sous les sassanides,* Paris, 1884, pp. 106 and 127. On the role of the wind, see also pp. 94, 102.

Casartelli, op. cit.. p. 127.

concerning the probability of current contacts between India and Iran during the centuries around the beginning of the Christian era, may be applied here. The Iranians and the Indians do not have only a common heritage from the pre-historic times, they also have in common a number of ideas which they have shared because of prolonged cultural relations and it is precisely each time the ideas were in accord with the old traditional notions held in common that the two peoples could have easily accepted together the later developments which had been given them separately.

We will, therefore, not examine here in detail the numerous *rapprochements* which can be made between the notions found only in the Middle-Iranian texts and in the Sanskrit works later than the Vedic epoch. We will limit ourselves to draw two conclusions from the comparison of the Vedic ideas relating to medicine with the corresponding ones in Iran. In the Indo-Iranian period, there does not seem to have existed any medical system which the Vedic Aryans could have brought with them into India. On the other hand, right from the Indo-Iranian period, several general notions concerning the cosmic rôle of the natural elements, such as the waters, the fire, the wind, had come into being. At the same time an idea of the correspondence between these elements and the constituent principles of the body had been developed and this must have prepared the latter-day development of the two parallel physiologies and cosmologies.

CHAPTER THREE

THE DATA OF THE VEDIC SAMHITAS ON PATHOLOGY

The Vedic literature contains, in all its parts, numerous references to the various parts of the body, to diseases and even to the functioning of the organism. In its oldest stratum, in the Saṁhitās, these references are fortuitous and they do not furnish us with enough data on the knowledge of the period. The Saṁhitās, being only the collections of hymns, of liturgical songs and of magical and ritual pieces, were in no way suited for descriptive accounts of the rudiments, which one could have acquired at that time, of anatomy, physiology and medicine. The references found in the most recent data of the Vedic literature in the essentially "brahmanic" stratum, that is in the Brāhmaṇas and in the Upaniṣads are more important for the contemporary state of science. There, often, the cosmo-physiological speculations are discussed in a way, which though not at all systematic, allows us at least to have an idea of the same. But the indications of the Saṁhitās, thanks to their antiquity, are also quite precious. Moreover, their comparison with more recent data allows us to observe either their agreement or their disagreement with the latter ones. It is, therefore, possible to distinguish between the notions which go back to the oldest texts and those which appear at a later date and to fix certain points of relative chronology in the formation of the medical science of India.

There is quite an amount of temptation to stick on here. Yet, the difficult problem of the absolute chronology of the Vedic texts cannot be avoided here. The position of the scientific ideas of ancient India in relation to those of the anterior and neighbouring civilisations can be studied only if it is possible to bring these texts, if not to the dates, at least to the periods of general chronology. To decide, for example, if a certain Indian notion is anterior, contemporary or posterior to a corresponding Greek notion, it is evident that it is not sufficient to state with precision the stratum of Vedic literature from which it is found, but it is equally essential to know at least the approximate epoch to which it appertains.

The existence of the Vedic literature is supposed by all other known literatures of India. Buddhism and Jainism, founded in the VIth century B. C., refer, in their ancient traditions, to the Brahmins and to their religion. It is certain that before their time, the essential part of the Brahmanic literature had been constituted and this had taken place a long time ago. Two concordant facts prove it. Firstly the language of these Brahmanic texts is not the language which had been in use during the centuries preceding the Christian era; it is much more archaic. Towards the end of IVth century B. C., at the time of the Expedition of Alexander and of the Seleucid Embassies to Central India, the current language was no longer the ancient Indian, the Sanskrit, it was already a form of middle-Indian; the forms of geographical names or of the names of men reproduced by the Greek sources, clearly establish this point. Moreover, in the totality of the Brahmanic literature, there are several successive strata of different ages as is shown by the evolution of terms or of the habitudes of style. Now this is the second fact which establishes the antiquity of the Brahmanic literature—the geographical horizon of the texts belonging to the oldest stratum is in the West of India whereas that of the linguistically more recent stratum, progressively extends itself towards the East. The authors of the oldest book, the *Ṛgveda,* belong to a circle of conquerors, the Aryas, fighting the indigenous people. The texts belonging to latter epochs thus lay out the stages of the conquest going from the West to the East, the conquest, which in the times of the Buddha and of Mahāvīra, had not only attained the East, but had also permeated the entire population for centuries, because the Sanskrit language, brought in at the time of the conquest and still used in the Brahmanic texts (which refer to it) had already transformed itself into middle-Indian.

Efforts have been made to have an idea of the time which must have passed between the successive literary strata, in which the Vedic and the Brahmanical texts can be chronologically spread out. These are of the *Ṛgveda,* of the other Vedas, of the Brāhmaṇas, of the liturgical commentaries, of the Āraṇyakas, "books of the forest" for the use of sages who have retired into the jungle, of the Upaniṣads, speculative texts generally attached to the Brāhmaṇas and the Āraṇyakas, and lastly the Sūtras, manuals of ritual and religious legality, associated with other technical manuals on grammar, prosody and astronomy which together form the group of *Vedāṅga* or parts of the Veda. Long ago Max Müller had proposed to calculate in roughly two hundred years the duration of each of the earlier periods corresponding to the first stratum, the last one having taken a longer time and having been possibly elaborated (in part), even a long time after the beginning of Buddhism. Certain savants have thought that this period of two hundred years was too short, others as too long and Max Müller himself said that his choice was altogether arbitrary.[1] He put it forward not as probable, but simply as being reasonably adopted for fixing the ideas while waiting for better things. His calculations showed that the collection of the hymns of the *Ṛgveda* was constituted sometime between 1200 and 1000 B. C.

It is not possible to be content with such an hypothetical dating. That is why efforts have been made, as had been done much before Max Müller, to fix the absolute dates of the Vedic texts in the light of the astronomical indications contained therein. Unfortunately, neither the effort of Colebrooke, who started from an astronomical text, much later than the *Ṛgveda*, the *Jyotiṣavedāṅga*, nor those of H. Jacobi and of B. G. Tilak, based on the interpretation of certain data in the *Ṛgveda* and dating this text several thousand years before Christ, have been convincing. The interpretations of the proposed texts were not always convincing and even if they were certain, it was not possible to calculate therefrom sure dates of these texts. These latter can always reproduce the astronomical data which are not contemporary to them but which have been inherited by them from an ancient tradition. Their indications cannot be decisive without cross-checking.

There is another means of dating these texts, which, with-

[1] *Physical Religion*, London, 1891, p. 96. For a bibliography of similar calculations and of various efforts at dating the Vedic texts, cf. L. Renou, *Bibliographie védique*, pp. 158 and ff.

out being infallible, have at least the advantage of being based on passably credible historical data, namely the data of the Purāṇas which have been neglected and often discredited. The Purāṇas contain long geneological lists which have greatly deceived those who have utilised them. These lists deserve all the criticism that has been made of them. They are not of a very old date and are full of disagreements and incoherent statements which completely condemn them. But before rejecting them, one must remind oneself that it is these very lists which have furnished the key to Indian history. It is in the geneological lists of the *Bhāgavatapurāṇa*, read in the translation made by Maridas Pullé of a Tamil version, that de guignes had recognised in 1771[1], under the name of Sandragutten (Candragupta), the Indian king Sandrokottos mentioned by the Greek and Latin historians as a contemporary of Seleukos. These very lists, once again, in agreement with the Simhalese chronicles, describe the succession of the Mauryas, revealing that Aśoka was the grandson of Candragupta and permit us to utilise for the general chronology of India (before the IInd century B. C.) the synchronism of Aśoka and the Greek king mentioned in the inscriptions of the former. Hence everything is not false in the Purāṇas. They furnish us the means to calculate the probable epoch of king Parīkṣit, legendary but only half so, whose praise is sung in the *Atharvaveda* (XX, 127) as of a living prince. One could, therefore, determine the probable period of the *Atharvaveda*.

According to the *Viṣṇupurāṇa* (IV, XXIV, 32), 1015 years passed between the birth of Parīkṣita and the consecration of the Magadhan king, Nanda. The same period is calculated at 1115 years by the *Bhāgvatapurāṇa* (XII, 11, 26) and at 1050 years by the *Vāyu*-(XCIX, 415), the *Matsya*-and the *Brahmāṇḍa-purāṇas*.[2] According to these texts, the dynasty founded by

---

1 Date of the composition of the memoir which has revealed this discovery and which has been read at the Académie des Inscriptions et Belles-Lettres, in 1772 and published in 1778 in the *Mémoires de l'Acad. des Inscr. et Belles-Lettres,* Vol. XXXVIII, pp. 312-336.

2 cf., H. H. Wilson, *The Vishnu Purana,* Vol. IV, London, 1868, pp. 230-31; F. E. Pargiter, *The Purāṇa Text of the Dynasties of the Kali Age,* Oxford, 1913, pp. 60 & 74. The various variants manifestly go back to a common origin.

Nanda would have lasted a hundred years. Therefore, the Purāṇas, (leaving aside the somewhat aberrant data of the *Bhāgavata*) without agreeing on the exact figure, allow a period of eleven centuries between the birth of Parīkṣit and the end of the Nandas. Now this end of the Nandas dates from the time when Candragupta took over power in 313 B. C. It is, therefore, in the XVth century B. C., roughly towards 1400 B. C., that Parīkṣit of the *Atharvaveda* should be placed. A number of hymns of this Veda could be older still, as the hymn to Parīkṣit belongs to the most recent stratum of the collection.[1]

There are several facts to confirm the authenticity of the Puranic information on this point. First of all, the Purāṇas while calculating the time between Parīkṣit and Nanda, also fix the corresponding positions of the stars (*Viṣ. p.* IV, XXIV, 33). Now these astronomical positions suppose an impossible movement of the Great Bear around the Pole. They are merely arbitrary conceptions and at first view they seem to compromise the value of numerical data. But one must observe nevertheless that these astronomical observations, not being in any way the results of observation, could not have been traditional. They are the result of a clumsy effort at astronomically determining a given period of time. But this period of time has every chance of having been indicated by tradition and that of the Purāṇas can easily go back to an ancient period. The Purāṇas, in the form in which we have them, are quite late but several books of this name, which were most probably utilised as models, are already mentioned in ancient literature. Moreover, even in the epoch of Candragupta, the epoch which closes the period measured by the Purāṇas, Megasthenes has observed that the Indians possessed long geneologies of royal families which contained the names of 153 kings who ruled during 6042 years. Under such conditions, if it is remembered that the succession of the Magadhan kings, as given by the Purāṇas before and after Candragupta is confirmed by other sources and appears

1 Oldenberg had admitted that the hymn was contemporary to Parīkṣi (*ZDMG*, Vol. XLII, p. 238) but Bloomfield, after Roth, ha supposed that Parīkṣit could have been a purely legendary pseudc sovereign; cf., *Vedic Index*, under Parīkṣit.

2 Arrian, *Inde*, IX; Pliny, *Nat. Hist.*, VI, XXI, 5 (Littré's Edn.). Plin gives 154 kings and 6451 years and 3 months instead of 6042 years. Soli follows Pliny.

to be exact, it will not be showing oneself as too credulous as regards the Puranic tradition if we say that they have correct ideas on the succession of anterior kings.

On the other hand the same tradition will have us believe that the grandson of Parīkṣit, Śatānīka had studied the Veda at the feet of Yājñavalkya[1], a sage who is unanimously considered to be the first master of the White *Yajurveda*. Now it is perfectly plausible that the various recensions of the *Yajurveda* should belong to a period neighbouring the epoch of the composing of the *Atharvaveda*.[2] On the contrary, the Brāhmaṇas, the Āraṇyakas and the Upaniṣads belong to more recent times as is proved both by the state of the language in which they are edited as also by the fact that they suppose as existing the same Vedic texts. Now the *Bṛhadāraṇyaka-up.*, which belongs to the *Śatapathabrāhmaṇa* of the school of the White *Yajurveda*, accords a lot of importance to *Yājñavalkya* and asks him through an interlocutor as to what happened to the descendants of Parīkṣit, (III, 3, 1). This is quite a natural query if *Yājñavalkya* has been the preceptor of the grandson of Parīkṣit. It shows that the school of the *White Yajurveda* had a souvenir of the relations of its founder with the descendants of Parīkṣit.

It seems, therefore, quite well to situate the composition of the *Atharvaveda* and of the *Yajurveda* towards 1400 or a little afterwards[3] and that of the hymns of the *Ṛgveda*, being older, towards at least 1500. The rest of the Vedic literature which is more recent, is to be necessarily dated in the centuries which follow, in part before Buddhism and Jainism, which suppose its existence and almost entirely before the IVth century B. C., the probable epoch of the grammarian Pāṇini. This latter

---

1 *Viṣṇu. p.*, IV, 21, 2; *Bhāg. p.*, IX, XXII, 37.

2 The date of the *Sāmaveda* has not been discussed here; this text simply consists of the *Ṛgveda* passages, arranged in view of liturgical songs.

3 It need not be said that inside the Vedic schools, in the various "branches" (*Śākhā*), it has been possible to arrange, retouch, even enrich the texts a long time after their composition. If the hymn of praise to Parīkṣit of the *Atharvaveda* goes back, in all probability, to the time of Parīkṣit, it has been possible to put beside it other hymns which were comparatively recent. The scrupulous faith with which the texts have been passed on up to our time does, in no case, favour the hypothesis of a long period of the re-editing of the texts. Once the concurrent *Śākhās* had been constituted, the texts had to be fixed definitely.

writes in a language which particularly corresponds to that of the ancient Gṛhyasūtras[1], which constitute one of the last strata of the Vedic literature. We may consider that the Brāhmaṇas and the Upaniṣads, the books which contain the biggest share of the cosmo-physiological speculations studied by us and are chronologically placed between the Saṁhitās and the Sūtras, belong chiefly to the period between 1000 and 500 B. C.

The Medical Rôle of Divinities:—Many of the Vedic divinities play, at least, occasionally, a medical rôle, in the sense that they dispense remedies or on the contrary, provoke diseases. This, of course, is not the place to record all that is available on the subject in the Saṁhitās as the divinities do not have much of an importance in classical medicine, whose formation we are studying.[2] Only it is necessary to remind ourselves of the chief traits of the divine and the demoniacal medicine of the Veda in order to measure all that Āyurveda has rejected therefrom and the little that it has kept in an extremely restricted field

In the first rank of the Vedic healers are the twins Aśvins[3], the "ones provided with horses", who have been compared with Dioscuros and who are also known under the name of Nāsatyas. The hymn X, 39, 3b of *Ṛgveda* invokes them as follows: "You, O Nāsatyas, it is you who are called doctors of whosoever is blind, of whosoever is weak, of whosoever has had a fracture".[4] It is the last expression which is their most typical characteristic as *bhiṣaj*, a word which ordinarily signifies doctor or healer but in the *Ṛgveda* denotes more precisely the

---

1 cf., L. Renou, *La Durghaṭavṛt*. Vol I, pt. I., Paris, 1950, p.8.

2 The richest selection of passages of the Veda concerning the medical role of the gods is found in G. N. Mukhopādhyāya, *History of Indian Medicine*, Vol. I, Calcutta, 1923 (cf., *JA*, July-Dec., 1933, fasc. annexe, pp. 102 ff). The most typical of these passages had already been studied occasionally by Bergaigne in his *Rel. véd.* to which a reference can be made. The work of Mukhopādhyāya is interesting for having published the therapeutic formulae which in the medical texts are ascribed to the gods. Reference may be made to it once for all. See also Reinhold F. G. Muller, *Die Medizen im Ṛgveda* in *Asia Major*, Vol. VI, 1930. But this last follows the system of arbitrary interpretations of Hertel.

3 On the legends concerning the Aśvins one may consult C. Renel, *L'évolution d'un mythe Aśvins et Dioscures*, in *Ann. de l'Univ. de Lyon*, Paris, 1936, but the author is imbued with the prejudices of the Vedic interpretation of Regnaud.

4 ......*andhásya cin nāsatyā kṛśásya cid yuvām id āhur bhiṣájā rutásya cit.*

"bone-setter" because the hymn IX, 112, 1 proclaims: "Yes, all that is diversified, that are our thoughts, those are the things to whom men dedicate themselves; the carpenter desires what is cut down (wood), the *bhiṣaj* that which is fractured, the priest that which flows (soma)...."[1] In them one has even desired to see the first orthopaedists of India as they have given a "leg of iron" to a certain Viśpalā, but she seems to be most probably a mare who had won a race,[2] the apparel of prosthesis seems to vanish in a metaphor. Moreover a leg made entirely of iron would not have been of much utility because of its weight; it is certain that the Indians of the Vedic epoch did not fabricate any such thing.

In the Veda, the Aśvins are often the protectors or the rescuers of the blind, the decrepit and old and of persons fallen into a pit. The literature of the epics has also sometimes accorded them this speciality. The *Mahābhārata* (I,715 ff.) narrates the history of Upamanyu who, having become blind for having eaten the plant "sun" *(arka)*, falls into a pit and who is rescued by the Aśvins after he had invoked them in a hymn as in the Veda.[3] In this *Mahābhārata*-passage (721) they are called the "doctors of the gods" (*devabhiṣaj)*, a title which brings to mind that of "divine doctors" *(daivyā bhiṣájā)* given to them in the *Ṛgveda*, VIII, 18, 8, and which is repeated in the *Yajurveda* (VS, XXVII, 9, *devānām bhiṣajā; Kāth*., XXVII, 4; *Maitr*., IV, 6, 2). Caraka describes them exactly in the same manner as the *Mahābhārata* and gives the following justification for the expression: "It is said that the Aśvins are the doctors of the gods, the conveyors of the sacrifice.[4] In fact they have replaced the severed head of Dakṣa, the broken teeth of Pūṣan and the lost eyes of Bhaga and it is they who have treated the paralysis of arm of the one who has the thunderbolt (Indra). They have treated the one who has the rabbit (the Moon) seized by the royal disease and thanks to them, the Moon of

---

1 *nā ānám vā u no dhíyo ví vratāni jánānām/tákṣā riṣṭám rutám bhiṣág brahmā sunvántam ichati...*

2 cf., R. Pischel, *Vedische studien,* 1,89, Vol. I, pp. 171-3.

3 On this hymn, L. Renou, *L'hymne aux Aśvins de l'Ādiparvan,* Eastern & Indian Studies in honour of F. W. Thomas.

4 cf., *RV.,* I, 15, 11, *yajñavāhasā.* Cakradatta, in his commentary of *Caraka* glosses *yajña-vāhau* by *yajñaṁ vahata iti.* They are the same words which are later on employed by Sāyaṇa for explaining the Vedic passage.

whom the *soma* (the element of virility) had fallen[1] has recovered his health. The son of Bhṛgu, Cyavana, an old lover, having become decrepit, was made lovely to look at and received, a lovely voice and became young once again. By these acts and many others they became the most eminent doctors of the Magnanimous ones such as Indra, etc., and to whom the utmost homage should be rendered. The men with two births prepare for them the libations of soma[2], the laudations, the formulae and all sorts of libations, the fumigations as also the beasts (to be sacrificed). In the morning, when the soma is pressed, Śakra partakes of the soma in the company of the Aśvins and on the occasion of the Sautrāmaṇi, the Blessed one (Indra) is happy in their company. It is Indra and Agni and the Aśvins who are mostly honoured by the twice-born; they honour them with the words of the Veda, differently than other divinities."[3]

---

1 Variant pointed out by Cakradatta: *atipacita*, "too much cooked" but Cakradatta glosses: *tatrapy atipacanena somapānātiyogam darśayati*, "here by the expression 'excessive cooking', is shown the abusive use of soma as a drink". The cooking in question is a case of digestion, cf., the following two notes.

2 But Cakradatta: *grahāḥ somapānapātrāṇi*, "cups for drinking the *soma*".

3 Caraka, *Cik.*, I, 4, 40-47:

aśvinau devabhiṣajau yajñavāhāv iti smṛtau|
dakṣasya hi śiraś cchinnam punas tābhyām samāhitam| |40
praśīrṇā daśanāḥ pūṣṇo netre naṣṭe bhagasya ca|
vajriṇás ca bhujastambhas tābhyām eva cikitsitaḥ| |41
cikitsitaḥ śaśī tābhyām gṛhīto rājayakṣmaṇā|
somābhipatitaś candraḥ kṛtas tābhyām punaḥ sukhī| |42
bhārgavaś cyavanah kāmī vṛddhaḥ san vikṛtim gataḥ|
vītavarṇasvaropetaḥ kṛtas tābhyām punar yuvā| |43
etaiś cānyaiś ca bahubhiḥ karmabhir bhiṣagottamau|
babhūvatur bhṛśam pūjyau indrādīnām mahātmanām | |44
grahāḥ stotrāṇi mantrāṇi tathā nānā havīṁṣi ca|
dhūmrāś ca paśavas tābhyām prakalpyante dvijātibhiḥ| |45
prātaś ca savane somam śakró 'śvibnyām sahāśnute|
Sautrāmaṇyām ca bhagavān aśvibhyām saha modate | |46
indrāgnī cāśvinau caiva stūyante prāyaśo dvijaiḥ|
stūyante vedavākyeṣu na tathānyā hi devatāḥ| |47

As has been observed to me by Mr. Renou, it is necessary to read *cendraḥ* in the verse 42 and translate as follows: "and thanks to them, Indra, fallen ill because of *Soma...*" although the various editions do not give this reading. Similarly *atipacita* should be replaced by *atipavita* in the variant remarked in the note 4. In fact, the MSS. of the *Bibl. Nat., Sanscrt.* 1304 (collection by Cordier of a Kashmirian MS.) reads: *somātipavitaś cenduḥ*, the original reading of the last word must be clearly *cendraḥ*. *atipavita* responds to the Vedic expression *Somātipūta* applied to Indra meaning "excessively purified by the *soma*", "having received too many libations of soma." It is all the more normal that Caraka refers to the episode of the healing of the drunken Indra, when in the ancient ritual there is a form of *sautrāmaṇī* which has the name of Caraka.

This beautiful tribute shows that, for Caraka, the Aśvins are the gods of another age and this was also the feeling of the editor of the legend of Upamanyu in the *Mahābhārata*, because he thought that they must be addressed in the antique style, whereas everywhere else, the hymns which dot the epic, are in classical Sanskrit. On his side, Suśruta describes the legend of the head of the sacrifice cut by Rudra and replaced by the Aśvins (*Sūtra*, 1, 14). We should, however, note that all the mythical facts thus mentioned in the classical medical texts are not already found in the *Ṛgveda*. The legend of Cyavana (Cyavāna in the *Ṛgveda)* is here implied, but it is evident and it was quite natural that the medical texts have received the legends concerning the Aśvins from other mythological sources, which can be placed between the *Ṛgveda* and them. The references of Caraka relate chiefly to the epic form of these legends, although the origin of the epic form sometimes goes back to the *Black Yajurveda* as is, for example, the case with the disease of Soma which we will discuss later and also with the replacement of the severed head of the sacrifice *(Taitt.* S, VI, 4,9; *Kāṭh.*, XXVII, 4; *Maitr.*, IV, 6, 2).

The mythological reputation of the Aśvins as the doctors of the gods has quite naturally designated them for fulfilling, as we have already seen, a rôle in the teaching of medicine to human beings, a science reputed to be of divine origin. This reputation was also the cause, especially from the epoch of the *Carakasaṁhitā*, of ascribing to them the revelation of various formulae, and still later, even of the composition of several works. Indra, to whom they are said to have taught medicine, is, on his side, reputed to be the author of various medicinal preparations. We have seen that, in the Indian tradition, he is included in the group of divine instructors and it is because of his relations with the Aśvins that he is specially regarded as a master of medicine, because by himself he does not have the reputation of a healer comparable to that of the Aśvins. Actually it cannot be said that in the Veda he is a doctor-god. Only in some of the passages (Bergaigne, II, p. 495) is he presented as a rescuer like the Aśvins and often he is asosciated with them, they being called Nāsatyas on such occasions. By chance we even know that this association existed at a very early date even outside India. The well-known treaty between the king of the Mitanni and Subiluliuma, the king of the Hittites (dated in approximately 1380 B. C.) enumerates in a list of divinities "the gods Mitras, the gods Uruwana, the god Indara and the gods Nasattiyas", that is to say, Mitra and Varuṇa, Indra and the Nāsatyas.[1]

By the side of the Aśvins and of Indra, the basically favourable gods, there is another whose character, as depicted in the Veda, is equivocal and which will remain the same in the Ayurveda : he is the powerful and terrible Rudra. He can come to the rescue but he is always ready to fly into a rage; "May we not make you furious, Rudra, by the adorations, or by a song of maleficent tribute, O Bull, neither by means of a concomitant invocation. Make our sons grow by means of remedies; I hear that you are the best among the doctors.[2]

This is one of those characteristics of Rudra which has developed most in the classical legends of Rudra-Śiva. The entire classical Sanskrit literature employs *krodha*, derived from the root *krudh*—(which figures in the Vedic passage just cited), to denote the state of frenzy of *Śiva* in his form of the destroyer. This is the normal state of Rudra; it is not, therefore, necessary to suppose along with Sāyaṇa that the adorations and other acts of cult described here are the incorrect forms of these acts of cult. All incitation, good or bad, can unleash Rudra. The Vedic invocation fortifying the magical power of the god to whom it is addressed, must be used with precaution when the god is as formidable as Rudra. But in his beneficent aspect, Rudra is, at other times, also celebrated as a doctor, notably in the *Yajurveda*, where he is the "first divine doctor" *(prathamo daivyo bhiṣak*, *Taitt. S.*, IV, 5, 1, 2; *Vāj. S.*, XVI, 5).

Rudra's sons, the Rudras, Rudriyas or the Maruts, have the same characteristics as he. On the one hand they are the gods of remedies while on the other they are terrible inasmuch as in their naturalistic aspect they represent the fury of

---

1 cf. among others, G. Furlani, *La religione degli Hittiti*, Bologne, 1936, p. 50. Lastly, Dumézil, *Naissances d'archanges*, Paris, 1945, p. 20. The plural number represents most probably the forms of dual numbers missing for the proper names in the language of the treaty. They are similar to the Avestan and Vedic ones which apply to two names constituting a couple. cf. Dumézil, op cit., p. 21.

2 *mā tvā rudra cukrudhāmā námobhir mā dúṣṭutī vṛṣabha mā sáhūtī | ún no vīramarpaya bheṣajébhir bhiṣáktamam tvā bhiṣájām śṛṇomi| |* RV., II, 33,4.

the storms. To their friendly forms are juxtaposed their maleficent forms (Berg., II, 401). Moreover, the author of the evil is the one who can cure it most easily as he is its master. Rudra himself heals the evils which he creates (Berg., III, p. 33) and the *Atharvaveda* at the end of a hymn consecrating an amulet against disease formally declares that: "One who has done, may he undo, it is he who is the chief among doctors; that he may therefore prepare for you the remedies through the intermediary of the human doctor; he the pure".[1]

Varuna, Sin and Disease:—Among the divinities having a medical rôle, Varuṇa is also worthy of being referred to. It is not so much for the rôle itself, which is small but because of his relations with an entity whose concept is a rudiment of the scientific notion, *ṛta*.

The *ṛta* is the regular order in general, being the moral rectitude, the ritural exactitude and the true law of the universe; in one word, it is the "Norm". Varuṇa is the Lord and the guardian of this "Norm". The concept of *ṛta* goes back to the Indo-Iranian period (see *supra*, p. 67); to the Vedic *ṛta* correspond exactly the Avestan *asa* and the Old-Persian *ṛta*. He has for basis the sentiment that all things are harmoniously regulated and are not left to chance in this universe. The fixity of the stellar figures, the periodical return of the mobile stars to similar positions, the evident verification of all the principal and regular phenomena of nature have, from a very early date, imposed this notion. Among the peoples inclined to explain the organism by the cosmos and the cosmos by the organism, this notion must have quickly extended itself from the sky to the earth, from the world to the living being. Although victim of innumerable accidents, the existence of this last one could not be conceived as being outside the orbit of the great cosmic law, as the same body was a little cosmos. If this is not, properly speaking, a scientific concept of natural law, it is at least an idea quite near the same. The scope of this idea is absolutely general because there is nothing which is not governed by *ṛta*, including the moral behaviour of man. Sometimes the Indian and the Iranian minds are blamed for having thus mixed

---

1 *yaś cakā·a sá niṣ karat sá evá súbhiṣaktamaḥ|*
sá evá túbhyam bheṣajāni kṛṇávad bhiṣájā śúciḥ| / *AV.*, 11, 9,5.

up the physical and the moral but it should also be recognised that this very mind has also raised above them a sufficiently large concept for covering both of them.

Oldenberg has carefully studied the *ṛta* and has very well observed that the origin of this concept lay in the spectacle of the regular movements of the sky, but he has not recognised that the generality of its application automatically brought in its extension to morals. In the simultaneous relationship of *ṛta* with the astronomical phenomena and moral behaviour he has only seen the double trace of an Indo-Iranian borrowing from the Semitics. Maintaining that Mitra, the habitual associate of Varuṇa, was the Sun and that Varuṇa was the Moon, he has supposed that the group of seven Ādityas, which is the culminating point of the two associates, was originally that of the Sun, the Moon and the five planets. Not finding among other Indo-European people the equivalent of a similar group, observing that the Indo-Iranians had another solar god and another lunar god and finding that they did not evince much interest for the planets, he thought that the group of Ādityas was by its origin a stranger to the Indo-Iranian mythology. He has supposed it to have been borrowed from the peoples who were more advanced in astronomy, that is, the Semitics. In the relationship of *ṛta* with the moral idea, he has seen a confirmation of his thesis because, he says, the Semitics seem to have raised themselves to a more mature concept of moral life earlier than the Indo-Europeans.[1] Such a building up of hypotheses without documentary support is astonishing when it comes from such a philologist as Oldenberg. Of course, it is plausible and one could look for new arguments to support it. One could observe, for example, that the name of Āditya signifying "son of Aditi", of the "Absence of link", would have fitted with the mobile heavenly bodies such as the planets (from the Indian point of view the Sun and the Moon are planets) in opposition to the stars, heavently bodies which seem to be permanently linked among themselves. But this only seems to reinforce the first hypothesis, which identifies the Ādityas with the planets, without rendering others less gratui-

1 *La religion du Veda,* French trans. by V. Henry, Paris, 1903, pp. 162-163.

tous, and all that one can learn of the Indo-European pre-history of Varuṇa by confrontation with Ouranos[1] is not favourable to the suppositions of Oldenberg. The essential characteristic of this god is that of being king and not Moon. In India, the god-Moon is a king surrounded by a group of constellations but Varuṇa is king in a larger sense and right from Indo-European pre-history itself; one cannot support its purely astral origin.

It was natural that the universal order, the notion whereof had been suggested by the regularity of cosmic phenomena, had been placed under the charge of a universal god-king and it is probably as his substitute that the Moon-god, Coryphaeus of the celestial procession, had received royal authority on this part of the domain of *ṛta* and royal authority in general therefrom. But these kings, Varuṇa in any case, are not capricious despots, Varuṇa makes the Norm prevail, he does not change it, either because he lacks the power to do so or because he does not have the desire for the same. *Ṛta* therefore, definitely appears as a quasi-scientific concept of celestial regularity, a concept extended to all the terrestrial and spiritual objects, which has been transformed into that of the universal Norm and has been influenced by the social representation of the monarchical organisation.[2]

---

[1] Oldenberg did not accept the equation Varuṇa—Ouranos, as correct.

[2] In a rectoral discourse published by M. Alsdorf after his death (*die magische Kraft der Wahrheit im alten Indien*, in *ZDMG*, 1944, pp. 1-14), Lüders has tried to give a new interpretation to the sense of *ṛta*. He maintains that in the post-Vedic epoch, when the word tends to disappear, it denotes "verity" and that this sense and this alone was the one which prevailed in the Veda. Its antonym *anṛta* would have always signified falsehood. The importance given to *ṛta* would come from the belief in the magical power of truth. This thesis appears to be unacceptable. Of course, truth has an eminent magical power in the Vedic ideas and the translation of *ṛta* by verity is satisfactory for the large part of the context. But this is due to the fact that the universal Norm is generally true, authentic. Otherwise it would not be the Norm in nature. If it were to happen that the moon were to rotate in the wrong direction, it will follow *anṛta,* it will make the Norm false, but as long as it does not happen, the Norm remains what it is and retains its permanent verity. The Norm is, therefore, precisely verity, but verity itself borrows its magic force from the Norm because all that is true fits in with it and works by its power. Darmesteter (*Ormazd et Ahriman*, p. 17), had well seen that the Vedic *ṛta* and the Avestan *asa* are simultaneously order and truth. Beside the opinion that in classical Sanskrit *ṛta* means only "verity" is not exact. This is the opinion of Indian lexicographers, because in the classical language, the sense has

In such like ideas disease is a phenomenon which does wrong to *ṛta*. In relation to the normal order disease is a disorder, and, as in the then current magical concept like brings in like, disease is linked with other disorders such as sin. Sin in its turn is a transgression of *ṛta* and it makes little difference whether this transgression is committed deliberately or by chance. Voluntary or not, the anamoly of behaviour or of thought brings in that of the organism. This does not mean that no importance is attached to intention; it aggravates the fault as it adds the anomaly of desire to physical or ritual disorder. But the responsibility is automatic, it is not effected by the purity of intention; hazard brings in baneful consequences just as effectively as they are brought in by pre-meditated perverse action. This concept has remained effective in the whole of classical India. The Epic and Puranic legends are full of stories where an accidental shortcoming is punished as a crime and the Jaina ascetics take extremely detailed precautions to avoid the unconscious destruction of minute beings which they do not at all see and thus save themselves from the fatal consequences of unsuspected deaths. In the texts of the classical period, *dharma* substitutes *ṛta* but that is merely a change of vocabulary, *dharma* like *ṛta* is the universal normal order and starting from the *Ṛgveda* itself, the *dharman* of *Varuṇa* is several times mentioned in place of *ṛta*.[1]

Although the concept of Norm has guided Indian thought and even Indo-Iranian thought from early times towards an outline of the scientific interpretation of the word regulated by an immutable law rather than by the caprices of divine personalities, scientific medicine of the classical period has not preserved the old simplistic assimilation made by the Veda of the disorders of health with the ritual, moral or other disorders.

---

specialised itself in that of verity or justice, but *ṛteṇa* is sometimes used in late rituals as an equivalent of *vidhinā*, "according to rules". Moreover, in the Veda, the word alternates with *dharman* which has specialised itself in the sense of "order". Lastly, it is not at all possible to separate *ṛta* from *ṛtu* which denotes assuredly real phenomena but chiefly regular ones: the seasons and the menses. Besides if verity was the force which moves the word, it would be nothing but its Law or its Norm.

1 Similarly also the *dhāman*, the "law" of Varuṇa. In classical Sanskrit *dharma* has, by the passage of the consonantic stem *dharman*—to the stem in—*a*, finally prevailed.

This medicine was too attentive to the multiple causes of various disorders, causes observed by it directly or inferred from observations and according to its theories. But under the stress of beliefs prevalent among the non-medical circles, it has admitted, at a sufficiently late hour, the automatic influence of pernicious acts, especially when they are voluntary; because in this case they have a more serious effect on the creation of diseases.[1]

If in the Veda the responsibility of acts or of intentions, not in conformity with the Norm of the world, is automatic, the application of consequences is often effected by Varuṇa, the guardian of this Norm. Varuṇa "ties" the sinner to his "ties". The oldest hymns do not explicity state the effect produced by them but the *Atharvaveda* drops a hint and the Brahmanical texts declare formally that the sinner tied down by Varuṇa is attacked by dropsy.[2] This is in accordance with the fact that Varuṇa who, in the classical literature, will become the god of the waters or of the oceans or will be reduced to this secondary rôle, is already in the *Ṛgveda* frequently in relation with the waters.[3]

Dropsy is a special disease, a special punishment of Varuṇa, but all sorts of other diseases spring from the infringement of the *ṛta* of any one of the natures. This is proved by the fact that Varuṇa, Lord of the Norm is, because of this link, the opponent of all diseases. He is invoked as the "guardian of the liquid of immortality"[4] and he is told: "A hundred, a thousand remedies do you have, O king. Great, profound be your benevolence. Remove far off perdition, far far off. All sins committed, remove them from us".[5] The number of remedies ascribed to him has little importance because the

---

1 This then concerns chiefly acts done in an earlier life. cf., *Un chapitre de la Hāritasaṁhitā sur la rétribution des actes*, in *JA.*, July-Sept., 1934, pp. 125-39.

2 For example, *AV.*, IV, 16, 7; *Ait. brah.*, VII, 15 (the texts employ "seizes" in place of "ties": *atha haikṣvākam varuṇo jagrāha, tasya hodaram jajñe...*, seized the descendant of *Ikṣvāku* and to this descendant was born a stomach...").

3 cf., Berg.. III, pp. 122 & ff and chiefly, the hymn, *RV.*, V, 63.

4 *RV.*, VIII, 42, 2: *amṛtasya gopām...*

5 *śatám te rājan bhiṣájaḥ sahásram urvī gabhīrā sumatiṣ ṭe astu| bādhasva dūré nirṛtim parācaíḥ kṛtám cid énaḥ prá mumugdhy asmát* *RV.*, 1, 24, 9.

formula which mentions them is a stock phrase applicable to other gods. But their very mention indicates that in his invocation the poet thinks of the disease and of the return of health when he demands the removal of "Perdition" and of sin. Now the "Perdition", *Nirṛti* has a name, which, by means of a sort of word-play, evokes the negation (preposition *niḥ*) of *ṛta;* it is also in some way "Anomaly" in general, which implies that all the diseases and sins depend on it.

Besides, the disease denoted by the most general terms like *ámīvā* and *yákṣma*, is formally put in relation with the sin. The *Atharvaveda*, taking up the hemistitches of the *Ṛgveda*, groups them in two verses, which illustrates very well the close relationship between physical trouble and sin, ritual or moral shortcoming, intentional or involuntary: "O Soma and Rudra, chase out the one who spreads herself everywhere, the disease *(ámīvā)* has penetrated into our house. Remove far away the "Perdition", far far away. All sins committed, remove them from us. Soma and Rudra, you, in us, in our bodies, deposit all the remedies. Untie, remove from us, whichever it might have been, the sin committed (by us) and attached to our bodies."[1] Elsewhere, he has said that the medicinal plants chase, from each limb of the body, the "evil of sin", that is to say, coming from sin or attached to it *(yákṣmam enasyám)*.[2] Similarly all sorts of anomalies which engender physical troubles are rather associated with sin or *Nirṛti*. The *grāhi* which, we have already seen, taking hold of the man, on whom *Tṛta* has wiped off the sin of gods *(supra*, p. 43*)*, is the type of seizing demons who can possess human beings. Among these are the *rákṣas* to whom are applied such epithets as "devourers" *(astrín)*, who particularly cause miscarriages and whose co-relation with the *grāhi* is attested by the fact that the *Atharva-*

---

1 *AV.*, VII, 42, 1-2:
sómārudrā ví vṛhatam viṣūcīm ámīvā
yā no gáyam āvivéśa|
bādhethām dūrám nirṛtim parācaiḥ kṛtám cid énaḥ prá mumuktam asmát | | 1 | |
somārudrā yuvám etāny asmád víśvā tanūṣu bheṣajāni dhattam|
ava syatam muñcátam yán no ásat tanūṣu baddhám kṛtám éno asmát | | 2 | |

2 *AV.*, VIII, 7, 3. The preceding verse invokes the plants against the "evil sent by the gods"...*yákṣmād devéṣitād*...It is precisely the disorder of sin because such an evil has passed from the gods to human beings by the intermediary of *Tṛta* (cf., *supra*, p. 36).

veda asks for the delivery of a man simultaneously from the one and the other (II, 9, 1). These *rákṣas* are themselves, in co-relation with the sorcerer-demons, the *yātudhānas* (cf., *supra*, p. 46). The nightmare (*dusvápnya)* is also, along with *Nirṛti* and the *rákṣas*, a cause of disorders because it is said: "that the stone for pressing (the soma), by talking may push back the *rákṣas*, the nightmare, *Nirṛti*, all that devours. . ."[1] Lastly, bad luck, materialised in the form of the black-bird, of bad omen, *śakuna* or *śakuni*, brings down, in association with *Nirṛti*, the sin on the human being or "wipes" it on him with the mouth of *Nirṛti (AV*., VII, 64, 1-2). All the causes of disorders are, therefore, related or allied; they belong to the domain of the sin, to the violation of the Norm and they affect, for most of the time, the healthy being like an impurity wiped off on him. That is why efforts are often made to treat them by the ritual of wiping off or of effacement as also by means of prayers.

These ideas have survived in classical medicine but not in the focal points of its doctrines. They have been preserved mainly in the common beliefs and have been introduced in the medical texts by the pressure of the latter without being integrated in their systems of more scientific explanations. The seizing demons, the *grahas*, the heirs of the *grāhi* attack specially children, just as the *rakṣas* attack the embryos, and, among other demons, certain *śakunis* are said to provoke diseases, studied by classical medicine in special chapters, separately and in addition to ordinary diseases about which it has to learn.[2] The she-demon related to the *grahas* and who are given the auspicious name of "mothers", the *mātṛkās*, play, in the same texts of the classical medicine, a rôle of the first order. They are also attached though this time indirectly to Vedic souvenirs because they form a part of the pan-demonium grouped around Śiva who, undoubtedly of the extra-Vedic origin, already appears in the hymns in the forms, already seen by us, of Rudra.[3] In any case, whereas classical medicine had

1 *grāvā vádann ápa rákṣāṁsi sedhatu duṣvápnyam nírṛtim víśvam atríṇam... (RV*., X, 36, 4).

2 cf., *Le Kumāratantra de Rāvaṇa*, pp. 62 ff., 177-8, On Śakuni, see the index of this book.

3 ibid., cf., Index, see the words Śiva, Rudra, Skanda.

to embark upon the path of the detailed explanation of morbid causes, in the eopch of the Vedic texts, it was thought to be enough if a relationship could be established between the pathological phenomena and all that appeared to be contrary to the Norm of the world if its origin could be ascribed to shortcoming and to fault, so that they could be fitted back in a general and familiar determinism.

Various Diseases: As our religious texts do not furnish us with systematic descriptions of the morbid states, the identification of these states is quite often uncertain and generally vague. The references made therein are, in any case, frequently sufficient to enable us to have an idea of the majority of the ailments mentioned therein. Moreover, every time we come across the name of a disease common to the Veda and to the manuals of classical medicine, we can try to apply the classical sense of this name to that passage of the Veda containing it; if this sense fits in well with the context and mainly with various contexts where that name comes in many a time, we have the right to admit that probably that sense is exact. This is the method which was used by Bergaigne for the determination of the sense of the Vedic words.[1] It is true that here it could be objected that the sense of the name of a disease is not at all comparable to a commonplace term. Scientific nosology keeps old terms for an indefinite period of time, but being in progress all the time and subject to ceaseless modifications, it frequently changes the concepts covered by these terms. Various words like "leprosy" or "asthma" have no relation whatsoever with *lepra* or *asthma* [of the Greek language] and it will be false to use them today in the translation of a Greek text without pointing out that they are meant in a sense altogether different than in the actual usage. Similarly, when a term of the Veda, is also found in the *Āyurveda*, one cannot be sure, *a priori* that it possessed the same sense in the Veda as it had in the *Ayurvedic* texts. Here it may be pointed out that the possibilities of the evolution of senses should not be exaggerated. *Lepra* [in Greek] denoted all sorts of non-classified cutaneous ailments, whereas leprosy today is an individualised disease, defined by a certain group of symptoms and it is bacteriologi-

1 *Etudes sur le lexique du Ṛg-veda*, Paris, 1884, p. III.

cally characterised. Similarly *Asthma* denoted all sorts of breathlessness whereas asthma today is a dyspnoea of the expiratory type coming on by fits and characterised by the cytological formula of expectoration. But asthma and leprosy still remain the ailments whose essential manifestations are respectively respiratory and cutaneous. If, therefore, in ignorance of the exact sense which the Greeks gave to the word *lepra,* the sense of "leprosy" as known to the modern doctors, were given to it, one would be ascribing to the Greeks an exact knowledge which they did not at all possess. But if one were to be content with the supposition that among the Greeks *lepra* signified a serious cutaneous disease, that will be quite exact. One could undoubtedly find examples of more complete changes of sense than those which have come in the case of *lepra* and "leprosy" and *asthma* and "asthma", but it will be difficult to find any which be such that nothing common exists any longer between the old and the modern connotation. Under such conditions, when a disease known to classical texts is found as mentioned in the Veda, if we do not have the right to believe that the Vedic authors knew it as it is taught by the Ayurvedic practitioners, we have, at least, the right of admitting that in the Veda also it is a disease of the same type as in the *Āyurveda*. Moreover the changes of sense between the Vedic period and the classical period could not have been as considerable as they have been between the Hellenic epoch and the modern period where medicine has profoundly renovated, thanks to modern discoveries, the significance of the old terminology preserved by it. Moreover, the terms common to the Veda and to the *Āyurveda* denote chiefly the states without specificity such as cachexy or isolated symptoms such as the lancinating pain. These states and these symptoms belong more to the domain of common experience than to that of medical diagnosis; their names are therefore more of commonplace expressions than technical terms whose significance would be subject to conventional changes.

One of the most important names of diseases in the Veda is *yákṣma* which we have already met with. This word appears not only in isolation but also in compound words such as *rājayakṣmá,* "royal disease", and *ajñātayakṣmá,* "unknown disease". These two compound words are found together in

RV., X, 161, 1: "I deliver you by means of oblation so that you may live, from the unknown disease and from the royal disease...".[1] *Yákṣma* is used in the plural in *RV.*, X, 85, 2, 31; *AV.*, IX, 8, 10, where the "poison of all the *yákṣmas*" is exorcised. The *White Yajurveda* counts a hundred *yákṣmas* (XII, 97) and it is clear that often it is a case of disease or diseases in a general sense.

The classical medical literature well knows the word to which it often gives a consonantic stem: *yakṣman*. In it the word *rājayakṣma* denoted the cachexy resulting from various consumptive diseases, among which we may recognise pulmonary tuberculosis. It is called *śoṣa*, "drying up" and *kṣaya*, "diminution". The *Uttaratantra* of the *Suśruta-saṁhitā* describes it as follows: "Followed by many disorders, coming in the wake of many disorders, difficult to know, difficult to push back, the 'drying up' is a disease of great strength. Because of the drying up of the organic juices... (which it provokes) it is called "drying up" and because it provokes the diminution of activity it is known as "diminution". Because it was, as is known, the disease of the Moon-king, certain persons still call it the "royal disease".[2] One should, therefore, understand by *yakṣman*, a state of decay, cachexy if it is a generalised disease and undoubtedly, an atrophy, a paralysis or even necroses, as we will see, if it is localised in an organ.

The denomination of *rājayakṣma* is explained by the Vedic legend which says that Soma, the Moon, the king of plants, of heavenly bodies and of the Brahmins, had been attacked by decay, wasting away. This legend is found in the *Yajurveda*

---

1 *muñcāmi tvā haviṣā jīvanaya kám ajñātayakṣamād utá rājayakṣmāt//* See also *AV.*, III, 11, 1.

2 *Utt.*, XI-I: *anekarogānugato bahurogapurogamaḥ*
durvijñeyo durnivāraḥ śoṣo vyādhir mahābalaḥ //3//
saṁśoṣanād rasādīnāṃ śoṣo ityabhidhīyate/
kriyākṣayakaratvāc ca kṣaya ity ucyate punaḥ//4//
rājñaś candramaso yasmad abhūd eṣa kilāmayaḥ/
tasmāt taṁ rājayakṣmeti kecid āhuḥ punar janāḥ//5//

Dalhaṇa glosses *kriyākṣayakaratvāt* as follows: *kriyā cikitsā kāyavāṅmānasam vā karma tasya kṣayakaratvāt/*, "*kriyā* is the therapeutics or the activity of the body, of speech and of mind, this is what is referred to by *kṣayakaratvāt*". The first term of the alternative is not creditable, yet Vāgbhaṭa (*Aṣṭāṅgasaṁgraha* & *Aṣṭ.-hṛd.*, *Nidāna*, V, 3) takes up, with slight modifications, this passage and declares that the disease in question is called *kṣaya* on account of its reducing action on the body and on medicines (*dehauṣadhakṣayakṛteḥ*).

(*Taitt.*, II, 3, 5, 2; *Maitr.*, II, 2, 7; *Kāṭh.*, XI, 3). Prajāpati had given his daughters to the king Soma. The *Taittirīya-saṁhitā* states more precisely that they were thirty-three in number and others say that they were the *nakṣatras*. But Soma was interested only in Rohiṇī. Others left him and he was attacked by *rājayakṣma*.

Interpreting this story is a delicate matter. The notion of the union of the Moon-god seems to be attested right from the verse of the *Ṛgveda* "... and Soma is established in the bosom of these *nakṣatras*".[1] This is one of those rare passages where Soma is already, as is regularly the case in more recent mythology, identified with the Moon (cf., Bergaigne, *Rel. vəd.*, I, 158). The hymn where he figures is an epithalamium of *Soma* and *Sūryā*, the daughter of the Sun, or the Sun in a feminine form, but the word *upastha*, which denotes "bosom, lap" in a vague sense, had soon taken the sense of "female genital organs" which it has right from the *Yajurveda* (*Vājas.*, XIX, 92). It has, therefore, been possible from a very early date to interpret the Vedic hymn as signifying that Soma, solemnly married to Sūryā, was also the husband of the *nakṣatras*. Now in the XIIIth book of the *Atharvaveda*, (1, 22, 23), appears a cow Rohiṇī, wife of the Sun-bull, Rohita. An assimilation has, therefore, taken place between Sūryā and Rohiṇī, the two feminine Suns. As regards the *nakṣatras*, they are the constellations. In the classical literature it is commonplace to proclaim that *Soma* is their king, (his bulk confers this rank on him) and to say that he "shines", *rājati*, and to call him in addition *rājā*, "king", by a play of words.[2] But the *nakṣatras* are also, in a more special sense, the twenty-seven or the twenty-eight constellations which lie along the monthly course of the Moon and Rohiṇī is one among them right from the *Atharvaveda* (XIX, 7, 2) and the *Yajurveda* (*Taitt.*, IV, 4, 10). Although the *Taittirīya-saṁhitā* says that the daughters of Prajāpati were thirty-three in number, they have to be identified with the *nakṣatras* marking the stages of the Moon as the other *saṁhitās* affirm that these daughters are the *nakṣatras*.

---

1 X., 85, 2, : *átho nákṣatrāṇām eṣām upásthe sôma āhitaḥ*

2 cf., for example, *Rāmāyaṇa* (Bombay), V, 2, 54: *candro ..tārāganair .. virājan...*, "The Moon...shining...along with his group of stars...". Also Caraka, *Cik.*, VIII, 8: *sa vimuktagrahaś candro virarāja viseṣataḥ*.

From this point onwards, it is difficult to understand the legend. It is difficult to understand why Rohiṇī, the co-wife of Soma along with other constellations, is said to be his favourite one, as the Moon, in the course of his revolution, successively covers the celestial spaces determined by these various constellations without specially stopping anywhere.[1] On one side, the decay of the king Soma seems to correspond necessarily to the waning of the Moon and this undoubtedly provides the key to the myth, on condition that we admit that the favourite of Soma, originally, was not the constellation Rohiṇī but the feminine Sun Rohiṇī which has been mixed up with the other because of homonymy. Actually as the Moon approaches the Sun, it wanes to disappear finally before the new Moon, this corresponding with her conjunction with the Sun. The Moon gets back its greatness and its brilliance as it gets away from the Sun, to sit enthroned, the full Moon in opposition, in the midst of the constellations of might. But Soma does not take much time in returning to Rohiṇī and to fall a victim to consumption once again. This schematic explanation is not, in any case, exhaustive because there are other complications in the legend. The *Yajurveda* (*Taitt.*, VII, 1, 6, 2) describes a "red" (*rohiṇī*) cow who is asked to come out of the waters for Soma; in souvenir thereof one must buy the soma with a red cow as its price. As Soma-Moon, the soma plant and sacrificial drink is in co-relation with a *rohiṇī*. The link of this ritualistic aspect of the question with the astronomical aspect is to be looked for in the mythical relations of the lunar heavenly body with the celestial drink of immortality and the terrestrial libation of soma.[2] We cannot stop here to discuss

---

1 Besides, this is what observes the *Maitrāyaṇis*. II, 2, 7. Seized by the *rājayakṣma*, Soma "*rushes* to *Prajāpati*". Prajāpati says to him, "say what is normal". He said thus what was normal, "That I may remain in all equally". That is why he remains equally in all (*sa vai prajāpatim evopadhāvat, tam prajāpatir abravīd ṛtam brūhiti sa ṛtam abravīd, yathā sarvasveva samāvad vasānīti, tasmād eṣa sarvasveva samāvad vasati*).

2 Another complication lies in the fact that *Taitt.*, II, 5, 6, 4 makes the nights of the fortnight to be the wives of Soma. He will be attained by disease as he does not co-habit with them during the night of the new Moon nor during that of the full Moon. The night of the new Moon being that of its conjunction with the Sun, therein lies a confirmation of the explanation given above, But that abstention during the night of the full Moon, when precisely it is in the midst of the constellations, raises difficulties. As the text has just now said that a woman should be approached neither during the night of the new Moon nor during

this problem any further but from only the preceding indications it appears clearly that *rājayakṣma*, in so far it is a disease affecting the king Moon, is an emaciation comparable to progressive cachexy and that if it attacks the soma drink, it must be, in all probability, a case of a decay of the energy inherent therein. It is therefore surely because of the violation of the Norm that the king Soma is siezed in the Vedic legend by *rājayakṣma*. In the *Maitrāyaṇī-saṁhitā*, Prajāpati makes Soma himself announce the name of the Norm infringed by him[1] and the *Kāṭhaka* is equally clear: "He inhabited Rohiṇī; this being an anomaly, the *yakṣma* seized him".[2]

The Vedic legend has been preserved in the classical medical texts. The *Caraka-saṁhitā* (*Cik.*, VIII, 1-11) describes it with certain modifications, befitting a text having a scientific purpose. It starts by saying that "the body of the god Moon, too much attached to Rohiṇī and not taking care of his organism, starts to wither away because of amourous exhaustion".[3] This is a natural explanation of the consumptive disease given in advance. Later it gives a version similar to that of the *Yajurveda*. The neglected wives complain to their father who becomes furious and turns out his anger with his breath. This anger attacks the god Moon who comes to demand succour from Prajāpati. Prajāpati permits the Aśvins to treat him and the text adds "Anger, *yakṣman*, fever, disorder (are the evils which) have only one signification: misery". As this disease had, first of all, attacked a king, it is considered as "royal *yakṣman*". The *yakṣman* exorcised by the Aśvins, reached the world of humans; it took hold of men due to four causes: effort out of proportion with force, overwork, exhaustion, the

---

that of the full Moon, one should probably see in the myth of Soma and his wives indicated immediately afterwards, the transposition of a religious interdiction. In any case, the myth in question does not agree with the one which is given a little earlier in the same text; this shows that this text is based on a complicated past of ritual and mythical speculations.

1 cf., Note 1 on p. 102.

2 XI, 3... *sá rohiṇyām evāvasat, tám tásminn ánṛte yákṣmo 'gṛhṇāc....*

3 *rohiṇyām atisaktasya śarīram nānurakṣataḥ| ājagāmālapatām indor dehaḥ snehaparikṣayāt||*—*Cik.* VIII, 2, cf. the translation (in French) of the entire passage in J. Filliozat, *Magie et médecine*, Paris, 1943, p. 42. The notion that amorous excesses are the cause of *rāja-yakṣman* is passed on to the classical literature, cf., *Bhāgavatapurāṇa*, IX, XXII, 23.

fourth cause of *yakṣman* being—let it be noted—irregular alimentation."

It thus appears that the medical text narrates the legend of Soma and Rohiṇī mainly to provide an etymology of the term *rājayakṣman* that it makes of the disease thus specified, a general consumptive ailment and it recognises for the same certain causes which are essentially natural ones. But in its version of the Vedic legend, it makes the *yakṣman* a seizing (*graha*, verse 8) demon, born of the anger of Prajāpati and it is by the power of the thought of Prajāpati's anger that this *graha* has been created because Prajāpati is a *guru*, a spiritual master. The Vedic forms of the legend did not contain these particular details which, on the contrary, are quite commonplace in the epics and in the *Purāṇas* and this can lead us to think that the Vedic legend has come to medical tradition through a Puranic intermediary. The verse which introduces the account in the *Caraka-saṁhitā* seems to confirm it: "The ṛṣis have heard a story from the inhabitants of the sky, while it was being told, a story of amorous passion, an old one and concerning the Moon".[1] *Paurāṇī*, "old", can also denote "Puranic". It is true that the principal Purāṇas only refer to the legend in question and that besides, they are much more recent than the *Caraka-saṁhitā* which could not have been inspired by them. But it is well known that old Purāṇas have been lost or that at least a mass of legends grouped under the name of Purāṇas existed in the Brahmanic period.[2] It is from these Purāṇas or from the body of the "Puranic" legends that the *Caraka-saṁhitā* has drawn inspiration.

In any case medical tradition has retained the idea that *rājayakṣman* is in correlation with sin as Dalhaṇa, commenting on the passage quoted above (*Suśruta-saṁhitā*, *Utt.*, XLI, 2-4), concludes by saying: "It being so, it appears that the disease

---

1 *krodho yakṣmā jvaro roga eko 'rtho duḥkhasamjñitaḥ|*
yasmāt sa rājñaḥ prāg āsīd rājayakṣmā tato mataḥ||9||.
sa yakṣmā huṅkṛto 'śvibhyāṃ mānuṣam lokam āgataḥ|
labdhvā caturvidhaṃ hetuṃ samāviśati mānavān||10||
ayathābalam ārambham vegasamdhāraṇakṣayam|
yakṣamaṇaḥ kāraṇam vidyāc caturtham viṣamāśanam||11||
divaukasām kathayatām ṛṣibhir vai śrutā kathā|
kāmavyasanasaṁyuktā paurāṇī śaśinam prati||—Cik., VIII. 1.

2 cf. Eug. Burnouf, *Le Bhāgavata-Purāṇa*, Vol., 1, 1840, pp. XX ff & *supra*, p. 83.

(in question) is born of a fault in one's acts".[1] Of course, it can be the result of physical activity but the expression *karmadoṣa* has a moral resonance which cannot be mistaken. On another side, tradition without losing sight of the notion that *rājayaksman* is so called because the king Moon had been its first victim, also gives another interpretation of this name. Vāgbhaṭa (*Asṭ.-s.* and *Ast-hṛd., Nidāna*, V, 1-2) says that *rājayaksman* is called "diminution, drying up and the king of disorders". As the king of constellations and of the twice-born had it in olden times and as it is king and *yaksman*, it is considered as *rājayaksman*.[2] It will be, therefore, necessary to translate this last expression as signifying *yaksmānām rājā*, "king of consumptions". In his commentary on the *Ṛgveda*, Sāyaṇa also gives an abusive interpretation of the word as signifying *yaksmānām rājā*, "king of consumptions", which corresponds to the expression, "king of diseases" (*rogarāja*) of Vāgbhaṭa.

As regards the form *ajñātayaksma*, it does not appear to occur in the classical medical literature, but the idea represented thereby seems to be present in the epithet *durvijñeya*, "difficult to know", which we have seen being applied in the *Uttaratantra* to cachexy. This epithet, as also undoubtedly the expression *ajñātayaksma*, have quite a natural explanation. Decay is not a determined disease, clear in its origin like the one which provokes a wound; it is a mysterious invasion, a disorder with an uncertain evolution. There is nothing, therefore, to prevent us from admitting that the term *yaksma* has the same sense of "decay" or "consumptive disease" in Vedic as in classical medicine, subject to the reservation that it should not be supposed that the medical notions developed in the Āyurveda around this term were already familiar to the Vedic authors.

Decay is not necessarily general; it may remain localised in a part of the body; this is the least that seems to result from the examination of some terms whose use is associated with that of *yaksma*.

In the two references which it makes to the legend of the

---

1 *evam ca sati karmadoṣajo vyādhir iti darśitam.*

2 *rājayakṣmā kṣayaḥ śoṣo rogarāḍ iti ca smṛtaḥ//1//*
nakṣatrāṇām dvijānām ca rājño 'bhūd yad ayam purā/
yac ca rājā ca yakṣmā ca rājāyakṣmā tato mataḥ//2//

Soma attacked by decay, the *Taittirīya-saṁhitā* declares that Soma has contracted this disease because of his wives (*jāyā*), from where the birth of the disease is called *jāyənya*.[1] It is possible that originally this *jāyəṅya* was not identical with the disease of Soma and had been brought near the latter one only to explain its name by an etymological play of words. But it is quite possible that *jāyənya* had been conceived as at least analogous to *yaksma*, which would justify the relationship. The *Atharvaveda* possesses a similar term, *jāyānya*, identified by the commentary with jāyənya and with *rājayaksma*.[2] The hymn VII, 76, contains a conjuration against this *jāyānya*: "One who breaks the bones to pieces, who keeps himself under the sole of the feet, one, no matter who he be, who sits atop (of the head); I have chased all *jāyānyas*. The winged one, the *jāyānya* flies, it enters men. Here is the remedy of the two, of one who is intact and of one who is well-broken. We know your origin, O *jāyānya*, from where you are born, *jāyānya*. How will you, therefore, attack there (that man) in whose house we offer the oblation?"[3] The hymn XIX, 44, which exalts the virtues of an unguent (*añjana*) sheds a ray of light which specifies the term *jāyānya*: "You are the rescuer of life, you are known as the remedy of all, (produce) therefore, O you unguent, well-being. Waters, produce well-being and security. One who is young, the *jāyānya*, the dissection of limbs, the *viśalyaka*, that the unguent push away all consumptive trouble (*yaksma*) out of

---

[1] II, 3, 5, 2 and 5, 6, 5.

[2] Bloomfield, *Hymns of the Atharvaveda*, in *SBE*, XLII, p. 561.

[3] *Yáḥ kīkasāḥ prásṛṇāti taḷīdyám avatíṣṭhati|*
nirāstam sárvam jāyānyam yáḥ káś ca kakúdi śritáḥ||3||
pakṣī jāyānyaḥ patati sá ā viśati pūruṣam|
tád ákṣitasya bheṣajám ubháyoḥ súkṣatasya ca||4||
vidmá vaí te jāyānya jānam yáto jāyānya jāyase|
kathám ha tátra tvám hano yásya kṛṇmó havír gṛhé||5||
kīkasa signifies "bones" in classical Sanskrit and can specially denote the vertebral. Bloomfield interprets *ākṣita* as "boil or sore, not caused by cutting" (*Kauś.-s.*, p. XLIII, Also *Am. J. Ph.*, p. 320) by reading *akṣata* because Dārila, commenting on *Kaus-s.*, XXXIII, 11 refers to *akṣata-bhaiṣajya*, "remedy of the *akṣata*" (cf., also *Kauś. s.*, XXXII, 11) and thus seems to take it as a special disease. But it is much simpler to take *akṣita* or *akṣata* in its normal sense of "intact". Caland in *Kauś-s.*, XXXI, 11, justly renders *akṣata* as "nicht gebrochene (Tumor)". The *akṣata-bhaiṣajya* is quite naturally the "remedy of that which is intact", that is to say, of the non-open collection.

the limbs...".[1] What immediately comes out of these texts is as follows: the *jāyānya* is a disease with superficial manifestations, which is treated with unguents, which can be ulcerated or not, which can be had anywhere because a formula expels it from the limbs and another points to its presence in the feet and in the head (even if it may not be understood to mean that it can go from the feet to the head) and in the last place which can provoke the necrosis of the bones. The term therefore stands for all types of suppurative ailments and of ulcers appearing externally. It is, therefore, quite understandable that this disease be included among the *yaksmas*, the consumptive ailments, because the consumptive ailments bring in their wake a rapid atrophy of the neighbouring parts and sometimes even cachexy; the abcesses of the bones particularly provoke a veritable melting of muscles which cannot remain unperceived by even the least attentive observers. In other words, the *jāyānya* is to the *rājayaksma* what a "phthisis" (and not "tuberculosis") is to general consumption. But if it comes near *rājayaksma* one may tend to believe that it had no relation with the *ajñātayaksma*, the "unknown consumptive ailment", because the Atharvanic sorcerer says to it that he knows it. However, it seems that the sorcerer boasts of himself either for imposing himself or for encouraging his patient.

The terms, which in the hymn referred to last of all accompany that of *jāyānya*, seem surely to denote the ailments of the same type, they being also treated by means of an unguent and being grouped under the generic name of *yaksma.*

Harimán, "the yellow", is naturally taken to be jaundice, which goes well with *yaksma*, the jaundice which is regularly accompanied by thinning and asthma.. On other occasions the *Atharvaveda* exercises the same, specially in the hymn, I, 22. It is sent back to the Sun conjointly with the "brilliance which is in the heart" (*hṛdyotá*), that is to say, apparently, the supposed cause of jaundice: an internal flash of yellow colour, like that of the

---

1 *āyuṣo 'si pratáraṇam viśvábheṣajam ucyase|*
tád āñjana tvám śamtātim śámāpo ábhayam kṛta||1||
yó harimā jāyānyo 'ṅgabhedó viśályakaḥ|
sárvam te yákṣmam áṅgebhyo bahír nírhantv āñjanam||2||
For the translation of the 2nd verse of the 1st stana, cf. notes of Whitney, *Translation of the Atharvaveda,* p. 966.

Sun and which radiates outwards through the skin and the eyes (principally the eyes if the skin is dark). The same hymn also sends jaundice to the birds, parrots and others, of whom certain varieties are yellow.[1] One could also admit that *harimán* can stand for copper or fawn-coloured spots on the skin like the ones produced by leprosy.

Aṅgabhedá is ordinarily understood in the sense of "pain rending the limbs asunder"; however in its correct sense this compound denotes the "section of limbs'. It can, therefore, designate the spontaneous mutilations provoked by leprosy and it would be natural to see beside an ailment which causes necrosis in the bones as the *jāyānya,* another which makes the limbs fall off.

Viśalyaka is more difficult to explain. The commentary of Sāyaṇa followed by Shankar Pandit, reads *viśalpaka* or *visarpaka*[2] and it would mean erysipelas, the serpiginous disease. This reading is quite possible because in various Indian scripts the groups *lpa* and *lya* are easily mixed together. On the other hand, in an enumeration of diseases *viśalyaka* is found alongside *aṅgabheda* and *aṅgajvara,* the "fever of limbs", (evidently the local fever of lymphangitis, *AV.,* IX, 8, 5).

[1] cf., V. Henry, *La Magie dans l'Inde antique,* 2nd edn., Paris, 1909, p. 182. *RV.,* I, 50, 11, 12, invokes the Sun, *Sūrya,* against the "ailment of the heart", *hṛdroga* and jaundice and contains the verse taken up by the *AV.* for sending jaundice to the parrots, etc. The substitution in the *AV.* of *hṛdyotá* by *hṛdrogá* of the *RV.,* clarifies the innate uncertain sense of *hṛdrogá*. This term has been interpreted as designating "cardialgia" whose mention in correlation with jaundice will be quite out of place. It is more probable that in the *RV.,* the Sun is invoked directly for chasing away the disease because it is he who causes it as proved to the Vedic sorcerers by the analogy of the morbid tint with that of his brilliance, It is true that a linking up of *hṛdyotá* to the root *dyut,* "to break", which is said to be found in the *AV.,* IV, 12, 2; 23, 5 and XII, 3, 22, is desired here, but another interpretation of the passages, by means of *dyut,* "to shine" (in a pejorative sense), is also possible. Besides if *hṛdyotá* were "the pain which breaks the heart", how is it that jaundice is brought alongside this disease, Sāyaṇa in his commentary says that *hṛdyotá* "burns the heart" (*hṛdayam santāpayati*) which seems to indicate that he recognises in the word rather the root *dyut,* "to shine", than the root *dyut,* "to break"; however *santāpayati* can also be understood in the sense of "torments". Whitney adopts the translation "heartburn". Beside *hṛdyotá* is found, several times, in the *AV., hṛdayāmayá* as a synonym.

[2] Bloomfield, *Hymns,* pp. 531, 601.

Erysipelas would be quite in place beside it.[1] However, the same word *viśalyaka* is found in other enumerations where neighbouring terms denote diseases of another type and chiefly, *viśalpaka* is a *lectio facilior*, whose authenticity is not certain. Bloomfield has rendered *viśalyaka* as "neuralgia" and this translation would be creditable if the neighbouring word *aṅgabheda* did certainly stand for a harrowing pain, all the more because *AV.*, IX, 8, 2, places "ear-ache", *karṇaśūla*, immediately before *viśalyaka*. But the analysis of the word itself remains embarrassing. One could suppose that this is a case of an adjectival formation in *ya* on *visala* or *bisala*, "shoot, bud", of the same type as *dantya* from *danta* with the extra addition of the suffix *ka* (quite frequent in the names of diseases). The word *bisa* exists in the vocabulary of classical medicine in *bisavartma* (*Suśr.*, *Utt.*, III, 26), "the eyelid in the form of a lotus-stalk" which is defined as below: "Is considered like the eyelid in the form of lotus-stalk, the eyelid which is swollen and has many small holes like the lotus-stalk inside water".[2] This aspect can be realised by glandular abcesses or by multiple styes causing oedema and opening out by as many small orifices. *Viśalyaka* could, therefore, even designate a disease "with buds" which would belong to the same category as the *jāyānya*.

The *jāyānya* is again quite near to the better defined lesions called, the *apacits*, "adenopathies". The 1st and 2nd stanzas of the hymn VII, 76 of *Atharvaveda* (whose 3rd to 5th stanzas constitute a conjuration against the *jáyānya*) are employed against the *apacits*. As has been quite well shown by Bloomfield,[3] *apacit* represents the disease known in classical medicine as *apaci*. Suśruta describes it quite clearly: "The *kapha* transforms the fat accumulated in the maxilliary, axilliary,

1 In the *AV.*, VI, 127, 1, *viśályaka* figures beside *vidradhá* "abcess", of *balāsa*, "oedematic ailment" (*infra*, p. 117. The stanza 2 of the *AV.*, VI, 127, indicates that *balāsa* is located in the cavity of the arm-pit", *yáu te balāsa tíṣṭhataḥ kákṣe muṣkāv ápaśritau*) and of *lohita* "the red" (undoubtedly a lympangitis). A distinction is made among three types of the same: those of the limbs (*aṅgya*), that of the ears (*karṇya*) and that of the two eyes (*akṣṇoḥ*). These special localisations fit in quite well with the hypothesis that *visályaka* is erysipelas.

2 *śūnam yad vartma bahūbhiḥ sūkṣmaiś chidraiḥ samanvitam|*
bisam antarjala iva bisavartmeti tan matam||

3 cf., Bloomfield, *Hymns*, p. 472 and *Am. J. Phil.*, XI, pp. 327 & ff. On the forms *apacit*, *apacī*, cf. L. Renou, *Grammaire Sanscrite*, p. 191.

claviculary (*fossa supraclaricularis*) and brachial (elbow) joints, in the neck and in the throat as a hard nodule, round or long, fluctuating and causing little pain. This nodule, increasing in size because of other nodules of the size of the myrobalan-stone, resembling the eggs of the fish and others of the same (aspect) and being of the same colour (as the chief nodule) is called, because of the pre-eminence of the pile: *apaci*".[1] It is, therefore, clearly a case of adenopathies, presenting themselves first in the form of isolated nodules (*granthi*), then becoming confluents (*apaci*) and which, of course, can be suppurating: "The ones, pruriginous, causing little pain, once crushed, disappear and others persist. This disease, coming certainly from the fat and the *kapha*, is difficult to vanquish; it continues for a number of years".[2]

The *Atharvaveda* (VII, 76, 2) localises them, as Suśruta, in the neck and in the armpits[3] (*upakaksyā* "which are under the wings", the translation of Whitney: "along the sides", faithfully follows the commentary and definitely gives the same sense), but he also places them in a region of the body, which is completely enigmatic, the *vijāman* intrepreted by the commentary, without mentioning the authority followed, as the region of genital organs (*guhya-pradeśa*). Probability would lead one to think of the inguinal regions, curiously omitted as the possible seat of *apacī* in Suśruta and it can only be a twin-organ, the exact sense being "twin". Two incantations against adenopathies distinguish a black adenopath, mother of the neighbouring adenopathies: "Of the red adenopathies, the black one is the mother, have we heard"[4] and in VI, 83, 3,

---

1 *Nid.*, XI, 8,9:
hanvasthikakṣākṣakabāhusandhimanyāgaleṣūpacitam tu medas/granthim sthiram vṛttam athāyatam vā snigdham kaphaś cālparujam karoti//8//
tam granthibhistvāmalakāsthimātrair matsyāṇḍajālapratimais tathānyaiḥ/
ananyavarṇair upacīyamānam cayaprakarṣād apacīm vadanti//9//
snigdha, literally "greasy" is the opposite of *sthira*, "hard", and designates evidently the adenopathies tending towards fluctuosity. The etymology given by Suśruta has a play on the word *upacīyamana* and the use of *caya* helps to show that *apacī* is considered as a derivative of the root *ci*, "to gather"; but habitually this root with the preposition *apa* signifies "to diminish"; it is with *upa* that it signifies "to grow".

2 ibid., *kaṇḍūyutās te'lparujaḥ prabhinnāḥ sravanti naśyanti bhavanti cānye/ medaḥkaphābhyām khalu roga eṣa sudustaro varṣagaṇānubandhī//10//*

3 *AV.*, VI, 25, 1-3, localises them in the neck, in the throat and in the shoulders (arm-pits).

4 *AV.*, VII-74. 1: *apacitām lohinīnām kṛṣṇā māteti śuśruma.*

adenopathy is called "mother of the black one" (*rāmāyaṇī*). The notion of a nodule, different from others, accompanied by others only as we have just seen in Suśruta, is apparently based on the observation that in a case of adenopathy with multiple cells, one of these, more developed and generally older, is the first to turn itself into an abcess. A little before the rupture of the thinned skin, it takes on a purplish-blue tinge, gangrenous. In this really appears a blackish tumefaction in the centre of others, which are simply red. Suśruta specified that the nodules accompanying the principal one have the same colour. This difference with the *Atharvaveda* is easily explained by the fact that in the beginning it is as described by Suśruta, whereas the *Atharvaveda* considers it (in its incantations) in the period when they run or are about to do so.[1]

V. Henry has conjectured that *jāyānya* was the general diathesis of which the *apacits* were the external manifestations[2], the *jāyánya* designating the inflammation of the osseous tissue, ulcers, etc., as we have seen, cannot be a diathesis. The relation it has with the *apacits* consists simply in that the *apacits* are a more individualised type of ailment since they are the ganglionic suppurations and not just any suppuration.[3]

V. Henry has also conjectured and at the same time Bloomfield too, that *jāyānya*, because of its derivation from the root *jan*, "to beget", or of a theme like *jāyā*, "wife", could designate a congenital disease, or better still, a venereal disease[4], and both of them have identified it definitely as

---

1 ibid., 1-2, the sorcerer declares that he pierces them (*vidhyāmi*). It is true that *AV*., VII,76,1, calls them "dry" but this is precisely because the stanza anounces beforehand the hoped-for result, to force it to produce itself. cf., V. Henry, *Livre* VII, p. 97.

2 Book VII of the *Atharvaveda*, Paris, 1892, p. 98 and *Magie*..., p. 192.

3 The abcesses and the inflammations of the cellular tissue are designated in the *AV*., VI, 127,1; IX,8,20, as *vidradhá*, in classical medicine *vidradhi* which includes the common abcesses and the purulent visceral collections. The difference between *jāyānya* and *vidradhá* seems to lie in that the first word designates all sorts of suppurant ailments, hot or cold, accompanied by local emaciation and the second, the collection of severe abcesses. In talking of the *apacits*, Bloomfield and V. Henry call it quite often "pustuls", although they make of it, rightly, the scrofulous disease, the scrofula. The use of the word "pustuls" not only does not come up to reality but also does not conform even with the idea they have of the disease in question.

4 V. Henry, *Livre*, VII, p. 98; *Magie*... p. 192; Bloomfield, *Hymns*... cf. also Zimmer, *Altindisch Leben*, p. 377.

syphilis. Bloomfield has brought in favour of this identification, an argument which is more pleasing than solid. The *Kauśika-sūtra* (32, 11-13), in the ritual indicated by it against *jāyānya* prescribes the attachment (to the patient) of an amulet tied with a cord of the lute (more exactly of *vīṇā*) and where also enters another organ of the same musical instrument as a component. From this Bloomfield supposes that the pieces of *vīṇā* are the substitutes of "nautch-girls" which must have produced the disease and that the charm is a homeopathic one.[1] To suppose that the Atharvanic sorcerers were capable of recognising a relation of cause and effect between the frequentation of prostitutes and the appearance of the abcesses affecting the bones or of ulcers, is to credit too highly their spirit of observation and their clinical sense. Even today, laboratory tests are not sufficient for proving the etiological relations of this type. As regards the idea that *jāyānya* can designate a congenital disease, it is not very probable, there being nothing to allow us to believe that the *jāyánya* in the *Atharvaveda* can be considered as appearing from birth and how could one then believe it to be congenital when it did not appear from that very moment?

The Profoundly Morbid Impregnations:—Another ailment or category of ailments is often taken to be not only congenital but even hereditary. The disease called, *ksetriyá*, "belonging to a field", is conceived by the Vedic commentators as hereditary or passing in the family, sometimes having been contracted during the period of embryo.[2] The hymns of the *Atharvaveda* where the *ksetriyá* is exorcised (II, 8 & 10; III, 7) do not enable

---

[1] *Hymns...* p. 561, where *jāyā*, whose correct sense is "wife, one who gives birth to children", is rendered by "woman" in this case. Besides there is nothing to prove formally that venereal diseases were known as such from the *AV*. The *Kauśikasūtra* (27, 32) does specify the recitation of the hymn III, 11, along with the ingestion of boiled rice with rotten fish in case of the "disease of coitus" (*grāmya*) explained by Ḍārila: *grāmyo vyādhir mithuna-saṁyogāt*, "the *grāmya* disease results from coitus". Now Hymn III, 11, begins with an invocation against *rājayakṣmá* and *ajñātayakṣmá* (cf., supra, p. 98) and Keśava also, in his commentary on the *Kauś.-s.*, declares that all this is the remedy in case of "consumption by coitus", *maithuna-rāja-yakṣman* (Bloomfield, *Hymns...*, 341). Most probably, this remedy is meant for cases of exhaustion due to sexual excesses (as interpreted by V. Henry, *Magie...*, p. 20) and not for diseases, which are probably speaking, venereal diseases.

[2] Bloomfield, *Hymns,...* pp. 286 ff. Ed. of the *Kauśikasūtra*, p. XLIV.

us to know its symptoms, but consider it as a bond (*pāśa*) of which two stars, the "unfastenings" (*vicṛt*) can deliver and they associate it with Nirṛti and with the bond of Varuṇa. In classical medicine the term does not seem to have been employed, but in a comparison, the matrix is represented by the "field", *ksetra* (Suśr., *Śār.*, II-33). It is, therefore, conceivable that the commentators have been able to think that *ksetriya* was a disease arising in the foetus or, better, coming from the matrix, hence hereditary.

The grammar of Pāṇini explains the word by means of an equivocal phrase: "*ksetriya* is one to be treated in (or: for, concerning) another field (the field of another, of others)".[1] The commentators are in doubt. The *Mahābhāsya*[2] says that *ksetriya* is an abnormal form (*nipāta*) formed by the elision of the word *para*, "other". In short *ksetriya* stands for *paraksetriya*. But the *Mahābhāsya* does not give the sense of this term. Later still, the *Kāśikāvṛtti*,[3] after reproducing the grammatical notes of the *Mahābhāsya* gives examples of the use of the word *ksetriya* as attributive adjective and offers several explanations to choose from "...the disease *ksetriya*, *ksetriya* leprosy. The *paraksetra* is the body of another birth (a new body after transmigration); it is for[4] this (body) that the *ksetriya* is to be treated. It is said that it is an incurable disease, which cannot be opposed, that is to say (that it does not) cease as long as one is not dead. Or *ksetriya* is the venom; it is treated by being

---

1 *kṣetriyaḥ parakṣetre cikitsyaḥ*, V-2-92.

2 Ed., Kielhorn, Vol. II, p. 390.

3 *...kṣetriyo vyādhiḥ kṣetriyam kuṣṭham/parakṣetram janmāntaraśarīram/ tatra cikitsyaḥ kṣetriyaḥ/asādhyo 'pratyākhyeyo vyādhir ucyate/ nāmṛtasya nivartana ityarthaḥ/athavā kṣetriyam viṣam/yat parakṣetre paraśarīre saṁkramayya cikitsyate/athavā kṣetriyāṇi tṛṇāni/yāni sasyārthe kṣetre jātāni/cikitsyāni nāśayitavyāni/athavā kṣetriyaḥ paradārikaḥ/paradārāḥ parakṣetram/tatra cikitsyaḥ nigrahītavyaḥ/sarvam caitat pramāṇam//*

4 Bohtlingk, whose interpretation has been deemed as authoritative, has translated the sūtra of Pāṇini as follows: "kṣetriya bedeutet "erst in einem andern Korper zu heilen" d.i. "in diesem Leben "unheilbar".This interpretation, though grammatically impeccable, is logically contestable. If *kṣetriya* is incurable in the present life, it cannot be said that it will be curable in another because that life, when it occurs, will be, in its turn, a present life. It is true that one can suppose that Pāṇini did not see this difficulty. But another interpretation is possible. If it is found that the disease ceases only on death, it is perfectly natural to say it should be treated *for* another body, so that it does not accompany in transmigration.

transferred to another field, i.e., to another body. Or the *ksetriya* are the herbs. When they have appeared in a field understood as in "a field of other plants because of the cereals they must be treated,[1] that is to say that they must be destroyed. Or the *ksetriya* is the adulterous lover, the wives of others are the *paraksetra*, it is regarding this (*paraksetra*), that it should be treated, (that is to say) that he should be punished. And all this is deemed authoritative".

The association made by the *Kāśikāvṛtti* with leprosy enables us to understand easily the idea it had of this word. *Kusṭha* translated here by "leprosy", denotes in classical medicine all sorts of dermatoses, leprosy being one of the severe forms of the same. There is a decisive passage on it in Suśruta: "When a woman and a man have (respectively) the blood and the sperm vitiated by the impurity of leprosy, the child born of them, is itself—it should be known—affected by leprosy. Leprosy in one, who has control over oneself, is curable, when it spreads to the skin, the blood or the flesh. When it has reached the fat, it is possible that it may be cured, but when it has reached beyond it, it becomes incurable. It is said that leprosy, a disease of sin, comes from acts such as the assassination of a Brahmin, of a woman, or of good persons or because of the appropriation of the goods belonging to another. If death takes place because of leprosy, it accompanies (the victim) even in his next birth and as there is no worse disease (*kasṭatara*), it is called *kusṭha*. When a patient takes a vow to observe the rules of life prescribed in regard to food and conduct, he may obtain release from this disease by means of best medicine and of austerities and can obtain a more favourable station (in the next life).[2] Evidently it is with notions contained in this passage that the author of the *Kāśikāvṛtti* wrote his explanation

---

1 It is evident that *cikitsya* must not be translated as "to treat" or "to be cured". *Cikitsya*, the desiderative form of the root *cit.*, "to think", signifies "to take into consideration, of which one must occupy oneself." It is by means of a current specialisation that it is often taken to mean "treatable" or "to treat", the sense which mixes itself with that of "curable" because it is a principle of classical medicine that only curable ailments should be treated.

2 Suśr., *Nid.*, V:
strīpuṁsayoḥ kuṣṭhadoṣād duṣṭaśoṇitaśukrayoḥ/
yad apatyam tayor jātam jñeyam tad api kuṣṭhitam//23//
kuṣṭham ātmavataḥ (cf., *27) sādhyam tvagraktapiśitāśritam/*
medogatam bhaved yāpyam asādhyam ata uttaram//24//

and since for Pāṇini *ksetriya* designates a disease, this word should be understood in the sense which results from these notions. Particularly, one must understand not that the disease in question will be cured in a new body, but that it must be treated as much by recourse to religion as to medicine so that the new body (of the next birth) may be free therefrom.

We cannot know if, in the *Atharvaveda, ksetriya* represents *para-ksetriya* as in Pāṇini and we do not have the guarantee that the notion of transmigration was allowed in the circle where this Veda was elaborated, although, most probably, this notion appertains to the pre-Aryan, anterior basis of this text. But it is clear that the correct significance of the name, "one who appertains to the field", gives an extremely plausible sense in accordance with what Suśruta has to say of the incurable dermatoses, which penetrate not only the skin, the blood and the flesh, but the entire body right up to its last elements. And, because it is a "bond" associated with the bond of Varuṇa, it must be definitely a "disease of sin", as is leprosy according to Suśruta, and as are the majority of ailments just studied by us. Thus it appears to be absolutely possible that *ksetriya* in the *Atharvaveda* designated diseases which completely impregnated the organism, such as the incurable leprosy. The fact that the *Atharvaveda* tries to cure it, proves nothing against this last point and must not lead us into supposing that its cure was necessarily expected only after transmigration. It is only the classical medicine, with sufficient experience to lay down with certitude the progonostics of incurability, which ordains the abandonment of incurable diseases. Hope and doubt justified the intervention of the Vedic magician and besides, we have seen that Suśruta himself gave prescriptions for treating cases of advanced leprosy and if not with a view to curing them, then at least for preventing their return after transmigration.

The Fevers:—By the side of major ailments which result

---

brahmastrīsajjanavadhaparasvaharaṇādibhiḥ (cf., Hārīta, in *JA*, July-Sept., 1935, p. 136)/
karmabhiḥ pāparogasya prāhuḥ kuṣṭhasya sambhavam//25//
mriyate yadi kuṣṭhena punarjāte 'pi gacchati/
nātaḥ kaṣṭhataro rogo yathā kuṣṭham prakīrtitam//26//
āhārācārayoḥ proktām āsthāya mahatīm kriyām/
auṣadhīnām viśiṣṭānām tapasaś ca niṣevaṇāt (cf., *Mahabh* , XII, 5967)
yas tena mucyate jantuḥ sa puṇyām gatim āpnuyāt//27//.

from the insidious ascendancy of the abnormal on the body and which are, therefore, more or less related to the guardian of the Norm, Varuṇa, one should also mention fever which can be precisely the child of Varuṇa. The *Atharvaveda* calls it *takmán*.[1] It clearly indicates in details its intermittent forms:

1. When fire (Agni) has burnt the water by penetrating them, there where those who observe the Norm make adorations, that is, it is said, the place of origin *par excellence* (of the fever). Knowing us well, spare us, O Fever!
2. Whether you are the flame or the heat or the one who aims the chips [of wood] (fire) be your place of origin, your name is Hrūdu, O god of the yellow. Knowing us well....
3. Whether you are heat or the burning heat or the son of the king Varuṇa, your name is Hrūdu....
4. Adoration to the cold fever. I bow to the burning Heat. To the fever which approaches once a day, once in two days, to one (who approaches) every third day, adoration be done.[2]

There can be no hesitation in recognising the shiver of the paludal attack (cold fever), its stage of intense heat, its various forms, daily, once in three days, once in four days.[3] Another

---

[1] The name of fever in classical Sanskrit is *jvara* which is known in the *Atharvaveda* as the second member of the compound *aṅga-jvara*, "fever of the limbs", which we have already met with and which undoubtedly has already occurred in the *Ṛg-veda*, I, 4.2-8, in the compound *nava-jvara*. There is a great deal of literature on *takmán* which before being recognised as fever, was seen to represent the least expected diseases. cf., V. Grohmann, *Medicinesches aus dem Atharva-Veda mit besonderem Bezug auf den Takman*; V. Henry, *Magie...*; Macdonell-Keith, *Vedic Index*, etc. Lastly, Reinhold F.C. Muller, "Der Takman des Atharva-veda", in *Artibus Asiae*, VI, 1937, pp. 230 ff. The article of P. Regnaud, *Notes d'exégèse védique, Détermination du sens de "tan", "tman" et "takman"*, in *Congr. Or.* 1897, appertains to a series of systematic conceptions which are not acceptable.

[2] I, 25:
yád agnír āpo ádahat praviśya yátrākṛṇavan dharmadhṛto námāṁsi/
tátra ta áhuḥ paramám janítram sá naḥ saṁvidvān pári vṛndhi takman//1//
yády arcír yádi vāsi śocíḥ śakalyeṣí yádi vā te janítram/
hrūḍur nāmāsi haritasya deva sá naḥ...//2//
yádi śokó yádi vābhiśokó yádi vā rājño váruṇasyāsi putráḥ/
hrúḍur..//3//
námaḥ śītāya takmáne námo rūrāya śocíṣe kṛṇomi/
yó anyedyúr ubhayadyúr abhyéti tṛtīyakāya námo astu takmáne//4//
On *hrūḍu* cf. V. Henry, *Magie...*, 184; Barth, *Oeuvres*, Vol. II, p. 254.

[3] In classical medicine *tṛtīyaka* denotes the fever which comes every third day (counting that of the first attack as the first), therefore the *tṛtīyaka* fever. Therefore the fever that comes every fourth day is called *caturthaka* and there is no mention of a fever between the daily (*anyedyuṣka*) and the *tṛtīyaka* (Suśr., *Utt.*, XXXIX, 67-8; Car., *Cik.*, III-34). But here, *tṛtīyaka* coming after the daily and the one coming every third day, can only be the one that comes every fourth day, the one that attacks every fourth day, excluding the day of first attack.

hymn invokes the cure of all the types of known fevers: "Destroy the fever that comes every third day, one that does not come every third day, the continuous and the autumnal, the cold fever, the hot one, the one that comes in summer and the one that comes in the season of rains.[1] Against this fever are invoked (V, 22-1) Agni, Soma and Varuṇa, and the same hymn (st. 12) relates it to other ailments: his brother is *balāśa*, his cousin the *pāmán*, his sister is cough (*kāśikā*).

Balāsa designates in medicine several ailments possessing the common characteristic of manifesting themselves in the shape of swelling and the word also serves as a synonym of *kapha* and *śleṣman*, which denote the aqueous element of the organism. The *balāsaka* (equivalent of *balāsa*) is, according to Suśruta (*Utt.*, IV-8), an ailment affecting the white of the eye, wherein can be easily recognised the superficial cyst of the conjunction.[2] The *balāsa* of the *Atharvaveda* can have no relation with this cyst. The *balāsa* represents once again in Suśruta (*Nid.*, XVI-53) the suffocating oedema of the throat.[3] Lastly among fevers, Suśruta knows one, which he does not describe but which he calls *vāta-balāsaka*[4] and which, he says,

Moreover, classical medicine knows also this sense of *tṛtīyaka*. The *Śārṅgadharasaṁhitā*, for example, differentiates between the intermittent fevers under question by describing them as *aikāhika*, "daily"; *dvitīyaka*, "coming every second day" and *tṛtīyaka* "coming every third day" (2, II, 54-5).

1 *AV.*, V, 22-13:
tṛtīyakam vitṛtīyam sadamdim utá śāradám|
takmānam śītám rūrám graiṣmam nāśaya vārṣikam||
vitṛtīyá has received several conjectural interpretations; the simplest one sees in it the fever, opposite to the *tṛtīyaka*, (i.e., which is simultaneously the daily and the *tṛtīyaka*); this interpretation here is quite natural, where the exorcism looks like a complete list of fevers in which the daily and the *tṛtīyaka* have been mentioned in abridged form.

2 *kāṁsyābho bhavati site, mbubindutulyaḥ, sa jñeyo mṛdur arujo balāsakākhyaḥ*, "There exists on the white (of the eye) something like a drop of water, shining like copper, hard, indolent. It is to be known by the name of *balāsaka*". According to a variant it is covered with blood-vessels (*sirāvṛta*). The text followed here is that of Jadavji Trikamji (verse No. 9).

3 *gale ca śopham kurutaḥ prvṛddhau śleṣmānilau śvāsarujopapannam|*
marmacchidam dustaram etad āhur balāsasaṁjñam nipuṇā vikāram||
"*Śleṣman* and wind in excess provoke in the throat a tumefaction accompanied by breathlessness and pain and which injures the vulnerable points (of the throat); it is difficult to vanquish; the experts give this disorder the name of *balāsa*.

4 Suśr., *Utt.*, XXXIX, 55 (*Vāta-balāśaka* in the edition of Jībānand Vidyāsāgar, but-*sa* in the edition of Jadavji Trikamji, Bombay, 1931 (verse No. 58). Jolly was the first to point out the probable relation between the *balāsa* of the *AV.* and the *vāta-balāśaka* (*Medicin*, p. 72).

is due to an excess of *kapha*. The *Mādhava-nidāna* defines the same fever as follows: "A patient having a slow fever permanently (a continuous fever), who is dried up, swollen (who) suffers because of this, has his limbs stiffened, has lots of *śleṣman*, suffers from *vāta-balāsaka*".[1] This definition enables us to understand the reason why this disease has the name of *vāta-balāsaka*, literally, "one pertaining to wind and to *balāsa* (*śleṣman*)"; the epithet *rūkṣa*, "dried up", which figures among the symptoms, is characteristic of the action of wind[2], the swelling comes from *balāsa*, the aqueous element of the organism. In the designation of this fever, *balāsa* is, therefore, a reminder of its pathogeny. One may conclude, therefore, that right from the *Atharvaveda*, *balāsa* had the sense of the aqueous element of the organism and was applied to a febrile ailment only to call attention to the pathogeny already conceived in the same manner in classical medicine. Nothing is farther from probability. The *balāsas* are a type of oedematic ailments; it is, therefore, quite possible that *balāsa* started with denoting the symptom of swelling and it is only secondarily that, after the theory of the classical medicine had been constituted, it became the synonym of *śleṣman*, the swelling being the essential manifestations of *śleṣman*, those in which can be seen directly in action the aqueous element of the organism.

A hymn of the *Atharvaveda* could, in any case, lead one to think that *balāsa*, far from being in this text, a "swelling", denotes a mutilating and necrotizing disease. The hymn IV, 14 begins, in fact, as if seeming to qualify the *balāsa* of "the fixed trouble in the heart (or internal trouble) which breaks the bones (*asthi-sraṁsá*), which breaks the joints (*paruḥ-sraṁsá*)".[3] In the light of this definition, one is tempted to put aside the identification of *balāsa* with swelling but, on the contrary, this identification is confirmed by a deeper examination of the

---

1 *nityam mandajvaro rūkṣaḥ śūnakas tena sīdati/*
*stabdhāṅgaḥ śleṣmabhūyiṣṭho naro vātabalāsakī//*II, 40.

2 Caraka, *Sūtr.*, XII-4. The epithet of "dried up" seems to contradict that of "swollen" but there is no such conflict. It is common knowledge in clinical practice that a part of the body, the upper part, for example, appears thin and dry when there exist also liquid discharge and oedemi.

3 *asthisraṁsám paruḥsraṁsám āsthitaṁ hṛdayāmayám/balāsam...*

adjectives *asthi-sraṁsá* and *paruḥ-sraṁsá*. The root *sraṁsa* does possess the sense of "falling to pieces, of being detached" but in classical Sanskrit, when limbs are referred to, its general sense is "to release, to fall down because of heaviness." *Srastāṅga* denotes "(one whose) limbs are disjointed".[1] The *Atharvaveda* itself makes use of this root in this very sense, in a slightly modified form, in *udaram śraṁśayitvā*, "by making the stomach hang down", (IV, 16-7) and this concerns justly the stomach of the sinner, which hangs down because it is swollen, because of the bonds of Varuṇa. It is, therefore, quite natural to admit that the root *sraṁs* in *asthi-sraṁsá* and *paruḥ-sraṁsá* evokes the heaviness of the limbs and the disjunction of the articulations, as a result of the synovial swelling and discharge. Moreover, tradition has preserved the idea that the hymn IV, 14 did refer to swelling, because Keśava, commenting upon the *Kauśikasūtra* (XXXIX, 30), which teaches the ritual use of this hymn, has this to say regarding the use in question: "It is said to be the remedy for *śleṣman*".[2] He, thus, understood *balāsa* as the aqueous element of the organism precisely in connection with the hymn where *balāsa* is called *asthi* and *paruḥ-sraṁsá*.

We will discuss a little later, the word *pāmán* in connection with skin diseases. The fever *takmán* along with the related ailments called *balāsa*, *pāmán* and *kāsikā* is sent, by the exorcisms of the same hymn, which names them together (*AV*, V-22) to the barbarian woman (*dāsī*, st. 6-7) and to the various stranger people having names which are mostly identifiable: the Bāhlīkas (Bactrians), the Aṅgas (Bengal), the Magadhas (Bihar), the Gandhāris (Peshawar District). Others are less easy to situate, they are the Mujavants and the Mahāvṛṣas. The Mujavant is the mountain, *par excellence*, from where comes the soma, destined for sacrifice.[3] The *Mahābhārata* (X, 785) makes it (in all possibility it is the same mountain) the place where Bhava (Śiva) practises austerities and it is known that the ascetic Śiva stays chiefly in the

1 cf., various references in *PW* under *sraṁs*, in the lower part of the column 1399; *Kumāratantra de Rāvaṇa*, p. 181, column 1, under *lus lhod*, "relaxation of the body" which renders *srastāṅgatva*, "the falling down of limbs" in Tibetan.

2 *śleṣma-bhaiṣajyam ucyate*.

3 Caland-Henry, *L'Agniṣṭoma*, Paris, 1906, Vol. I, p. 44; *RV.*, X-34-1.

Himalayas, in the North. The *Mahāvṛṣas*, "those who have big bulls", seem to belong to lower Panjab.[1] This hymn against fever has been, most probably, composed in Central India, the Madhyadeśa, say between Delhi and Allahabad, because all the stranger people named therein surround precisely this region.

We may also remark that the *dāsī*, literally the "woman-slave", is the woman belonging to stranger people, hostile to the Vedic society and that the Mujavants are particularly despised. The Merchant of soma, who brings the plant from the mount Mujavant, is a being who is chased away by being beaten with batons, once the soma has been delivered.[2] It is, therefore, natural that in Vedic ideas, fever is sought to be discharged on such persons. The word *takmán*, for its formation, is attached either to the roots *tañc* or *tak*. The former denotes "to contract, to coagulate" and is found only in the texts on grammar; it is, however, represented in usage by the forms *ātañcana*, "that which makes the milk curdle", *abhyātañc*, "curdling for another", *upātaṅkya* (that which makes the milk curdle). It is difficult to see the possibility of the semantic passage. *Takmán* shows itself as an agent-name and a word denoting "Coagulator" is not well-suited for designating fever. On the other hand, *takmán* could, more probably, be derived from *tak*, which indicates a rapid movement, the passage in the sense of "provoking a dash" in one "which causes a fit." This will explain that the word has been used to denote fever.[3] Although this etymology is plausible, one may as well ask if it is not a loan-word. In fact, it can be observed that the *Atharvaveda*, (V-22—we have summarised its contents above) declares: "The Mujavants are its abode, the Mahāvṛṣas are its abode; from the moment of your birth, O

---

1 A. Foucher thought, as he had very kindly indicated to me, that the Mahavṛṣas should be looked for there, because of the magnificent bovine race of Hissar, taller than man. It is the same race whose specimens were sent by Alexander to Greece.

2 *L'Agniṣṭoma*, I, p. 47—The merchant is included among those whose food must not be eaten because of their abject condition, *Yājñavalkya*, I-165.

3 The root *tak* gives as derivatives *páritakmya* (*RV.*), denoting "one who dashes around", and *paritakmyā*, "peregrination, revolution"; this confirms that *takmán* must have been derived from the same root.

Takman, you derive pleasure in living among the Bāhlikas".[1] It is, therefore, not only because one desires to banish it to stranger countries, that it is sent there, but also because it is a disease of theirs and it cannot be excluded, *á priori* that its name current in the country, where it was endemic, has been used. In any case, the word *takmán* has not survived in classical medicine[2], where, however, the study of classical medicine has had a big development. Only the names of its intermittent forms, as we have seen, have been preserved. We may also point out in this regard that it will be extremely misleading to date the medical notions according to the dates of the texts of the classical tradition in which they are arrested. The intermittent fevers are studied in the *Suśruta-saṁhitā* only in the *Uttaratantra*, suspected to have been appended at a later date and yet their notion was possessed from the time of the *Atharvaveda*. The silence of the older part of the *Suśruta* is explained by a simple lacuna in the editing of this text.

Isolated Morbid Phenomena:— The majority of other ailments which are named in the *Ṛgveda* and the *Atharvaveda* are isolated morbid phenomena. No effort is made for discerning across the groupings of these phenomena, the diseases of which they represent only the symptoms. In the presence of patients suffering from cephalitis, vomitting and constipation, we are used to evoke immediately the diagnosis of meningitis. The Vedic healer saw therein three disorders occurring simultaneously or, if he knew that these disorders were interconnected because of their co-existence and were connected with others which do not fail to accompany them, the disease that caused them to occur together was not

1 *óko asya mūjavanta óko asya mahāvṛṣāḥ|*
yāvaj jātás takmams tāvān asi báhlikeṣu nyocaráh||5||
It is possible that on account of a certain assonance, the memory of the *takmán* has probably given the sense of "fever" to the word *ātaṅka* which normally denotes "torment" and is derived from the root *taṅk* [known only to the grammarians as also its other derivatives, except *prataṅkam* (*AV.*) which has the sense of "furtively"]. *Ātaṅka* is used by Caraka (*Cik.*, III-11) and Vāgbhaṭa (A.H., *Nid.*, I-2), etc., in the sense of "torments" or of "disease". Only the *Rājanighaṇṭu* and certain lexicographers make it a synonym of *jvara*, but the *Rājani.* itself (XX-1) takes it in the sense of "disease". Caraka and Vāgbhaṭa, in the passage quoted above, also use it as a synonym of *jvara* but this is because they understand once *jvara* in the sense of "disease".

determined for him and did not constitute for him a definite clinical entity. Behind the concrete lesions and evidently morbid accidents, he did not individualise the syndroms.

Expressions such as *śīrśaktí* and *śīrsāmayá* seem to denote the "pains in the head" whose precise nature cannot be determined by us because the *Atharva* does not let us guess their characteristics. *Pṛṣṭyāmayá* (*AV.*, XIX, 34-10), "disease in the back", denotes lumbago as is apparently proved by a comparison with the *Ṛgveda*, I, 105-18: "He raises himself up like a carpenter suffering from pains in the back" (. . . *uj jihīte nicāyyā tásṭeva pṛsṭyāmayī* . . .)." The "flux", *āsrāva*, is simultaneously polyuria or even the normal flux of urine, diarrhoea, Haemorrhage, the excessive discharge of all that can normally or abnormally flow from the body. *Śūla* denotes the lancinating pain in *karṇa-śūlá*, "pain in the ear" (*AV.*, IX, 8-1). The names of skin-diseases, of which several are mentioned, seem to be only the simple names of morbid symptoms.

Alají, mentioned in a list of exorcised diseases[1] is well known to Suśruta under the orthography of *alajī*. It is not a characteristic disease, but a type of morbid element, appearing in various diseases. It is one of the ten vesicular ailments (*piḍaka*) appearing as a complication in patients suffering from the "alteration of urines" (*prameha*), "alajī is red, white, pustulous, painful".[2] It can arise in the penis and can be, in that case, due to *Śūka*, concerning whose causal nature the commentators have different hypotheses[3]; it has, in any case, the same characteristics when it complicates the "alteration of urines". Lastly, *alajī* is also the name of the vesicles of sclero-corneal limb: "It should be known that *parvaṇī* is a type of swelling coming from blood, round, copper-coloured, short, accompanied by heat and lancinating pain, caused by a union of the black and the white (of the eye); there can be at this very (localisation) the *alajī* defined by the symptoms described

1 *AV.*, IX, 8-20: *viśalyásya vidradhásya vātīkārásya vālajéḥ/*
yákṣmāṇam sárveṣām viṣám nir avocam ahám tvát//
—"of the Erysipelas (cf. *Supra*, p. 108) of the abcess or of that which produces wind, of *alajī*, the poison, of all the weakening ailments, I have chased them out of you, by speech".

2 *raktā sitā sphoṭavatī dāruṇā tv alajī bhavet.*—Suśr., *Nid.*, VI-12.

3 Suśr., *Nid.*, XIV, 1 & 5.

above (i.e., according to the commentator Dalhaṇa, defined by the same symptoms as the *parvaṇī* from which it differs only by additional thickness).[1] The most probable old sense is, therefore, "vesicle", in any case the name is that of a morbid form and not that of a disease.

Kilāsa is found in the *Atharvaveda* along with *palitá*, denoting "pale", but is classically applied to hair turned white by age or pain[2] and the exorcism of the hymn I, 23, aims to restore the normal colouring, weakened by *kilāsa* and *palitá*. This hymn is important enough to be examined in its entirety:

1. You are born at night, O sombre plant, black and dark. O *rajanī*, colour this *Kilāsa*.
2. And make disappear from here that which is spotted, the *kilāsa* and the pale. That the colour which is its (the colour of that which is white) may penetrate you. Chase the whites away.
3. Devoid of white is your solution, your station is devoid of white, you are dark, O plant, make disappear, from here that which is spotted.
4. By incantation I have destroyed the white spot which is in the skin, of the *kilāsa* born from the bones, born from the body, produced by malefice.[3]

In classical medicine the word *rajanī* denotes sometimes

---

1 *tāmrā tanvī dāhaśūlopapannā raktā jñeyā parvaṇī vṛttaśophā|*
jātā sandhau kṛṣṇaśukle 'lajī syāt tasminn eva khyāpitā purvaliṅgaiḥ||
—*Utt.*, II, 6.
The "vesicles of the limb" are not the veritable limbs, yet they resemble them and that is why we call them so. It is because of this resemblance which, in India as in Europe, has caused the use of the same word for denoting them as also the real vesicles.

2 Suśr., *Nid.*, XIII, 32-3.

3 *naktam jātāsy oṣadhe rāme kṛṣṇe ásikni ca|*
idám rajanì rajaya kilāsam palitám ca yát||1||
kilāsam ca palitám ca nír itó nāśayā pṛṣat|
ā tvā svó viśatām várṇaḥ párā śuklāni pātaya||2||
ásitam te praláyanam āsthānam ásitam táva|
ásikny asy oṣadhe nír itó nāśayā pṛṣat||3||
asthijāsya kilāsasya tanujásya ca yát tvaci|
dūṣyā kṛtásya bráhmaṇā lákṣma śvetám anīnaśam||4||
V. Henry, *Manuel védique*, p. 135, note, remarks in connection with st. 3 that *praláyana* is derived from *pra-lī*, "to dissolve oneself"; He understands: "black is thy decoction (read: solution), black is thy station (on the stalk)". i.e., "dead or alive, thou art always black". This interpretation, however, is uncertain. One can also read: "Devoid of white (when) thou art in the lying position . . ." which signifies "dead (pulled out) or (yet standing) you are black". In the same work V. Henry interprets *svo varṇaḥ* of st. 2, as applicable to the plant and understands it as follows: "take the proper colour (O plant, in the patient's body)", i.e., "become there dark, and thereafter, darken him." It is more natural to think that the aim of the formula is to transfer the pale spots to the plant, because it is black in essence, it will absorb that white.

the curcuma and at others the indigo. Curcuma being of clearyellow shade cannot be in question in this hymn; Indigo, on the contrary, can be, with equal facility, qualified with black inasmuch as the same names are employed in Sanskrit to denote the black and the dark blue and it is we who, according to propriety, translate them as "blue" or "black". On the other hand, indigo is obtained by leaving the indigo plant to be fermented in water; therefore it seems likely that the word *pralấyanà*, "dissolution", refers to this process of extraction. In any case, *kilāsa* is evidently a disease of the skin which is characterised by decoloration; it is, therefore, an achromatism, a morbid phenomenon which can be produced by different causes and which is clearly described by the text by being associated with *kilāsa* and *palitá*, the "pale". Classical medicine ranges *kilāsa* among the *kuṣṭhas*, that is to say, skin-diseases (and not only leprosy, contrary to the common translation given by the dictionaries). Suśruta characterises it as follows: "The *kilāsa* also is a variety of skin-disease. It is of three types, due to wind, due to *pitta* and due to *śleṣman*. The difference between the skin-disease (the most serious, leprosy properly called) and *kilāsa* lies in the fact that *kilāsa* attains (only) the skin and does not ooze out. The one due to wind is circular, rose, rugose and disintegrates a great deal (desquamates). The one due to *pitta* is like the leaf of the rose-coloured lotus and is encircled by inflammation. The one which is due to śleṣman is white, smooth, thick and pruriginous. Among (all) these the one which appears in confluent circles, develops at an extremity and has red hair, is incurable as also the one which is burned by fire (cicatrisation of burning)".[1]

The precise indication given by this text concerning the difference existing between *kilāsa* and leprosy shows us clearly that one must not identify these two diseases. The form of *kilāsa* due to the wind seems to be psoriasis which has nothing

---

[1] *kilāsam api kuṣṭhavikalpa eva|*
rat trividham, vātena pittena śleṣmaṇā ceti|
kuṣṭhakilāsayor antaram tvaggatam eva kilāsam aparisrāvi ca|
tad vātena maṇḍalam aruṇam paruṣam paridhvaṁsi|
ca pittena padmapatra-pratīkāśam saparidāham ca śleṣmaṇāpi śvetam snigdham bahulam kaṇḍūmacca|
teṣu sambaddhamaṇḍalam ante jātam raktaroma cāsādhyam agnidagdham ca||—Suśr., *Nid.*, V-14.

to do with leprosy. The two other forms do not appear to have any corresponding forms in our nosology but are also not of leprous nature. The fact that *kilāsa* is a purely superficial disease in Suśruta, does not accord with the data of the *Atharvaveda* which, though it situates the white spot of *kilāsa* in the skin, declares that *kilāsa* can come from the bones or from the "body". The *kilāsa* of the *Atharvaveda* cannot, therefore, be the same disease as that described in Suśruta and one may ask oneself if it does not represent, as is generally believed, a name of leprosy. Later, in classical medicine, this name could have been deflected from its older meaning, to be applied to more superficial types of dermatoses and of a different nature. But first of all, it must be observed that even in classical medicine there exist several forms which are very near *kilāsa* but which can be more profound. In fact, on the above-quoted passage of Suśruta, the commentator Dalhaṇa observes that according to the teaching of Viśvāmitra: "(The disease), which attaining the skin, does not cause oozing, is called *kilāsa*. When it crosses the skin and penetrates (the constitutive) elements (of the body), leaving the name of *kilāsa*, it should receive the name of *Śvitra*".[1] It is, therefore, possible that in the *Atharvaveda*, *kilāsa* already denoted the same disease which is found later in other classical authors. These later authors, however, do not distinguish the exclusively cutaneous form of the disease, which is accompanied by deeper lesions. The only difference that will persist after all, will be due to the fact that the Vedic text considers the disease as coming out from the depth on to the surface, whereas the classical doctors recognise an inverse sense in its clinical evolution, which is more reasonable and is explained quite naturally by a better knowledge of pathological facts.

Moreover, whether *kilāsa* has changed or not changed its sense between the *Atharvaveda* and classical medicine, in the hymn translated above, it is considered only as a disorder of the coloration of the skin due to malefices and it is sought to be suppressed by a tincture and by incantations. We know

1 *tvaggatam tu yad asrāvi kilāsam tat prakīrtitam|*
yadā tvacam atikramya tad dhātūn avagāhate|
hitvā kilāsasaṁjñām ca śvitrasaṁjñām labheta tat||

well that achromy often exists along with leprosy but the Vedic sorcerer limits himself to stating the superficial symptom and to perceiving at the most that it can hold on to deeper lesions. There is nothing to attest that he conceived it as a simple manifestation of a polymorphic clinical entity and as a complex one like the one called "leprosy".

The word *pāmán*, which figures in the Avesta as in the Veda and denotes a "cousin" of fever, has already been studied (*supra*, p. 52). The disease known as *kumbhīkā* in the *Atharvaveda* is also related to skin-diseases, concerning which the context gives us no information, but which is well-known in classical medicine. Like *alajī*, it is a morbid form which can be met with at the penis as also in the eyelids. In the first case[1], it is compared to the stone of the rose-apple fruit, in the second it is said thereof that "the vesicles resembling the grains of Pistia stratiotes L., which arise on the eyelids, provoke swelling: when they burst, they are the vesicles *kumbhīkā*".[2] The same hymn of the *Atharvaveda* mentions along with *kumbhīkā dūṣīkā* which denotes "conjunctival secretion".

Vedic pathology gives a large place to wounds, to poisons and to parasitic worms but we are given information only regarding the magical exorcisms used to oppose them. It should also be recognised that the *Ṛgveda* and the *Atharvaveda*,

---

1 *kumbhīkā rakta-pittotthā jāmbavāsthi-nibhāśubhā*—"the *k.* comes from the blood and *pitta*, it resembles a stone of the rose-apple fruit and has a bad aspect"—Suśr. *Nid.*, XIV, 4b. Ḍalhaṇa takes *aśubhā* in the sense of "black".

2 *kumbhīka-bīja-pratimāḥ piḍakā yās tu vartmajāḥ|*
ādhmāpayanti bhinnā yāḥ kumbhīka-piḍakās tu tāḥ||—Suśr., *Utt.*, III-8.
The etymology of *kumbhīkā*, manifestly derived from *kumbhī*, "pitcher", "vase", and literally denoting "small pitcher", is well-explained by the fact that once the vesicles are open, they transform themselves, especially when they are situated on a swollen tissue, into small craters—comparable to small receptacles. It cannot be admitted that they have received the name *kumbhīkā* because of their analogy, at the commencement of their evolution (when they are still a protrusion) with the grains of the *kumbhīkā* plant because the other quoted passage of Suśruta compares them to a totally different type of grain, even though it gives them the same name. Moreover, the use of *kumbhīkā* as the name of a disease as also the use of *kumbhī* to denote the pitcher goes back to the *Atharvaveda*, whereas its use in Botany does not seem to be known before Suśruta. It is rather the name which has caused the grains of *kumbhīkā* to be selected as the element of comparison. The grains of *kumbhīkā* are simply the extremely small grains of a gigantic lentil of water resembling a lettuce.

being collections of hymns, are not books of medicine and did not have to explain the contemporary pathology. Useful indications are only accidental; the data of classical medicine, when it relates to diseases, whose names were already in use in the Veda and when this data are in accord with Vedic indications, enables us to have some idea of the diseases known to the Veda. But where the indications are too vague and where the medical tradition is silent, we are left only with etymological conjectures, which, by themselves, are not plausible. Moreover, whether possible or not, they do not have any interest for the history of medicine. Even when the older sense of the word, supposed by its etymology, is clear, it is not sure if it applies to the passage where it is found to be employed. The Veda, though ancient, is not an ancient book in which only forged words have been inserted intentionally. Sufficient time must have passed between the formation of medical terms (those alone interest us here) and their insertion in the Veda to enable all sorts of deviations of sense and the specialisations of usage. Moreover, the medical names are quite often deflected from their sense right from the time of their formation itself. These terms are habitually drawn from banal ones denoting objects with which is compared the disease or one of its salient characteristics. The name of the lancinating pain, *śūla*, is, for example, the same word which denotes "lance", slightly deflected from its original meaning. Here the deviation is insignificant, but sometimes the deviation is so great that the secondary meaning retains only an extremely vague relation with the original meaning and the latter does not enable one to comprehend the former. It is in this manner that one of the last words examined by us, *kumbhīkā*, has as its older meaning, "small vase or small jar". According to this meaning it could be supposed that a plant of this name is a gourd and all sorts of hypotheses could be made regarding a disease, called *kumbhīkā*, imagining it to dig petty holes under the skin as it really does. But one could rather imagine it in the form of fistulised liquid-containing pockets or even as cysts looking like small jars. Thus one would run the risk of completely misleading oneself. We will, therefore, leave aside a series of morbid phenomena till we obtain more information regarding them, as we can have some idea of their nature only by means of etymological considerations of doubtful value.

The disease *apvā* is chased away from the interior of the abdomen (*AV.*, IX, 8-9), and in an incantation of the black-magic found in the *Ṛgveda* (X, 103-12), an *apvā* is called upon to trouble the spirit of the enemies, seize their limbs and burn their hearts. This does not enable us to identify it.[1] The disease *viklíndu* (*AV.*, XII, 4-5) attacks the man guilty of keeping a cow instead of giving it to Brahmins. *Gláu* and *galuntá* (*AV.*, VI, 83-3), *Udyugá* (*AV.*, V, 22-11), *Nirāla* (*AV.*, VI, 16-3) cannot be as yet seriously identified even if they were diseases. *Vilohitá* (*AV.*, IX, 8-1; XII, 4-4) according to the manner of the formation of the word, probably denotes a flux of the blood (of the nose?—Bloomfield), the decomposition of blood (V. Henry) or anaemia (Whitney). *Pramóta* probably denotes the dumb (*AV.*, IX, 8-4), *Viśará* (*AV.*, II, 4-2), *Víśarīka* and *āśarīka* (*AV.*, XIX, 34-10) are evidently derived from the root *śṛ*, "to break"; probably they denote various forms of contusive pains, but *visara* appears in a list of names having the chance of being applied to provocative demons of diseases rather than to the diseases themselves. These names are (*AV.*, II, 4-2), *jambha*, from the root *jabh* "to pound", which signifies "tooth" in the *Ṛgveda* and later "jaws",[2] *víṣkandha* and *abhiśócana*. Other names of the same type are found elsewhere: *sáṁskandha* (with the new *víṣkandha*, *AV.*, XIX, 34-5), *Sipada*[3] (in *aśipadá*, with a privative particle, *RV.*, VII, 51-4), *Śímidā* (*AV.*, IV, 25-4 and in *aśimidá*, *RV.*, VII, 51-4). For all these words one can only resort to etymological conjectures which, though linguistically sure, are of no value, in the

---

1 Oldenberg, although doubtful, translates "diarrhoea" (*Rél. du Veda*, p. 425) which cannot be defended in the presence of the passage of the *Ṛgveda*, which Oldenberg had before him when he made the translation. In the passage in question, it could also refer to something else than a disease (cf., Bloomfield, *Hymns*, 327; V. Henry, *Manuel védique*, index which proposes "panic, rout").

2 All sorts of conjectures have been made regarding the disease provoked by the demon Jambha who attacks children and who is a *rakṣas* (Ḍārila on *Kauś. S.*, XXXII, 1). Zimmer and V. Henry had thought it to be the crisis of dentition; Bloomfield took it for a crisis of convulsions and Caland that of *trismus*. It is not possible at present to settle the question.

3 The commentator Sāyaṇa recognises therein the disease. *śipada;* unfortunately this disease is not known elsewhere. He probably thought of *ślīpada* which is the elephantiasis.

absence of decisive context, for fixing the sense in which they are used.

Demons and Abortion: Certain names of Vedic diseases can also be the names of demons already referred to by us. Many of their misdeeds do not directly interest us, but the *rakṣas* already encountered by us and who specialise in provoking abortion seem, according to a hymn of the *Ṛgveda*, to be considered capable of causing the death of the child during the different stages of confinement. This hymn is interesting to study as it thus seems to attest that the different stages of confinement as also the risks run by the child during this period, had been noted.

1. That with the help of the incantation, Agni, killer of *rakṣas*, push away from here one who, being ill, having a sinister name, sits in thy foetus, in thy womb.
2. That, which being disease, having a sinister name, sits in thy foetus, in thy womb, (he) the eater of flesh[1], with incantation Agni has expelled it.
3. The one, who kills thy (foetus), which is about to descend, which is seated, one who (kills it) when it slips fast, who wants to kill it when born, we suppress it from here.
4. The one who separates thy thighs, who lies down between husband and wife, who licks the womb inside, we suppress it from here.
5. The one, who having become a brother, a husband, having become a lover, lies down with you, the one who desires to kill thy progeny, we suppress it from here,
6. The one who lies down with you, having misled you by means of sleep, of obscurity, him who desires to kill thy progeny, we suppress it from here".[2]

---

1 *kravyādam* in the accusative refers to a demon, causing abortions and this is not the only example of a similar use. But frequently Agni itself receives the epithet of "eater of flesh", *kravyād*. In this case, it refers specially to the fire of the funeral pyre (cf., V. Henry, *Magie . . .* p. 217). Here then is another example of antagonistic forms, assumed by the same entities. Here, Agni, the Fire, chases the *kravyād;* elsewhere he himself is the *kravyād* (cf., Oldenberg, *Ṛgveda . . . Noten*, Berlin, 1912 on X, 16-9-11).

2 *RV.*, X, 162:
brāhmaṇāgniḥ samvidāno rakṣohā bādhatām itáḥ/
ámīvā yás te gárbham durṇāmā yónim āśáye//1//
yás te gárbham ámīvā durṇāmā yónim āśáye/
agnís tám brāhmaṇā sahá níṣ kravyādam anīnaśat//2//
yás te hánti patáyantam niṣatsnúm yah sarīsṛpám/
jātám yás te jighāṅsati tám itó nāśayāmasi//3//
yás ta ūrū viháraty antarā dámpatī śáye/
yónim yó antar āreḷi tám itó nāśayāmasi//4//
yás tvā bhrātā pátir bhūtvā jāró bhūtvā nipádyate/
prajām yás te jighāṅsati tám itó nāśayāmasi//5//

It seems that verse 3 alludes to the different periods of confinement. If the foetus can be killed when it is descending, this is during its entry into and passage of the pelvic canal where it can die in case of prolonged labours. The seated foetus appears to be one that presents itself by its seat. If this manner of presentation is not the most dangerous, it is at least the most frequent of abnormal presentations. Lastly it is at the time of coming out that the child slips fast because of the last contractions which no longer meet with any resistance, and because of the viscous coating covering the child. There also the child is exposed to dangers such as a violent fall or a serious drawing of the cord.

Generally the verse has been interpreted a little differently. Mr. Reinhold Müller, latest of all (*Asia Major*, Vol. VI, p.343) understands the term just translated by us as "one who is about to descend" as denoting "hurrying itself" (*eilenden*) because the root *pat*, from where the term of the text *patáyantam* is derived, denotes "to fly" (in the *Ṛgveda*). But right from the *Atharvaveda* itself, *pat* takes the sense of "to fall" (hence the translation given)[1] and the present hymn can be considered as belonging to an epoch neighbouring that of the Atharvanic incantations of the same type. It is true that, in the *Atharvaveda*, *patay* continues, as a general rule, to denote "to fly". But since the sense of a Vedic word can be determined essentially according to the conformity with the context and the accord with later tradition, it should be possible to admit that the meaning of "to fall down" is already attested in the *Ṛgveda* (our hymn), because it is the only plausible meaning. "To fly" in the literal sense, would be absurd. "To hurry" or "to precipitate" are secondary senses in the same way as "to fall down" and cannot be preferred to the latter. Moreover, regardless of the understanding that the foetus is descending or that it is hurrying, it should be recognised that, in the two cases, an allusion is made to the first period of parturition. It is, therefore, righ that we have

---

yás tvā svápnena támasā mohayitvā nipádyate|
prajām yás te jíghāṅsati tám itó nāśayāmasi||6||
The Hymn, *AV.*, VIII-6, takes up a part of these verses, and largely develops these very themes, giving numerous names of demons.

1 Although the sense of "to fly" remains very much alive (e.g., *AV.*, I, 11-6; *yathā pátanti pakṣiṇaḥ*, "as fly the birds").

therein evidence guaranteeing that the Vedic authors had observed and distinguished the phases of confinement and the corresponding accidents; this, however, does not prove the existence of an advanced obstetrics. Hence once again we find a pathological fact in the Veda, but only in a stage purely rudimentary, but which shall be later taken up with considerable progress in classical medicine, because Indian obstetrics, specially that of Suśruta, is one of the most complete and one of the most audacious of antiquity.

THERAPEUTICS

In the Vedic *saṁhitās* therapeutics appears essentially as consisting of incantations, magical practices and prayers. As such, it could have only a slight echo in classical medicine, based on the knowledge of diseases and the determination of their causes.

The majority of hymns used in curative charms, whether they belong to the *Ṛgveda* or to the *Atharva*. are formulae of exorcism of this type, irrespective of the fact whether the disease aimed at is presented as being caused by the action of a demon or not. But it is certain that the recitation of hymns did not suffice. It was accompanied by a ritual, which has not been preserved for us in the oldest texts but by others like the *Kauśikasūtra* attached to the *Atharvaveda*. This Sūtra has probably modified the ceremonies in usage in the epoch of the *Atharvaveda* but it certainly contains ancient traditional data and gives an extremely exact general idea of Vedic therapeutics. This therapeutics is essentially magical. We have, incidentally, picked up some of its traits, which show that it has little to do with the really medical.[1] The numerous plants mentioned in the hymns manifestly assume the rôle of magical ingredients rather than that of veritable drugs. We have already seen the use of *rajanī*, "colouring", which, because of its dark colour, is used to re-dye the decolourised skin and will absorb the decolorisation, of which it is antagonistic. This is not a truly medical use. One of the chief remedies mentioned (*RV*., I, 43-4, VII, 295; *AV*., II-27-6, VI-57), the remedy *par excellence*

For more details, cf., V. Henry, *Magie . . .*; Caland, *Altindischen Zauberritual*, Amsterdam, 1900.

of Rudra, *jālāsa* is, according to Bloomfield, only urine, who interprets in this manner the indications of the *Kauśikasūtra*, or rain-water conceived as cosmic urine according to Geldner:[1] in any case it is not a real remedy. But, *á priori* one must think that in the Vedic epoch, one could not have helped observing the medicinal properties of certain plants and of their products, but these are not generally these properties which appear in the hymns. The bdellium (*guggulu* or *gulgulu*), for example, to which classical medicine attributes medicinal properties, figures in the *Atharvaveda* only as an odorous product, suitable for chasing away bad influences; it retains this characteristic in the field of exorcism right up to more recent epochs.[2] The hymn, XIX, 38, is addressed to the bdellium of Sindh and to that of the ocean, that is to say, brought in by maritime commerce.

Along with bdellium, the hymn addresses itself to a certain *Arundhatī*. Often this name denotes a certain star, but here a vegetable product is meant, also mentioned in the *Atharvaveda*, which calls it *lākṣā* too (*AV*., V, 5-7). Now *lākṣā* is the resin known as "lac" which flows out as a result of pricking caused by an insect, called Coccus lacca, in the branches of various types of trees, of whom the chief are Ficus religiosa, Ficus indica, Rhamnus jujuba and Butea frondosa. Hymn V says, in verse 5, to *Arundhatī*: "You come out of the good Ficus infectoria, from Ficus religiosa, from Acacia catechu, from Grislea tomentosa, from the good Ficus indica and from Butea frondosa".[4] Acacia catechu gives the black

---

1 cf., Macdonell-Keith, *Vedic Index*, see *jalāsa-bhesaja*.

2 *Kumāratantra de Rāvaṇa*, pp. 14 ff., 40, n. 1.

3 cf., Zimmer, *Altindische Leben*, Berlin, 1879, p. 28.

4 *Bhadrāt plaksān nis tisṭhasy aśvatthāt khadirād dhavāt/bhadrān nyagródhāt parṇāt. . .*
The translators have always supposed that *arundhatī* denoted a creeper, which attaches itself to certain types of trees (cf., *Vedic Index*, see the word). It is said that it climbs the trees (*V*., V, 5-3) but the trails of resin run on the bark as the stalks of creepers, with which they can be compared. The names of trees from which it "comes out" remove all doubt. Moreover *Arundhatī* receives the name of *lomaśa-vakṣanā* (*AV*., V, 5-7) which has been translated by Roth as: "am Leibe behaart" and which is included in the *Vedic Index* as signifying one which has "a hairy stem". But these interpretations are based only on the supposition that it is a plant. The root *vakṣ* denotes "to grow; to shoot up" (Ger. Wachsen, etc.). The word should therefore be understood to mean "one which has a growth of

catechu which is obtained not by incision as the gums, but by boiling the bark; the incision of the bark furnishes a certain gum. Grislea tomentosa produces a variety of honey in its flowers (red in colour and used in dyes like the lac), its wood is succulent and eatable. There is every reason to believe that the resins and gums grouped under the names of *arundhatī* or *lākṣā*[1] were not solely those which are produced under the action of the Coccus lacca and which form the red lac but also those which are produced from those very trees by means of incision. In fact, in hymn V, 5 (st. 6 & 7), it is said that *arundhatī* has the colour of gold (*hiraṇya-varṇa*) and that of the Sun (*sūrya-varṇa*) which can be correctly applied to resins but not to the red lac.

Arundhatī is used to obtain the cicatrisation of wounds and heal up that which is broken. V. Henry believed that it owed its virtues solely to the speculation of popular grammar on the etymology of its name, *arun* . . . might have signified *arus*, "wound", and *-dhatī* might have suggested the idea of the root *dhā*, "to heal".[2] He put aside deliberately the hypothesis that recognised healing properties might have given it its name. The case where the name of a thing commands its use in magic is extremely common and many Indian plants or vegetable products draw their properties from an etymological hypothesis or from a popular etymology.[3] But here etymology has had no rôle to play. Once *arundhatī* is recognised as the resin-gum, the reason of its use as a healer becomes evident; this gum which comes to fill up the incisions in the trunks of trees and stops them by hardening is the

hair", i.e., which grows from the trunk as hair from limbs, or better still, "one which has a growth of hair", i.e., which grows in trails comparable to hair if *loman*, in this compound, can have the rare but proven sense of "hair" (cf., Aufrecht, *Lomaśātana*, in *ZDMG*, 1877, Vol. XXXI, p. 768). Lastly verse 2 of hymn V, 5 says: "one who drinks you, lives . . .", *yás tvā píbati jīvati* . . . , which cannot be said of a creeper but can very well be explained when understood as referring to a resin as shown by the rite referred to hereafter.

1 *lākṣā* is the term from which the word *lac* is derived by means of the Persian-Arabic *lak* or *lakk* and the Latin (mediaeval) *lacca. The Periplus of the Erythrean Sea* (6) mentions *lac* as *lakhkhos*. The two forms of Persian-Arabic are the exact transcriptions of Indian forms. In Mid-Indian, *lākṣā* had to change into *lākhā* (attested in Pali) or *lakkhtā* (on the final vowel cf. J. Bloch, *Indo-Aryen*, Paris, 1934, p. 41).

2 *Magie* . . . , p. 180.

3 *Kumāratantra* . . . , pp. 32-3.

healing type. In the ritual of the *Kauśikasūtra*, where the translators have, this time, recognised the real nature of the product, appearing one under the name of *lākṣā*, this *lākṣā* is dissolved in boiling water, mixed with milk and given to the patient to drink.[1] In another practice taught by the same text and its commentaries,[2] the wound is washed with a solution of lac, which is also given to the wounded person to drink. One can easily understand the sense of this curative rite. If the wound is bloody, it is probably a homeopathic rite if the lac used is red as supposed by Caland and Henry,[3] but lac is chiefly given for drinking to repair the wound of the patient by the same process as that of the tree. Because the resin which springs in the wound fills it up and closes it, comes from the interior of the tree.

Despite the mystical character of Vedic therapeutics, one may ask oneself if in certain passages, one should not recognise references to methods of treatment that are really medical. These could have been used in practice but concerning them the hymns, because of their character, can only rarely provide any information. One may ask oneself, for example, if vesical cathterism was not known. Hymn I, 3 of the *Atharvaveda*, used as an exorcism against the retention of urine, actually refers to a reed (*śara*) which could serve as a sound, because verse 7 says: "I break thy urethra as the dyke of a pond . . .[4]" and it is quite natural to think that an operation for making the urine flow was really performed by means of the reed. Hymn I, 2, on its side, says: "We have recognised as the father of the reed ("or of the arrow" made from the reed) Parjanya (god of rain) who nourishes abundantly; we have recognised for its mother, Earth which has numerous aspects. . . just as the shaft of an arrow stands between the Sky and the Earth, that similarly may this cane stand between the disease and the flux".[5] The cane in question is a hollow stalk of a

1 XXVIII, 14.

2 XXVIII, 5-6.

3 *Magie . . .*, p. 181, n. 1.

4 *prá te bhinadmi méhanam vártram vecantyā iva/*

5 *vidmā śarásya pitáram parjányam bhūridhāyasam/*
vidmó ṣvasya mātáram pṛthivīm bhūrivarpasam//
yáthā dyām ca pṛthivīm cāntás tíṣṭhati téjanam/
evā rógam cāsrāvám cāntás tiṣṭhatu múñja ít//

plant similar to the sugar-cane, the Saccharum munja. It can, therefore, be said that it relates to a sound made from a similar stalk. This sound, once in place, is well situated between the painful vesical globe and the flux of urine which flows out at its other end. Unfortunately a difficulty renders this interpretation doubtful. First of all, it is not clear if an extremely fine stalk of the Saccharum munja can be hollowed and used as a sound. Only a sufficiently voluminous stalk can be emptied of its internal sap, while keeping its sides sufficiently resistant, but then it is impossible to employ it as an urethral catheter. Possibly this referred only to a symbolic operation. The hollow cane has been used without being introduced in the urethra for mimicking and leading by means of initiative magic the flow, which it was desired to be produced by the urethral canal.

We cannot pursue the examination of innumerable magical practices, which constitute Vedic therapeutics as they have no rôle in the formation of the scientific medicine of the classical epoch. Of course, it is admitted that magic prepares the appearance of science and furnishes it within its first elements. But it seems to be an illusion. Certainly medical magic starts to treat all sorts of ailments, thus providing the magician with an occasion to observe them. Besides, the curative charms comprise the use of a large number of plants and of products which, leaving aside their supposed magical virtue, can have a real physiological action. From there it is readily concluded that the magician ends up by acquiring, more or less in spite of himself, exact notions of pathology and of therapeutics. But this is too vulgar a manner of conceiving the formation of scientific notions. A notion can be called scientific only if it comprises a rational element, the rudiments of the natural explanation of a phenomenon or of the justification of an observed property. When the healer observes a disease, if he contents himself with only observing the symptoms of the disease, he makes neither science nor magic; he does not get out of pure empiricism. If he tries to explain the observed disease, two things can happen. Either he joins it immediately to a system of phenomena with which the disorder shows some analogy, allowing its participation in this system of phenomena without trying to find out any reason thereof; in that case he poses a magical relationship. Or, by means of reasoning he relates it to a group of understood facts. It is only then that he establishes or sketches out a scientific explanation. It is possible that the same man, who has, at first, posed a magical relation, later on conceives a scientific explanation, but the latter does not result from the former. On the contrary, the latter could only have been delayed by the former. The right path does not lie in the prolongation of the wrong route. A person, who after losing his way, finds it, does not owe his success to his former mistake; he owes it to his research. Similarly, if the healer finds a truly medical explanation of pathological facts, it is not because he has at first tried a magical speculation, he has continued the research from which the former would have led him away.

Historically, the magical interpretations are tried before scientific explanations because they are simpler to elaborate, but to believe that the former have prepared the second is to allow oneself to be duped by the sophism, *post hoc ergo propter hoc*.[1]

In the domain of therapeutics, the magical use of drugs is still less conducive to their rational utilisation. To enable a magician to recognise the natural efficacity of a magically used drug, two conditions need to be fulfilled. Firstly, the magical use should take place under those special conditions which may enable the manifestation of efficacity. Secondly the magician, observing the success, should stop linking it with his magical rite, that is to say, should precisely stop thinking as a magician.

Only this much can be easily admitted that in the case where the magician sees his rite succeeds, when an accident interrupts its normal cause, he can be put on the way of recognising that the efficacity did not depend on that rite but was the result of the virtue inherent in the element employed. Experience can, then, confirm to him the existence of this virtue in that element. Thus, by an accident of the magical operation, a real property can, certainly, be discovered. But still, this is not the scientifically recognised property; it is merely an empirical datum, accidentally acquired. It is true

---

[1] cf., J. Filliozat, *Magie et médicine*, specially pp. 129 ff; pp. 140 ff.

that this datum can be precious and that it is essentially medical but it is not even then scientific because practical medicine contains a large part of empiricism. Science comes in only from the moment when the efficacity of the remedy is systematically explained and where its properties are rationally applied.

Once again magic, which in spite of itself serves empiricism and nothing but that, does not always furnish it with valid data. If, perchance, the magician can cease to attribute a curative action to magic and can relate it to drugs, it is certain that he cannot always, if he employs several drugs, discern the one which is really efficacious. In such a case he runs the risk of introducing false notions in empiricism, of as much overburdening it as of enriching it by others.

Classical Indian medicine claims to explain by means of a coherent system the pathogeny and applies its therapeutics as a function of its theories; its design is entirely scientific, even though many of its doctrines are, in fact, erroneous. It cannot, therefore, have its bases in the pathology and the therapeutics of the Veda. It does not, however, follow that the classical medical texts are not rich in Vedic souvenirs. We have seen that a number of Vedic names of diseases are explained by naturally climbing back from their meaning in classical medicine to the sense possessed by them in the Veda. But in the Veda, we have not found the prefiguration of ulterior pathological doctrines. Moreover, we will take up this problem in connection with physiological notions of the Veda.

As regards therapeutics, Vedic souvenirs do exist in classical medicine, but they are extremely limited. A number of the names of plants already attested in the Vedic saṁhitās reappear in classical texts. But they are mostly employed for dogmatic reasons or because their efficacy has been empirically recognised and not because they formed part of the magical arsenal of the Veda. One may, however, pick out in the medical saṁhitās prayers of the same type as those of the Vedic magicians. The *Suśruta-saṁhitā* notably contains a prayer destined to reinforce the effectiveness of emetics. First of all, the text declares that "among the emetic substances, fruits and others, the fruits of *madana* (Randia dumetorum Lam) are the best''.[1] It indicates, thereafter, with precision the preparation of potions, prepared from these fruits, whose emetic properties are, moreover, perfectly real.[2] But their use must be along ritual lines.

> "Facing the North, accompanied by the chanting of incantations, the patient should be made to drink it with his face turned to the East after he has recited this mantra: "that Brahman, Dakṣa, the Aśvins, Rudra, Indra, the Earth, the Moon, the Sun, Agni and the Wind, the *ṛṣis*, the groups of those who have the medicinal plants and the mass of spirits, guard you! That this remedy be unto you like the elixir of the *ṛṣis*, like the divine ambrosia, like the nectar of superior dragons".[3]

The *mantra* does not belong to Vedic poetry; it is in Sanskrit verse of the most common type. But by the purpose behind it, it constitutes the survival of the spirit of Vedic therapeutics. But this is only an indirect survival because formulae of this type have been perpetuated in those of later Hindu religion, particularly in the abundant literature of the *kavacas*, the "armour", which have been extremely popular right up to now and which itself prolongs the Vedic prayers only because of the general purpose which inspires it. It is, undoubtedly, rather by the pressure of beliefs current in non-medical circles than by a direct souvenir of the religious therapeutics of the Veda that this mantra has been introduced in the Āyurveda. There also it constitutes an exceptional case. As a general rule, the therapeutics of the *Āyurveda* does not comprise the use of any invocation.[4] Holy prescriptions are

---

1 *vamanadravyāṇām phalādyānām madanaphalāṇi śreṣṭhatamāni bhavanti* (*Sūtr.*, XLIII, 1).

2 cf., A.Dj. Achart, *Quinze cents plantes dans l'Inde*, Pondichéry, 1905, p. 373; K.N. Nadkarni, *The Indian Materia Medica*, Bombay, no date, (towards 1925), p. 737; Dr. Parmanand Mariadassou, *Le Jardin des simples de l'Inde*, Pondichéry, 1913, p 89.

3 *Brahmadakṣāśvirudrenndrabhūcandrārkānalānilāḥ|*
ṛṣayaḥ sauṣadhigrāmā bhūtasaṁghāśca pāntu te|2|
rasāyanam ivārṣīṇām devānām amṛtam yathā|
sudhevottamanāgānām bhaiṣajyam idam astu te|3| Suśr., *sūtr.*, XLIII, 2-3.

4 In the preparation of emetics, it has been, however, a traditional practice to use this *mantra*, corresponding to that of Suśruta *Kalpasthāna;* I, 16) and Vāgbhaṭa reproduces it (*Aṣṭ. S.*, *Sūtr.*, XXVII, Vol. I, p. 139; *Aṣṭ hṛ, sūtr.*, XVIII, 16-17) following it by a Buddhist *mantra* addressed to the Bhaiṣajya-guru Buddha (cf., *JA*. April-June, 1934, p. 303, n. 1).

found there, but they do not habitually constitute a part of medicine properly so called. They concern, for example, the ritual of birth, occasionally mentioned with reference to birth, but, evidently, they do not constitute an integral part of the obstetrical teaching.[1] At the most, one may find cases where the use of certain plants in therapeutics does not seem to be justified by their real properties and seems to be a survival of their utilisation in Vedic magic.[2]

1 cf. *Le Kumāratantra . . .*, pp. 28 ff.
ibid., pp. 32-33.

CHAPTER FOUR

THE DATA OF THE VEDIC SAṀHITĀS CONCERNING ANATOMY

THE number of anatomical terms found in the Vedic Saṁhitās is quite large. A large number of different parts of the body have each a special name and sometimes several names. Many of these names have passed from Vedic Sanskrit into classical Sanskrit and are consequently met with both in medical texts and in Vedic hymns, because they do not have a strictly technical value and their knowledge has never been limited to savants. The notions represented by them are quite rudimentary in so far as the internal organs are concerned, their anatomy, even in Europe, having been unravelled much later. Moreover, it is difficult to understand, by means of the Vedic texts, the manner in which the authors of these hymns understood the organs named by them. It goes without saying that the Vedic hymns contain no anatomical description; it is only accidentally that the different parts of the body are mentioned chiefly in magical incantations, where they are enumerated in order to chase away the disorders of each one of them or in the passages where the elements of the body are placed parallel to those of the universe. And, unfortunately, there are no precise anatomical descriptions in the medical books, lesser still the figures. In India, where oral instruction surpasses other forms, anatomy, which can be really learnt best only by direct examination, was certainly taught orally. The books contained only lists to help the memory. We cannot, therefore, always identify an organ, whose name is nevertheless employed both in the Vedic and Ayurvedic texts. Moreover, a certain number of names are found only in the Veda.

Much work has been done by R. Hoernle on one aspect of Indian anatomy, namely, Osteology.[1] But this part of

---

1 *Studies in the Medicine of Ancient India*, Part I: *Osteology . . .*,

anatomy is less important for the constitution of medical doctrines and the work of Hoernle is based on ruinous foundations. However, the credit, usually given to him, does not allow us to neglect an examination of his work.

Several hymns enumerate the limbs of the body of man or of the cow or of the celestial bull (*RV.*, X, 90 and 163; *AV.*, II, 33 almost identical to *RV.*, X, 163; *AV.*, IX, 7 & 8; X, 2 & 9; XI, 3 & 8, etc.). Hoernle had thought to have found in the Hymn X, 2 of the *Atharva*, a nomenclature of bones related to the one found in the *Caraka-saṁhitā* (*Śār.*, VII). Now the observed concordance does not imply any relation of dependence between the two texts. First of all it is abusive to claim that the hymn in question contains a nomenclature of bones. This hymn enumerates the limbs of the body of the Çosmic Man, asking, regarding each of them, its respective creator. Caraka, on his side, indicates the number of bones contained in each part of the body. It is not at all necessary to suppose that in the times of the *Atharvaveda*, there already existed a list comparable to that of Caraka and which, as believed by Hoernle, inspired the hymn in question. This hymn refers only to the most commonplace notions regarding the human body, and when two texts start enumerating the parts of the human body, the concordances, established perforce between them, do not suppose any imitation of one by the other. Besides, the Vedic hymn contains several terms which are entirely unknown to Caraka or which have been employed by him in other passages only. Without paying any heed to these facts, Hoernle has prepared a table (p. 112) where the words of the hymn and those of Caraka are put in correspondence, one against another, and are accepted as synonyms. But in order to maintain these similarities, he is forced to lend to the author of the Vedic hymn the strangest ideas. This is how he establishes a

Oxford. 1907, taking up the articles of *JRAS*, 1906, pp. 915 ff., & 1907, p. 1 & ff. This work has been very well received by the critics (cf., notably Barth, *Oeuvres*, pt. p. 296; A. B. Keith, *ZDMG*, 1908, p. 136), although his most excessive inductions have been challenged. The attention to minute detail and the erudition of the critical apparatus conceal at first sight the inanity of the basic hypotheses. We have already observed, pp. 8 & 9 that the conjectures of Hoernle on the History of the Āyurveda are unacceptablet correspondence between *stana*, "bosom", and *pārśvaka*, "side"; now the *Atharva* says: *káti stánau vyadadhuḥ* (st. 4), "How many (gods) have disposed (his) two breasts" and Hoernle feels obliged to understand that this refers to "the sides of the two breasts". He coldly supplies the word "side" in the translation.[1] One case of this type should have sufficed to warn him that the Vedic hymn did not have bones in view. He has not hesitated from changing the naturally attributable sense of certain terms of the hymn to find them a pendant in the medical list. For example, he puts *skandha* of the hymn (st. 4) as an equivalent of the word *grīvā*, "neck" of Caraka, which he translates as "neck-bones", but *skandha* in classical Sanskrit signifies "shoulder"; this word appears for the first time in the *Ṛgveda* (I, 32-5) in the form of *skandhas* having the ramifications (of the trunk of a tree). In our hymn it is in plural number; one may, therefore, think that it denotes the "ramifications (of the human trunk)", shoulders, neck etc; nothing allows us to suppose it as an equivalent of the word *grīvā* of Caraka, specially when *grīvā* is employed precisely in that first part of the stanza, where the other figures.[2] Hoernle also places the words *lalāṭa* and *kakāṭikā* with regard to the

---

1 How many disposed (the ribs of) the two breasts? p. 110.

2 Hoernle places along with *grīvā* of the *Atharva*, *jatru* of Caraka which he gives as an equivalent of *grīvā* (although *grīvā* also appears in the list of Caraka) and which he translates as "wind-pipe". The translation, which he has thought to justify by ten pages of discussion (*Osteology*, pp. 158-68) is inadmissible. He has, himself, shown clearly that *jatru* in singular denotes the base of the neck (p. 162) but he claims that it is also the synonym of *grīvā*, "neck", which (although denoting, once again according to him, the osseous cervical column) is ranged among the cartilages by Suśruta; it can, therefore, denote the "duct", hence the translation "duct" for *jatru*. But it is not exact that Suśruta "in his class-list of bones enumerating the cartilages, or tender bones (*taruṇa*), makes them to include "the nose, the ears, neck (*grīvā*) and eyeballs" (p. 160) because Suśruta says: *ghrāṇakarṇa-grīvākośeṣu taruṇam*, "the cartilages are in the nose, the ears, the neck and the coverings of the eyes." (*Śār.*, V, 17) as Hoernle had himself correctly understood at first (p. 77). Hoernle also says (p. 161) that in regard to the disease called *manyāstambha*, "hardening of the muscular mass of the neck" (torticollis and contraction), Caraka employs the expression *grīvā antarāyamyate*, "the neck becomes bent inward" (Car., *Cik.*, XXVIII, 41) whereas Vāgbhaṭa (*Aṣṭāṅga-hṛdaya*, *Nid.*, XV, 22) says *jatrur āyamyate* whence *grīvā=jatru*. *āyamyate* denotes "is drawn" (like a bow, the comparison in Vāgbhaṭa follows immediately) and it refers to the disease called *antarāyāma*, "tension inside" (that is to say here in flexion), a type of tetanus (emprosthotonos). The words of Caraka denote therefore that the neck is contracted (and therefore twisted as explained by the commentators, which Hoernle understands

compound of Caraka, *nāsikā-gaṇḍa-kūṭa-lalāṭa*, denoting together the bones of the nose, the cheek-bones and the arcs of the eyebrows. He imagines that *kakāṭikā* represents the bones of the nose and the cheek-bones conceived as an unique bone. But *kakāṭikā* is most naturally explained as a doublet or *kṛkāṭikā*[1] denoting "neck" and the stanza where it occurs can be translated: "Which is the god (among the gods) who, the first, has climbed the sky after having constructed his brain, his front, his neck, his cranium, that which is constructed on the jaws of man."[2] We cannot, therefore, confidently make use of the identifications proposed by Hoernle although they have been often accepted (*Vedic Index*, see word *Śarīra*, in part.; Dasgupta, *Ind. Phil.*, Vol. II, pp. 284 ff). On another side, the explanations of the Vedic commentators such as Sāyaṇa and Mahīdhara do not always deserve to be accepted. The enormous distance separating, in time, these commentators from the texts interpreted by them, creates the fear that they have not known the real meaning of

---

as if the verb *ā-yam* denotes to wring), those of Vāgbhaṭa that the base of the neck is contracted; it does not, however, follow that "neck" and "the base of the neck" are synonymous. In the form of tetanus described, the sterno-cléido-mestoids draw violently their attachments so that the osseous sterno-clavicular arc (which is the bone of the *jatru*) is drawn although little deformable, as a bow.

1 By the vocalisation of *ṛ* (cf., *víkaṭa*, *RV.*, X, 155-1; J. Block, *Indo-Aryen*, p. 35). The equivalence proposed by Hoernle will be justified only if the correspondence of the two lists had been established as necessary and absolute, but precisely he gives this equivalence as one of the proofs of the correspondence of the two lists. He, thus, argues in a vicious circle.

2 *mastiṣkam asya yatamó lalāṭam kakāṭikām prathamó yáḥ kapālam|citvā cítyam hánvoḥ pūruṣasya dívām ruroha katamáh sá deváḥ*. 8. *citya*, as has been observed by Senart (*Légende du Buddha*, Paris, 1882, p. 99, n. 3) has a double meaning, signifying "that which is to be constructed" and the "wood pyre, the pyre having the jaws of the cosmic Man as an image". V. Henry says (*Livres*, X, XI, & XII., p. 48) that the preceding verse shows the tongue as placed "on (between) the jaws" (*hánvor hí jihvām ádadhāt* . . .), and that in consequence *citya* must denote the tongue. In any case, this is in no way an anatomical term but a technical term of liturgy and at the same time a commonplace term used to denote simultaneously the organ which is between or over the jaws and the fire of the sacrifice represented by this organ. Hoernle sees therein the confirmation of his comparison with Caraka (p. 177) because he claims that the piling up on the jaws ["structure (pile) of the two jaws"] denotes the teeth, the alveolars, the osseous palate and the climbing branches of the lower maxillary. But the preoccupation of the author of the hymn is not that of the osteologist; he saw in the Cosmic Man something else than a skeleton —*lalāṭa* denotes ths lower part of the front, the arcs of the eyebrows.

many ancient words (especially of those which evoked no interest for the traditional religion). Often enough their explanations betray a profound ignorance of anatomy, even of classical anatomy known to the medical authors of their times. Lastly the etymology, although often clear and capable of attaining, by means of rigorous methods of the comparative Indo-European linguistics, a high degree of probability, indeed the certitude, cannot suffice to give the meaning of technical words such as the names of anatomy. The primitive meaning which can be restored, does not indicate quite surely the derivative meanings in which the words have been used in the texts. This is proved by numerous examples in our languages. A name like *pancreas*, whose primitive sense is undisputably "all fleshy", does not suit the organ which it denotes. This is the gland of the spongy aspect, in which no part of flesh enters. Even in antiquity it did not correspond, in its etymological meaning, with the organs so named by the medical authors. If we had only the etymological meaning of this word to give us some information on this organ, one could only propose false identifications.

Therefore the sense of many of the anatomical terms of the Veda must remain uncertain. It is, however, useful to compile an index of these terms, even if that were for drawing attention to them and eventually to provoke an improvement of their translation. It is also useful to include in this index those names which refer to the bodies of animals, often better known because these bodies were opened up under the knife of the butchers and the sacrificers. This review of the vocabulary will enable us to have an idea of the anatomical knowledge of the Vedic period and to see the reserve drawn upon by the authors who elaborated the Ayurvedic science.

Anatomical Nomenclature of the Vedic Saṁhitās[1]

áṁśa (m): shoulder.
amhubedī (f): vulva ("which has a narrow slit") *(VS)*.
ákṣi (n): eye. At the end of a compound, *akṣa*.
agrajihvá (n): tip of the tongue (*VS*, *MS*).

[1] The term anatomical has been taken in a wide sense, comprising in the Index even the names of the organic liquids or "organic breaths". Abbreviations used: V=Veda, all the saṁhitās; *RV*=Ṛgveda; *AV*=Atharvaveda; *YV*=Yajurveda=totality of *Taittirīya saṁhitā* (*TS*),

áṅga (n): limb, body, cf., *áṅgāparuṁṣi* (*TS*), "limbs and joints", corresponding respectively to the full and New Moons, whose totality constitutes the body of the year.
aṅguri (f): finger (*AV*) (*RV: su-aṅgurí*).
aṅgulá (m): finger (*V*) (at the end of a compound): (Cl.).
aṅguli (f): finger (*VS*., Cl.).
aṅgulī (f): finger (*AV*., Cl.).
áṅghri (m): foot (*VS*., Cl.).
atiruj (m, dual): bend of the knee (*VS*).
atīruj (m, dual): bend of the knee (*MS*).
adharhanu: cf., *hánu*.
aná (m): breath in *prāṇa* from *RV* and alone from Br. cf., *āna*.
anuvṛj (dual): (*KS*). cf., *anūvṛj*.
ánūka (m., n): cf., *anūkyá* (*AV*).
anūkyá (m, n, dual): spine regarded as a double bone (?) (*RV*, *AV*).
anūvṛj (m, f, dual): two fleshy elements near the back (Sāy.) (*TS*, *AV*). cf., *anuvṛj*.
antaḥpārśvyá (n): intercoastal muscles (*VS*); *antaḥpārśvā* (n) (*TS*).
antarā: name of organ (?) (*TS*).
antarodara (m): internal abdomen (interior of the abdomen) (*AV*).
apāná (m): breath directed downwards (V. except *RV*, Cl.) cf., *pāpavāta*.
apikakṣá (m): region of the armpit, shoulder (*RV*), cf., *kakṣa*.
apikarṇá (n): region of the ear (*RV*).
aratni (m, dual); elbow, fore-arm (cf. *aratní*=elbow) [*RV*, *VS*, (XX-8. Mahīdhara: *aratnī-hasta-deśau*, "the *aratnis* are the two regions of the hand")] cf., *hásta*.
ālgá (m, dual): groin (*MS*, *VS*).
ávaka (m): flesh in the form of *vallisueria* (an aquatic plant with sheath-like leaves (*TS*, *KS*).
avakrandá: organ of the cry (larynx?) (*VS*, *TS*, *MS*, *KS*).
áśru (n): tear.
aṣṭhīvánt (m): knee ("which has a stone", the rotula) (Cl.); also *aṣṭhivant*, cf., *ūrvaṣṭhīve* (n, dual); thigh and knee (*VS*).

Maitrāyaṇī-saṁhitā (*MS*), *Kāṭhaka-saṁhitā* (*KS*) and *Vājasaneyī-saṁhitā* (*VS*); Br =Brāhmaṇa; Cl.=Classical Sanskrit (including medical) Say. =Sāyaṇa; Mahī.=Mahīdhara. The absence of abbreviation at the end of the meaning of the word indicates that the meaning in question is common to the entire literature from the *RV*. to Classical Sanskrit.

asán (n): blood (*AV*, Cl.).
ásu (m): vital breath.
ásṛj (n): blood.
asthán, *ásthi* (n): bone. At the end of a compound—*astha*.
āṇi (m): In *RV*, "pin of the axle", but a prehistoric meaning of "knee" is proposed for the Indo-European by comparison (E. Benveniste, *Origines de la formation des noms en indo-européen*, p. 105): now *āṇi* in Suśruta (*Śār.*, VI, 28) denotes a vulnerable point (*marman*) constituted manifestly by popliteal sciatica after their division above the articulation of the knee.
āṇḍá (n, dual): testicle.
ātmán (m): (a) breath, soul, pneumatic entity; (b) body (in opposition to limbs) (*VS*, Cl).
āná (m): (a) mouth (*RV*, Sāy.: nose; cf., Cl. *ānana*); (b) breath (cf., *aná*) in *udāna*, *vyāna*, *samāna* from *AV*., rare Cl.
ānatá (n): region of the neck (Sāy., *TS*, *KS*).
āntrá (n, pl.): entrails, small intestine.
ās (n?): mouth (*RV*).
āsán (n): mouth (V).
āsyá (n): mouth.
ikṣu (m): lower eye-lashes (*VS*, *MS*, *TS*).
īrmá (n): front-foot of animal (*AV*).
uchalakhá: dual, hapax (?) (*AV*).
utá (n): eyebrows (*VS*, *MS*, *KS*, Br.).
uttarahanu: cf., *hánu*.
utsādá (m): protuberance (from the body of an animal) (*YV*).
udára (n): abdomen.
udaryá (n): flesh of the stomach (*YV*).
udāna (m): breath directed upwards (V. except *RV*, Cl).
—udhan: cf., under *ūdhan*.
upapakṣa (m): side (*TS*).
upás (m): upástha (*RV*).
upástha (m, n): genital organs (chiefly feminine)—"that which is held below", "foundation" (*VS*, *MS*, *KS*, Br. *RV*): figurative use supposing the sense of "lap", "bosom" (I, 146-1: *pitrór upásthe*," in the bosom of his parents").
uras (n): chest.
ulba (n): embryonic membranes (later Vedic: *amnios*, cf., *Kumāratantra*, p. 35).

uṣṇihā (f., dual, pl): cf. *uṣṇīsa(?);* cranial protuberations (parietal vertex and bosses) (*RV, AV*).

ūdhan, ūdhar, ūdhas (n): Mamma; also *udhan* in *tryudhan. RV ūdhan*, no Cl.

ūbadhya (n): contents of the entrails (undigested nourishment) cf., *ūvadhyu*.

ūru (m): thigh.

ūavdhya:- *RV* orthography of *ūbadhya*.

ṛkṣálā (f. pl.) vessels (or tendons) which are found above ankles (in the quadrupeds) [*VS* (Mahī. *gulphādhaḥsthā nāḍyaḥ*)].

ṛchárā (f., pl): cf. *ṛkṣálā* (*AV*).

ójas (n): corporeal vigour (Cl. medicine: vital sap).

oṇí (m): arm (*Neisser, Zum Worterbuch des Ṛgveda* (*RV*).

óṣṭha (m): lip.

kakāṭikā (f): neck, cf. *kṛkāṭa* (*AV*).

kakud (f): tourniquet (culminating point), bosse of Zebu, (*AV*), cf. *Śitikakud* (*TS*) and below *kākud*.

kákṣa (m): armpit (*AV*, Cl.) cf. *apikàkṣá*.

káṅkukha (m): cf. the following (*AV*. Paipp.).

káṅkūṣa (m, pl.): part of the head (?) (*AV*).

kaṇṭhá (m): throat, larynx (*AV*, in *sahákaṇṭhikā; MS/VS*, in *adharakaṇṭhá* & *śuṣkakaṇṭha;* alone: Cl.

káṇṭhya (n): flesh of the neck (*VS*).

kanānaka (m): apple of the eye (*TS*).

kanīnaka (m): apple of the eye (*VS*, Cl.).

kanīnika (m): apple of the eye (*MS*).

kanīnikā (f): apple of the eye (*AV, MS, TS, KS*, Cl.).

kapāla (n): cranium, flat bone (in the form of potsherd) (*AV*, IX, 8-22: *śīṛṣṇaḥ kapālāni*, Cl.) cf., *śīrṣakapāla*.

kapíñjala (m): pastern (*YV*).

káppṛth (m): penis ("which gives the pleasure") (*RV*).

kaphauḍá (m, dual, hapax): Böhtlingk-Roth "elbow"? (*AV*, X, 2-4). Appears in an enumeration of the parts of the body attached to the trunk. Could be brought near *kapola*, "cheek", which is more recent but the disaspiration will be unusual (cf., J. Bloch, *Indo-Aryen*, p. 59). One can not invoke the disaspiration of Pali *kapoṇi*=Skt. *kaphoṇi*, "elbow", given by Childers following *Abhidhānappadīpikā*, this reading not being found in the texts (communication of Helmer Smith). One could ask oneself if **kaphaula*, in the dual, would not designate two humid organs (*ola*) of phlegm (*kapha*) such as the lungs, but *kapha* is found only in the Cl. and *ola* in later lexicons.

kábandha (m, n): stomach (meaning derived from the primitive "tun" (*AV*). In Cl. "trunk", cf., Louis Renou, *JA*, July-Sept. 1939, p. 391.

kará (m): hand. All the texts, but the *RV* uncertain. In Cl. become secondarily "ray", cf., L. Renou, *JA*, July-Sept., 1939, p. 346.

karásna (m): fore-arm (*RV*), cf., L. Renou, *BSL*, 1937, p. 23; enlargement of *kará*.

karūkara (n): ? (*AV*, Br.).

kárṇa (m): exterior part of the ear.

kākud (f): palate [Cl. (Lexicons)], cf., *kakud* above.

kāśí (m): closed fist (*RV*).

kīkásā (f; *YV*, Cl. m): vertebra (Cl. "bone"), cf., under *jatru*.

kukṣí (m, dual and pl.): small pelvis, pelvic regions.

kulphá (m): *gulphá* (cf. *kusṭhā* & *kuhá*).

kuṣṭha (m, dual): big sciatic cut (*MS*, *VS*). (Mahī. *kakundara* and cf., Suśr. *Śār.*, VI, 31).

kuṣṭhā (dual): a part of the horse's body (*TS*). (Bloomfield, *Vedic Conc.* under *pratikramaṇam ku.*) cf. *gusṭhā*.

kuṣṭhikā (f., pl.): a part of the legs of the cow (?) (*AV*).

kusindha (n): trunk (described as one which is held by the thighs and supported by the shoulders) (*AV*, also Br.).

kuhá (m, dual): part of the horse's body (*TS*). (*Vedic Conc.* under *vīryam kuhābhyām*) cf., *guhá*.

kṛkāṭa (n): neck (*AV*, IX, 7-1) (opposed to *lalāṭa* as *kakāṭikā*).

keśa (m): hair [V. except *RV* (but *RV*: *keśin*, *kéśavant*, etc.), Cl.].

kośyá (n): two chunks of flesh situated on the covering of the heart (Mahī. *VS*, *TS*,) (*Padapāṭha*, *nikośya*).

kroḍá (m, Cl: n): breast (of horse) (*AV*, Cl.).

klóman (m, Cl. nl): probably lungs [V. except *RV* (*VS*, XXV-8: plural)]; sometimes right lung, more often totality of lungs (singular) or lungs (and their lobes) (pl.).

kṣíp (f, pl); finger, index? (*RV*).

ksīrá (n) milk.

khá (n): openings of the body (*AV*, Cl.).

khādá (m): molar tooth (*TS*, *KS*).

gábhasti (m): arm, hand (becomes Cl. "rays"; cf., L. Renou, JA.,

July-Sept., 1939, p. 345.)

gárbha (m): 1. womb; 2. embryo.

gavīní, ī- (f); ureter (?), two canals which collect the urine coming from the entrails (Sāy. on *AV*, I-3-6) TS (in the mantra corresponding to *AV*, I, 11-5) cf., *parīṇah.*

gāvīnikā (f): ureter (*AV*, I, 11-5) (Sāy. *gavīnike yoneḥ pārśvavartinyau nirgamanapratibandhike nāḍyau,*" the *g.* are the two canals situated on the sides of the uterus and hindering the expulsion" ?): IX, 8-7 (*yá ūrū anusárpaty átho eti gavīnike,* "the one—the disease—which creeps along the thighs and attains the *g.*").

gātra (n): limb.

gudá (n): 1. rectum (*TS*, Cl.); 2 vagina (*VS*).

gudā (f, often pl.): rectum, big intestines.

gulphá (m): ankles (V. except *RV*, Cl.)

guṣṭhā: cf., *kuṣṭhā* (*KS*).

guhá (dual): cf., *kuhá* (*KS*).

gṛdhrá (m): armpit [*TS* (Sāy. *kakṣá* but in pl.), *KS*].

grīvā (f): neck [V, generally pl., Cl., sing. and *grīva*, m. (cf., *grīvadaghná*, *TS*)].

glau (m, pl.): vessels of the heart (*MS, VS*, (Mahī. *hṛdaya-nāḍyaḥ*).

cákṣan (n. dual): eye (*AV*).

cákṣas (n): eye (*RV, AV*).

cákṣu (m) eye (*RV*, but *hapax cákṣos=cakṣusoḥ*).

cákṣus (n): eye.

cárman (n): skin, leather.

chavī (f): glow which attains the eye [*TS*. (Sāy. *netragatā kāntiḥ*), *KS*].

chubuka (n): chin (*RV*, Cl. *cibuka, cubuka*).

jaghána (m): posterior (in comp. also *jāghana*, q.v.).

jáṅghā (f): leg.

jaṭhára (n): abdomen.

jatru (m, pl.): clavicles and sternum, or clavicular and sternal regions (specially sub-claviculars and sub-sternals. Cl. base of neck, joint of neck and of the chest). In *Śat. Br.*, VIII, 6-2-10: *imā ubhayatra parśavo baddhāḥ kīkasāsu ca jatruṣu,*"his sides are attached on both hands to the *Kīkasās* and to the *jatrus*". Therefore, *k.*=vertebra, *j.*=sternum, to which are joined the clavicles.

jāghana; cf., *jaghána.*

jānu (n): knee, cf., *jñu.*

jāmbīla (n): stomach, but Mahī. *jānumadhya-bhāga,* "middle part of the knee" [*VS, MS, KS, TS* (Sāy. *āmāśaya,* a more probable interpretation than that of Mahī., because the context refers to teeth and tongue which pulverize the plant which is deposited in the stomach.)].

jámbha (m): 1. jaw (*RV, AV, VS,* Cl.); 2. teeth (Cl.).

jámbhya (m): teeth, specially lateral teeth (Sāy. on *TS,* V, 7-11, *YV*).

jarāyu (n): back-load, embryonic annexes, placenta (prop. "that which is cast off"). (Later Vedic sometimes "chorion", cf., *Kumāratantra* . . . . p. 37).

jihvā (f): tongue, cf., *agra-jihvá.*

juhū (f): tongue (of Agni, a metaphorical expression) (*RV*).

jñu=*jānu* at the end of a compd. and in *jñubādh* (*RV*).

takari, takarī (f): pelvic organ (?) indeterminate (*TS.* in the same formula *AV t.* is rephased by *mehana*),*KS*(*takari*),(*TS*).

tagarī (f)=takarī (*AV.* Paipp.).

tániman (n): liver (*TS,* Br.).

tanū (f): body.

tālu (n, rare. m): palate (*VS,* Cl.).

tedanī (f): blood (?) [*AV, VS.* (Mah. *tedanīm devatām*)].

tvác (f): skin.

°*da,* °*dant*: teeth in *ubhayāda* °*dant,* "one who has teeth on the two jaws" (*RV, AV, TS*).

dáṁṣṭra (m): canine tooth (*VS, MS, KS,* Cl.).

dánta (m, n): teeth.

danta-mūlá (n): dental root, better still, base of teeth (*VS,* Cl.).

dūṣikā (f): rheum (V. except *RV,* Cl.).

doṣán (n, dual): 1. lower part (of the fore-feet of an animal) (*AV*), 2. arm (*AV, TS*).

dós (n.m., *RV* once): arm.

dhamáni, -ī (f): vessel (relatively voluminous according to Sāy. cf., *Snāvan*) (*AV,* Cl.) cf., p. 130.

nakhá (n): nail.

nandáthu (m): sexual organ (*lit.,* "pleasure") (*TS, KS*).

nás (f): nose, nostrils (dual), cf., *nās.*

násya (n): vibrissa (*VS, MS KS*).

nāḍī (f): canal, vessel (*AV,* VI, 138-4, spermatic canals or cords;

yé te nāḍyau devákṛte yáyos tiṣṭhati vṛṣṇyam, "the two canals made by the gods, in which resides virility"; *KS*, Cl.). cf. *vṛṣṇya* and p. 158.

nābhi (f): Navel [V. except *RV*, (but *nābha* at the end of a compd. *RV*), Cl.].

nās (f): nose (*RV*, II, 39-6) cf., *nás*.

nāsā (f): nose, nostrils (*AV*, Cl.).

nāsikā (f, dual): nostrils.

nikośyá: cf., *kośya* & *śiṅgī*.

nipakṣati (f): second rib (cf., *pakṣati*) [*VS*, *TS*, (Sāy. rib adjacent to the *pakṣati*, second free rib?) *MS*, *KS*].

nirbādhá (m): protuberance (cranial ?) (*YV*).

pakṣá (m): side.

pakaṣati (f); first rib [*VS* (13 are mentioned for each side), *KS*, *MS*, *TS* (Sāy. *daksiṇa-pārśvasya mūle varttamānā yeyam vaṇkriḥ sā pakṣatiḥ*, "*p.* is the rib situated at the base of the right side", first free rib?)]

pákṣman (n): upper (eye) lash (*VS*, *MS*, *TS*, Cl. (eye) lashes).

pád (m) foot, cf. *pād*.

páyas (n) milk, eventually sperm.

parīṇah (a): corr. in *KS*, XIII-9 to *gavīṇyau* of *TS*, III, 3-10-1.

párus (n): joint (joint or, often, portion included between two joints, limb or member of the body) (V., Br.).

párvan (n): *ibidem*.

párśu (m): rib. (V., Br., Cl. *parśukā*).

páśas (n): penis (V. except *RV*., Br.).

pājasyá (n) ? [Sāy. on *RV*, chest, on *TS*.: heart; Mahī.=limb which is the cause of force in a quadruped; Geldner on *RV*="inguen" (abdominal coating?); V., Br. (in *RV*, *tri-pājasya*)].

pāṭūrá (m): totality of transversal apophyses [*VS*, *TS*, (Sāy. *etā vaṅkrayo yasmin pṛṣṭha-bhāgagate 'sthipārśvaśeṣe sambandhyante so'yam pāṭūraḥ*)].

pāṭora (m)=*pāṭūrá* (*KS*).

pāṇi (m)=hand.

pād=pad.

pāda (m): foot.

pādu (m): foot (*RV*).

pāpa-vāta (m): "bad wind" (*TS*, V, 7-23; Sāy.=*apāna*).

pāyu (m): anus (V. except *RV*, Cl.).

pārśvá (n., m): side.

pārṣṇi, ī (f.): heel.

pittá (n.): bile [V. except RV., cl.]

pības=*pīvas*.

pīvas (n): fat (*RV, AV*).

pucha (m, n): tail [*AV* (other expressions, X, 9-22 for tail of serpent, bird, etc.) Cl.].

puritát: cf. the following (*TS*).

purītát (n): pericardium [*AV, VS* (XXV-8, Mahī.: *purītad hṛdayācchādakam antram*, "*p.*=entrails which cover the heart")].

pulitat: pericardium (*KS*).

pulītat: pericardium (*MS*).

pṛṣṭi (f, pl.): vertebrae (V, Br.).

pṛṣṭha (n.): back.

pṛṣṭhā (f. (comp.), dual); flesh near the anus. ? (Sāy.), (*TS, KS*)

pratiṣṭhā (f): leg ("supporting point") (*AV*).

pratyāsá (m or n ?, dual): excrescence near the sexual organ (Sāy.) (*TS, KS*).

prápad (f): fore-foot (*AV*).

prápada (n, dual or pl.): fore-foot (animals). (*AV*).

praśādá (m): hymen ? [*TS* (Sāy. "sort of particle of flesh which falls at the time of defloration?", *viśasana-kāla-patito māṁsa-leśa-viśeṣaḥ*), *KS*]. cf., *viśasana*.

prāṇá (m): 1. vital breath; 2. breath of the anterior part of the body.

plāśí (m, sing.): urethra, penis? (Mahī. *śiśna*); pl. spermatic canals and urethra (excretary canals) (Mahī.: *śiśna-mūla-nāḍyaḥ*, "canals at the base of the penis") (V, Br.).

plīhán (n): spleen.

bársva (m): gum (Sāy.: *danta-mūla-māṁsa*, "flesh at the base of teeth") (*YV*).

balāsa: cf. *supra*, pp. 117-19.

bāhu (m, dual): arm.

bila (n) 1. orifice of sectioned vessels (*AV*); 2. excretory orifice (*AV*, I, 3-8, vastibila, "orifice of the bladder, urinary meatus").

bīja (n): sperm (*lit.*, "seed", "grain").

bháṁsas (n): anus ?, anterior part of the hip-bone (Macdonell-Keith, *Vedic Index*) (*RV, AV*).

bhasád (f): behind, vulva (V, Br, Sūtra).

bhāsad (m): behind, buttock (Mahī., *RV*, *AV*, *VS*) (Mahī. *nitambau*) (*MS*).

bhásman (n): part of the body ? (*YV*).

bhrū (f): eye-brow.

majján (m): marrow.

mátasna (m, n, dual): unindentified viscus [*RV*, (Sāy. *pārśvayor vartamānav āmraphalākṛtī vṛkkau*, "kidneys looking like mangoes, situated in the sides), *VS*. (Mahī.: *grīvādhastād-bhāgasthitahṛdayobhaya-pārśve asthinī*," bones—or "stones" or "mass" found on each side of the heart, below the neck), (*MS*, *KS*).

mányā (f, dual & pl.): muscular tendinous mass of the neck (V. except *RV*, Cl.).

mārman (n): vital point (essentially vulnerable) (V., Cl.).

malhá: which has excrescences at the neck (goat) [*TS* (Sāy. *galastana*, which, according to the *Vaidyakanighaṇṭu* quoted by Umesa Chandra Gupta, *Vaidyaka-śabda-śindhu* denotes *chagagalasthastana* "(appendix in the form of) udder found on the throat of the she-goat")].

mastíṣka (m, n): brain.

māṁsá (n, sing. & pl.) flesh.

mukha (n): mouth.

muská (m, dual): 1. testicles; 2. big lips (*AV*).

muṣṭí (m): fist.

mūtra (n): urine.

mūrdhán (m): head.

meḍhra (n) Penis, cf., *mehana*.

médas (n): fat.

méhana (n): 1. penis (as an urinary organ) (*RV*, Cl.); 2. urethra (*AV*, Cl.).

yakán (n): liver.

yákṛt (n): liver (V. except *RV*, Cl.).

yóni (f): womb, vagina.

rarāṭa (n): forehead (*VS*) cf. *lalāṭa*.

rása (m): fluid of life, organic sap, sexual secretion, cf., pp. 27, 165.

rétas (n): sperm.

róman (n): =loman.

romaśa (n): vulva (*lit*. "which has hair") (*RV*).

rбra (m, dual): articulation of shoulders (*VS, MS*).
lalāṭa (n): forehead (especially lower part of the forehead, arcade of the eyebrows). (*AV*) cf., *rarāṭa.*
lóman (n): hair.
lóhita (n): blood (V. except *RV*, Cl.).
vaksáṇā (f, pl.): breast, flanks (*RV*, *AV*). breast (womb) (*RV*, X, 27-16). But cf. Cl. *vaṅkṣaṇa,* groin.
vákṣas (n, sing and pl.): breast, chest.
vankri (f): rib.
vanaṁkáraṇa (n): organ of defecation (*RV*).
vaniṣṭū (m): cf. the following (*MS, KS*).
vaniṣṭhu (m): colon (V, Cl., *VS*, XIX-87: *kumbhó vaniṣṭhur janitā śácībhir yásminn ágre yónyām gárbho'ntaḥ,*" "the vase *vaniṣṭhu* is generator by assistance; in it, in the beginning, in the womb is the foetus", Mahī.: *sthūlāntra,* "big intestine". But, in a popular type of anatomy, confusion can arise between a big viscus shallow like the colon and the uterus, which being gravid, fills up the stomach.)
vapā (f): epiploon (specially the fatty epiploon of the bullock, the thin epiploon of the horse is not well-known, cf., P.E. Dumont, *L'Aśvamedha,* p. 185) [V. (*RV* in *vapāvant, vapodara*), Cl.].
vártas (m): eye-lash (*VS, MS*).
vártman (n): eye-lid (*AV*, Cl.).
vaśā: *vasā.*
vásā, vasā (f): fat of the muscles.
vastí (m, f): bladder (V. except *RV*, Cl.).
váha (m): shoulder (of the bullock, "the one which carries") (*AV, VS, TS*).
vājina (m): sperm (*MS*).
vāyu (m): breath (of the mythical bull=wind) (*AV*, IX, 7-4; Cl.: wind and wind of the organism=organic breath).
vāla (m): horsehair, mane, horse-tail (V. except *RV*, Cl.).
vāladhāna (n): tail (*TS*).
vijāman (n): genital organs (Sāy.), inguinal regions ? (cf. p. 110) (*AV*).
viśásana (n): vulva ("cut", "defloration" ? cf. *praśādá*). (*TS, KS*).
viṣāna (n): horn (crumbling. "which detaches itself") (*AV*).
vṛkká (m, dual): kidney (*AV, VS, MS*, Br., Sūtra).

vṛkya=*vṛkká* (*TS*).

vṛṣaṇa (m, dual): testicles (*VS*, Cl.).

vṛṣṇya (n): virility, but *AV*, VI, 138, 4, concrete sense, (virility residing in several canals, cf., *nāḍī*), therefore "sperm", cf., *vṛṣṇiya* "sperm" in *Vādhūlasūtra*, Caland, *Acta Or.*, IV, 1927, p. 184.

vaitasá (m): penis (metaphorically "which is related to the reed", cp. rod) (*RV*, *AV*, in lit. sense, Cl.).

vyātta (n): open mouth (*AV*, *VS*, *TS*, Br., cf., Cl. *vyattānana*, *vyāttāsya*).

vyāná (m): breath diffused in the body.

vríś (f): finger (*RV*).

śakunisādá (m): part of the horse's body? (*YV*).

śaptra (n): labial commissure ? (*KS*) cf., *snáptra*.

śaphá (m): hoof (of quadruped).

śárīra (n): 1. body; 2. parts of the body (pl.) (*RV*).

śárkara (m): granular bone, rugose (small bone of the face and of the cranium) [*TS*, V, 7-11 (Sāy. *śarkarāḥ tatsadṛśāni kaṭhināsthīni*)].

śākhā (f): finger (metaphorically, *RV*. denotes in Cl. the limbs by special use of the sense of "branch") cf., *skandhá*.

śikhaṇḍá (m or n, dual): flesh above the hips (Sāy.) (*TS*, *KS*).

śiṅgi (f): part of the entrails (*TS*, I, 4-3-1; but *VS*, XXXIX, 8: . . . *śiṅgīni kośyābhyām* . . ., Mahī.: *śingīni śingisaṁjñāni daivatāni*, "*ś*=the goddesses called *ś*.").

śitāman (n): according to *Nirukta* "arm", "womb", "liver", "fat" (*VS*), cf., śitīman.

śitīman (n, dual): excrescence near the sexual organ (Sāy.) [*TS*, *KS*, (°*mant*)] cf., *śitāman*.

śipí (m): in *śipiviṣṭa* (=*śepa*, *Nirukta*). Probably, skin, prepuce (*RV*, *TS*, *KS*).

śípra (n): lip ?, tooth ? (*RV*, *MS*).

śíprā (f, pl.): denture (*RV*).

śíras (n): head.

śiśná (n): 1. penis ? (*RV*, *AV*); 2. tail.

śīrṣá (n): head.

śīrṣán (n): head (V).

śīrṣakapālá (n): cranium, brainpan (head-bone in the form of potsherd) (*AV*, *TS*, Cl.).

śukrá (n): sperm.

śūpti (f): shoulder (according to the Avestan *supti*) but Sāy: mouth (*RV*).

śṛṅga (n): horn.

śépa (n): penis.

śepha (m): penis (*TS*).

śnáptra (n): labial commissure (Mahī. *VS*). cf., the following.

śnyáptra (n): labial commissure (*TS*). cf., *śaptra* and *śnáptra*.

śmáśru (n): beard.

śróṇi (f): hip (V, Cl. pelvi-perineal regions).

śrótra (n): ear (organ of hearing, not the external ear)., cf. *karṇa*.

samsīdá (n): cf. the following (*KS*).

saṁsūdá (n): nostril [*TS*, (Sāy.: *samtatakṣaraṇo nāsikādiḥ,* "continually flowing nostrils", etc.)].

sákhti (n, dual, pl.): thigh (*V*., Cl.) by euphemism "vulva" (V).

samtāná (m): tendon ? (*TS*).

saudhí (m): joint, articulation.

samāná (m): concentrated breath (V. except *RV*., Cl.).

sātu (m): womb (but an improbable conjecture) (*RV*).

sānu (m, n): back, rump (of *Vṛtra,* of Vala, of a horse, literally, "summit" "plateau", cf., Benveniste-Renou, *Vṛtra et Vṛthragna*, p. 135) (*RV*). cf. *snu*.

sīmán (m): vertex, line of the parting of hair and of the body (*AV*, Cl.).

sūtrī (f): womb (of the cow ?) [*AV*, IX, 7-4 (But the hymn refers to the mythical bull.)].

sṛkvan (m, n): labial commissure [*RV*, Cl. (Suśruta, *sṛkvanī*, f)].

séhu (m): indeterminate viscus (*AV*, *KS*).

skandhá (m, generally pl.): ramification of the trunk (cf. *skandhas*, *RV*, I, 32-5, referring to a tree) (V, Cl.), cf. *śākhā*.

stána (m, n): breast, udder, dug.

stukā (f): tuft of hair (on the head of a horse) (*RV*, *AV*), cf. the following.

stupá (m): tuft of hair (*VS*) cf. the preceding and the following.

stūpá (m): tuft of hair (*MS*) cf. the preceding.

straíṇa (n): vulva but exactly "that which is feminine", a sense which generally suffices (*AV*, VIII, 6-4 ?). All the texts: "that which is feminine".

sthūra (m, dual): fetlock-joint of a quadruped (*VS*, *TS*, *KS*, Cl.).

sthūragudā (f): big intestine (*TS, MS, KS*).
sthūlagudā (f): big intestine (*VS*).
snāvan, snāván (n): tendon (cf. Cl. *snāyu*) but Sāy. (on *AV*, II, 33-6) fine vessel (cf. *dhamani*) (*AV, VS, TS*).
snāvanyá (m or n, dual): base of five tendons (Sāy.) (*TS, KS*).
srákva (m or n): mouth of carnivorous animals ? (*RV*).
svéda (m): sweat.
hánu (f, dual): jaw (V, Cl.) cf. *uttarahanu*, "upper jaw" and *adharahanu*, "lower jaw" (*AV*).
hálīkṣṇa (m or n): (*AV*, II, 33-3; in *TS*, V, 7-23, name of animal).
hásta (m): hand, also fore-arm (cf., *aratní*); trunk of elephant.
hārdi (n. m): heart (*RV, AV*).
hirā (f): blood-vessel (*AV, VS, MS*, later Vedic *hitā*, Cl. *sirā*), (cf., p. 160.)
hṛd (n): heart.
hṛdaya (n): heart cf., *sthūlahṛdayá*, (*TS*). "big heart?"
hṛdayāgrá (n): point of the heart (*VS*, Cl).
hṛdayaupaśá (m): organic mass located near the heart (*YV*). The interpretations "aorta" (*VS*, XXV-8) or "heart and pericardium" (dual, *TS*, V, 7-16) proposed by Böhtlingk & Roth are not justified by the Commentaries. Mahī.: *hṛdaye upaśete hṛdaya-upaśam hṛdayastham māṁsam*, "flesh which lies on the heart, which is situated on the heart" and the aorta is not a "piece of flesh". One should rather take it as referring to the left auricle or to the fatty and conjunctive mass which cover the heart. On *TS*, Sāy.: *hṛdayamadhyam aṣṭadalam māṁsapadmam aupaśam tadveṣṭanam māṁsam*, "the centre of the heart is a lotus with eight petals, the *aupáśa* is the flesh which surrounds it". The heart is usually compared, in the classical period, to a lotus and in the *Chānd-up.*, VIII, 1, 1-2, but the description of the pericardium as flesh is not satisfactory.

The examination of numerous terms contained in the above list shows that many of these are metaphorical or periphrastic designations. They are not veritable terms, consecrated by the usage of the language. They are much less technical terms. Occasionally employed in the *mantras* of the ancient Saṁhitās, these designations have often remained in the vocabulary of the later Vedic texts, Brāhmaṇas, Āraṇyakas and Sūtras. This is how they are so frequently encountered, but it does not follow that they were never really in usage. It is quite natural that belonging as they did, to the fundamental *mantras,* they have often been taken up again in the literature devoted to the interpretation and the ritual application of these *mantras.* But they have not come out of the sacerdotal jargon and have not come into classical Sanskrit. Not possessing the value of the anatomical terms, they are not found in the medical texts. Moreover, a certain number of words used in the Vedic period have gone out of use during the centuries that passed between this epoch and that of the scientific manuals. On the other hand, in these manuals are to be found many other anatomical terms found from the Veda onwards. It is here that one finds terms which are quite often authentic and which have been preserved not because of the sacred character of the *mantras* containing them but following the preservation of the Vedic language itself in classical Sanskrit.

Leaving aside banal terms such as the ones which denote organs like the heart, feet or hands, there are certain others which deserve to be studied, because in medicine they have become technical terms, while retaining a great part of their old Vedic value. They correspond to Vedic notions which have remained as formative elements in the classical doctrines of the doctors. They can be divided in two groups: names of organs or of the regions of the body and names of the substances which compose the body. From the first group we will retain only those which denote the organs or regions playing a specially important and characteristic rôle in the physiological conceptions of Āyurveda: the canals and the vulnerable points.

The canals are denoted in the Vedic saṁhitās by the names of *nāḍī, dhamáni* and *hirā.* The first two have been preserved without any change in the Ayurvedic texts, the last one having been replaced there by the term, *sirā.*

The sense of *nāḍī* (written as *nāḷī*) in the oldest passage where it appears (*RV.*, X, 135-7) is "flute" or "straw": ". . . here is the seat of Yama which is called the residence of the gods; this flute of his is blown; it is prepared by the chants".[1] The root *dham*, used here for "blowing", is the one from which is derived *dhamáni* practically becoming a synonym of *nāḍī*, but which, in the *Ṛgveda* (II, 11-8), is a "breath"[2] ("sent by Indra," *indreṣitām dhamánim* . . .) and not a tube which conducts the breath. The term *nāḍī*, on the contrary, was definitely a conduit of air and it has remained the same in the anatomical exercises of the Yoga. But it has also been a "tube", capable of being filled up with any material. The *Atharvaveda* (VI, 138-4), regards as *nāḍī*, the two conduits of the human body, which are the spermatic ducts or the cordons (cf., p. 124). Moreover, the word *nāḍī* is to be met with as a derivative of *naḍa*, "reed".[3] Similarly, in the Ayurvedic texts, *nāḍī* does not exclusively denote "channel for air", but is commonly used to denote "channel" in general. This is how *nāḍī* has come to denote the nourishment-providing vessel of the umbilical cord: "the umbilical vessel of the embryo is connected with the maternal vessel carrying the organic sap".[4] It also denotes the tubulure of an inhalatory apparatus, an apparatus causing "vaporisation by tube", *nāḍīsveda*.[5] Therefore, the general notion of *nāḍī* in the classical medical texts is the same as it had been in the Vedic epoch.

In the epoch of the *Atharvaveda*, the mystical speculations on the similarity of the *nāḍī* of the human body with the cosmic regions had already commenced. But in this respect Ayurvedic medicine has not preserved the heritage, which has been passed on, in its entirety, first to the later Vedic texts and then to the texts of Yoga and Tantra. The hymn X, 7 on *skambha*, the "support" of the world poses, among other

---

1 *idám yamásya sādanam devamānám yád ycyáte|*
iyám asya dhamyate nā[ḷ]īr ayám gīrbhiḥ páriṣkṛtaḥ||
This sense of "flute" or "reed" is found elsewhere, for example, *Kāṭh.*, XXIII, 4, beside other names of musical instruments.

2 Sāyaṇa writes that it is the "voice" put forth by Indra. Actually it refers to the effect of thunder, voice, (and in consequence, breath) of the cloud.

3 *dhamáni* is, on its side, derived from *dhamana* given as a synonym of *naḍa*, "reed", in the *Amarakośa*, but *dhamana* is found quite late. Actually speaking it denotes "one who breathes in" (on the formation of the word, see Renou, *Grammaire Sanskrite*, p. 168).

4 *mātus tu khalu rasavahāyām nāḍyām garbhanābhināḍī pratibaddhā*, (Suśr., *Śār.*, III-27).

5 Suśr., *Utt.*, XXI-3, cf., "*nāḍī* in the form of the elephant's trunk" (*hasti-śuṇḍākārā n.*). *Cik.*, XXXII, 2; Car., *Sūtr.*, XIV-43; cf., J.L. Doreau, *Les bains dans l' Inde antique*, p. 84.

enigmas, the following: "The one, in whom, in the Man are closely reunited immortality and death, the one whose ocean and the canals are closely re-united in the Man, that support, utter its name, which one is it? The one of whom the four quarters are the main canals, the one on whom the sacrifice has advanced, that support, utter its name, which one is that?"[1] The Man referred to here is the Cosmic Man as also the man, both of whom have their basis in the same entity. From the macrocosmic view-point, the expression "canals" can be said to refer firstly to rivers and specially to celestial rivers and from the microcosmic point of view "ocean" can be said to refer to the totality of the organic liquids. The second mention of the "canals" implies that the canals of the body are understood as the currents of energy radiating from all sides in the world, such as the solar rays emitted in all directions, mentioned in the *Chāndogya-upaniṣad,* III-1, etc.

Dhamáni is met with in the *Atharvaveda* and has the precise meaning of "blood vessel", where the hymn, I,17 is an exorcism against haemorrhages. There it is an antonym of *hirā,* which, at first, seems to denote also blood vessels though of smaller calibre: " . . . if the smallest stops, let her stop, the big *dhamáni.* The middle ones of hundred *dhamánis,* of thousand *hirās* have stopped . . ."[2] The biggest vessels are the least numerous and Sāyaṇa commenting upon *AV,* II, 33-6 considers the *dhamánis* as the relatively voluminous vessels. However, another passage of the same Veda directly contradicts the one translated above: VII, 35-2 mentions a thousand *dhamánis* and of a hundred *hirās.* But Sāyaṇa agrees with the later Vedic literature which replaces *hirā* by *hitā* and recognises 72,000 vessels of this type,[3] defining them as *nāḍīs,* "like a hair split thousandfold".[4] The *dhamánis* are, therefore, to be understood as the big vessels. Moreover, in another passage,

---

[1] *yatrāmṛtam ca mṛtvúśca puruṣé'dhi samāhite/*
samudró yásya nāḍváḥ puruṣé'dhi samāhitā/
skambhám tám brūhi katamáḥ svi t eva saḥ//15//
yásya cátasraḥ pradíśo nāḍyás tíṣṭanti prathamāḥ/
yajñó yátra párākrānta skambhám . . .//16// *AV.*, X, 7-15-16.

[2] . . . *kaniṣṭhikā ca tíṣṭhati tiṣṭhād íd dhamánir mahī/2/*
śatásyá dhamánīnām sahásrasya hirāṇām/
asthurín madhyamā . . . (*AV.*, I, 17, 2-3).

[3] *Bṛhad-up*, II, 1, 19.

[4] ibid, IV, 2-3 &. 3, 20 (*yathā keśaḥ sahasradhā bhinnaḥ*).

the *Atharvaveda* refers once again to the hundred *dhamánis* (VI, 90-2). It is, therefore, the relatively smaller number which is preferably attributed to *dhamánis.*

Macdonell and Keith have thought that, in the *Atharvaveda, dhamáni* probably denoted "artery" or "vein", or more generally "intestinal canal".[1] Not one of these three translations can be accepted. There is nothing to prove that in Vedic times distinctions were observed between arteries and veins and, on the contrary, there is every reason to believe that these distinctions were not known because they are found missing in the Ayurvedic medicine itself, which is, however, much more advanced. Moreover, while employing the word "artery", an ambiguous term, it should be clearly explained whether it is to be understood in the old sense of "aerial canal" or in the modern sense of blood canal coming from the heart. As regards its translation as "intestinal canal", it contradicts both the contexts and the commentator[2] and agrees only imperfectly with the general sense of the word in Sanskrit.

The *Suśruta-saṁhitā* challenges an opinion current in its time, which took the *sirās,* the *dhamánis* (*sic*) and the *srotas* (conduits) to denote the one and the same thing. It, however, admits that their functions, even though distinct, are analogous.[3] The main *dhamánis* are 24 in number and are born at the navel from where they spread, ten upwards, ten downwards and four horizontally.[4]

---

1 *Vedic Index*, Vol. I, p. 390.

2 On *AV*, I, 17-3 Sāyaṇa explains that the *dhamánis* are the main *nāḍīs* which go to the heart (*hṛdayagatānām pradhāna-nādīnām*) and that the *hirās* are the *sirās* (classical form), the *nāḍīs* of the branches (*śākhā-nāḍīnām*), that is to say of the limbs; this implies that they, themselves, are the vascular ramifications. On II, 33-6, he explains *dha.* as denoting the thick *sirās* (*sthūlāḥ*). [The passage, II, 33-6 is found as a variant of XX, 96-22. Shankar Pandurang, Vol. IV, p. 794, *dhamáni* is found here after *snāva* which is rendered by Sāyaṇa as fine (*sūkṣmāḥ*) *sirās*]. On VI, 90-2, (Ed. Shankar, *Hymn*, 263-2), he simply replaces *dhamáni* by *nāḍyāḥ*. On VII. 35-2, an incantation for making a woman sterile, he interprets *hirās* as being the small vessels found inside for supporting the embryo *garbha-dhāraṇārtham antar avasthitāḥ sūkṣmāḥ*) and the *dh.* as the big vessels which are the external support for the womb (*avaṣṭambhikā bāhyāḥ sthūlāḥ*); it is however, in this passage that the *hirās* are 100 in number and the *dh.* 1000.

3 *vibhaktakarmaṇām apy avibhāga iva karmasu bhavati*, "even for those whose functions are distinct, there is something like an analogy as regards functions".—Suśr., *Śar.*, IX-1.

4 *tāsām tu nābhiprabhavāṇām dhamanīnām úrdhvagā daśa cādhogāminyás catasras tiryaggāḥ*—Suśr., *Śār.*, IX-2; also *Sūtra.*, XIX, Susr., *Sar.*, IX-2; also *Sūtr.*, XIV-1.

"Those which go upwards maintain the organism by carrying particular things: sound, touch, form, taste, smell, inhalation, exhalation, yawning, hunger, laughter, talking, crying, etc. They reach the heart and become three-fold, they are (then) thirty in number. Among them, ten carry two by two, the wind, the bile, the phlegm, the blood and the organic juice. By eight are seized the sounds, forms, tastes and smells. By two one talks, by two is uttered the loud cry, two are employed for sleep and two for awakening. And two carry tears, two which are located in the bosom carry the mother's milk. It is these two which carry the sperm coming from its two "udders".[1]

The following portion of the text similarly details the functions of the inferior and horizontal *dhamánis,* which carry in the body the entire matter of flow and circulation. The intestines, therefore, figure in the list of *dhamánis,* but the *dhamánis* are not, in general, the intestines; they are simply the canals of the organism. In the *Atharvaveda,* they are more particularly the vessels but the word must have had, from the beginning, the general sense of "canal" which it has in Āyurveda.

As regards *sirās* or *śirās,* they are sometimes, in classical medicine, understood as veins. A chapter of the *Suśruta-saṁhitā* (*Śār.*, VIII), devoted to blood-letting, is entitled *sirāvyādhavidhi,* "the technique of the cutting of the *sirās*". It follows, therefore, that those vessels, which we call "veins" are the *sirās,* but not that the latter always represent the veins. In fact, the word is, most of the time, a synonym of *dhamáni* and of *nāḍī.* Like the *dhamánis,* the *sirās* "have the navel for their root and they spread from there upwards, downwards and horizontally".[2] Like them, they carry the circulating organic

---

[1] *ūrdhvagāḥ śabdaśparśarūparūsagandhapraśvāsocchvāsa-jṛmbhita-kṣuddhasitakathitaruditādīn viśeṣān abhivahantyaḥ śarīram dhārayanti / tās tu hṛdayam abhiprapannās tridhā jāyante, tās triṁśat / tāsām tu vātapittakaphásoṇitarasān dve dve vahataḥ, tā daśa śabdarūparasagandhān aṣṭabhir gṛhṇīte / dvābhyām bhāṣate ca dvābhyām ghoṣam karoti dvābhyām svapiti dvābhyām pratibudhyate / dve cāśruvāhinyau dve stanyam striyā vahataḥ stanasaṁśrite / te eva śukram narasya stanābhyām abhivahataḥ* . . . (Suśr., *Śār.*, IX-3).

[2] *tāsām nābhir mūlam tataś ca prasaranty ūrdhvam adhas tiryak ca*— Suśr., *Śār.*, VII-1.

fluids, specially the wind, the bile, the phlegm and the blood.[1] Like them, they can carry everything: "There is no *sirā*, which carries only the wind, the bile or the phlegm. It is, therefore, said that they carry all. Since they are the fixed derivatives of the corrupted elements of trouble which develop and overflow and that is why it is said that they carry everything".[2] This, however, does not assimilate them completely to the *dhamánis* as it is only on the occasion of the corruption of the elements of trouble that they can transport something else than the four principal liquids.

According to medical texts, therefore, the *sirās* are, in principle, more specialised than the *dhamánis*. These latter are a type of quite big vessels whereas the former are more numerous, 700[3] instead of 24,[4] are finer and in them habitually circulate only extremely thin liquids. They have ramifications throughout the body. "By them, the body is like a garden or like a field with water-channels".[5]

From all these facts it follows that the anatomy of the classical texts of medicine is, in so far as the notions on the various canals and vessels of the body are concerned, a direct descendant of the Veda. It is equally from a Vedic conception in preserving the corresponding Vedic name that classical medicine has elaborated one of its most characteristic notions of anatomy, that of the vulnerable points or *marman*.

We do not have a special term for denoting the points of

---

1 Suśr., *Śār.*, VII-4. Here the text does not add the word *rasa*, the organic juice, but Mahīdhara, who is also a very late author, while commenting on the word *hirā* in the *VS*, XXV-8, says that they are the *nāḍīs* which carry nourishment (*annavāhinyo nāḍyaḥ*). Now nourishment circulates in the body in the form of the *rasa*, a form which it assumes by digestion . . . cf., *infra*, p. 165.

2 *na hi vātam sirāḥ kaścin na pittam kevalam tathā/*
*śleṣmāṇam vā vahanty etā ataḥ sarvavahāḥ smritāḥ/*14/
praduṣṭānām hi doṣāṇām, ucchṛtānām pradhāvatām/
dhruvam unmārgagamanam ataḥ sarvavahāḥ smṛtāḥ/15/—Suśr., *Śār.*, VII, 14-15.

3 Suśr., *Śār.*, VII-1: *Sapta sirāśatāni bhavanti.*

4 As we have seen, the *Atharvaveda* gives respectively the figures of 1000 and 100 except in a passage where the figures are reversed.

5 ibid., then follows: *yābhir idam śarīram ārāma iva jalahāriṇībhiḥ kedāra iva ca* . . . This justifies the explanation, given by Mahīdhara, of *hirā*, as "conduits carrying nourishment" (cf., note above). Even this is possible that Mahīdhara had this passage in mind because he gives an etymology of *hirā* by the root *har*, used here in the word "channel" *hāriṇī: haranty annarasam iti hirā*, "the *hirās* carry away the juice of the nourishment".

the body, whose wounding can either be fatal or particularly serious because it causes paralysis. The Veda calls these points *marman* which the *Ṛgveda* employs mostly in the references to the killing of Vṛtra by god Indra. The form is derived from the root *mṛ*, "to die", and it means above all a "mortal point".[1]

The Ayurvedic texts have an extremely detailed catalogue of the *marmans* and they are, in general, quite easily identifiable, thanks to the precisions that are furnished. They are most often the big vasculo-nervous packets or the tendons and the important nervous trunks. Because of haemorrhages which they determine or the paralyses or functional impotences they bring in, the wounds thereof are extremely serious. From its point of view, the *Suśruta-saṁhitā* sets out the reasons of this gravity: "The vessels of four types[2] which are in the body are ordinarily found to be contained in the *marmans*. Refreshing the tendons, the bones and the flesh as also the articulations, they protect the body. Also, when a *marman* is injured, the wind which is spread, diffuses itself all around. Now, the wind, spreading itself, propagates extremely serious ailments in the body" (*Śār.*, VI).[3] There is nothing to prove that right from the epoch of the *Ṛgveda*, the danger of the wounding of the *marmans* was thus conceived, nor even that they had been catalogued. But the notion of *marman*, like that of the *sirās*, had already been individualised. Medicine has not created this element of its anatomical representation; it has received the same from the Vedic tradition in a ready-made form and has only developed it.

The constituents of the body recognised by the Veda are those which Āyurveda has also recognised. The majority comes within the same sense and the notions concerning them are, properly speaking, not anatomical but commonplace. Such are the blood (*lohita*), the flesh (*māṁsa*), the bone (*asthi*), the narrow of the bone (*majjan*), the fat (*medas*) and the sperm

---

1 cf. L. Renou in E. Benveniste et L. Renou, *Vṛtra et Vrthragna*, p. 137.
2 The *sirās* carry the wind, the bile, the phlegm and the blood.
3 *caturvidhā yās tu sirāḥ śarīre prāyeṇa tā marmasu sanniviṣṭāḥ/*
snāyvasthimāṁsāni tathaiva sandhīn santarpya deham pratipālayanti/23/
tataḥ kṣate marmaṇi tāḥ pravṛddhāḥ samantato vāyur abhistṛṇoti/
vivardhamānas sa ca mātariśvā rujaḥ sutīvrāḥ pratanoti kaye/24/

(*śukra*). But others correspond less to the observations of the anatomists and are nearer the theoretical conceptions and the fact that they are found simultaneously in the Veda and in Āyurveda is quite characteristic of the rôle played by the old ideas of the former in the formation of the latter.

In classical medicine, *rasa* denotes, among other things, an organic juice of primordial necessity. "That which is called *rasa* is the essence produced by the extremely subtle fire of the rightly digested nourishment".[1] It is, therefore, chyle but in the organism it has a rôle which largely goes beyond that of chyle. It is found in the heart and from there it spreads through the 24 *dhamánis* in the entire organism. "It is aqueous, but on reaching the liver and the spleen, it becomes red,[2] and forms the blood. In this connection Suśruta quotes two verses: "the waters, reddened by the fire which has its seat in the human bodies, without being altered by the one which shines (in the external world), it is called 'blood'. Therefore, the blood of the woman called 'menses' comes from the organic juice (*rasa*) and (shows itself) from 12 years and disappears at fifty years".[3] In a long passage where he explains the conditions necessary for the formation of the embryo, Caraka insists on the importance of the *rasa* furnished by the mother: "This embryo is born from the mother; in fact, in the absence of *rasa,* the course of life of the mother is impossible".[4]

Now the *Ṛgveda* has a passage showing that the notion of *rasa* (*rása*) as the maternal contribution in the process of fecundation had already been established: "The wife clasps the

---

1 . . . *āhāryasya samyakpariṇatasya yas tejobhūtaḥ sāraḥ paramasūkṣmaḥ sa rasa ity ucyate* . . . Suśr , *Sūtr.*, XIV-1. Dalhaṇa explains *tejobhūtaḥ* as *vahnisambhūtaḥ;* It is actually under the action of the internal fire that the nourishment is digested. Thereafter Dalhaṇa gives other interpretations, which render *tejas* as *ghṛta,* "heated thing" (specialised in the sense of clarified butter, ghee) and *tejobhūta.* "equivalent to saying—become comparable to ghee".

2 *sa khalva āpyo raso yakṛtaplīhānau prāpya rāgam upaiti*—Suśr., *Sūtr.*, XIV-1, end.

3 *bhavataś cātra / rañjitas tejasā tu āpaḥ śarīrasthena dehinām/ apyāpannaḥ prasannena raktam ity abhidhīyate//rasād eva striyā raktam rajaḥsamjñam pravartate/tad varṣād dvadaśād ūrddhvam yāti pañcaśataḥ kṣayam//*—Suśr., *Sūtr.*, XIV-2. Dalhaṇa explains *prasannena* as *prakṛtisthena.*

4 *rasajaś cāyam garbhaḥ/ na hi rasād ṛte mātuḥ prāṇayātrāpi syāt* . . . Car., *Śār.*, III, 18.

husband in her arms, they spread the virile milk, in delivering herself she milks for herself the *rása* . . .".[1] This passage should be read in conjunction with those where a "semen" (*retas*) is attributed to the mother-Earth as also to the father-Sky (*RV.*, I-159; 2, et VI, 70, 1).[2] Hence the idea that the Indian medical men have formed of the rôle of the female *rasa* in generation has antecedents in the Veda. Moreover, in the hymns of the *Ṛgveda, rasa* is frequently associated with *soma*, whether it is a question of the *rasa* of the soma or that *rasa* be called "somic" (*somia*),[3] and the precise souvenir of this Vedic correlation has remained alive in medicine. The *Suśruta-saṁhitā* after having posed the problem of knowing whether the *rasa* is *saumya* or *taijasa* (igneous), affirms that it is *saumya* but is modified by the fire.[4] Of course, this epithet merely signifies that it is "somic", whether it refers to Soma as a mythical liquid or as a sacrificial liquor. All that it says is that its nature is humid; the echo of the Vedic tradition is equally clear here.

Another echo of the same type, and quite near, is to be found with reference to the organic element, which in the classical texts of the medicine is called *ojas*. The same word *ojas* signifies "force" in the Veda and designates, for example, sometimes the force of Indra; sometimes that of Vṛtra.[5] The word goes back to Indo-Iranian because it is found in the

---

1 . . . *ā jāyā yukte pátim / tuñjāte vṛṣṇyam payaḥ paridāya rásam duhe* . . . *RV.*, I, 105, 2. The group of words *vṛṣṇyampayaḥ duhe* is parallel to the formulae *śukram payaḥ duh* . . . (I, 160, 3; IX, 54, 1).

2 Bergaigne, *Rel. véd.*, I, 239, sees therein the effect of the mechanical vocal application of the same attribute to the two partners of a pair designated in the dual number, whereas this attribute fits only one of them. In fact he could not conceive that one could have believed that the woman delivered a "semen". But this was a banal belief of antiquity, not only in India but also in the Hellenic world (cf., Censorinus, *De die nataii,* VI, who attributes it to Alcmeon, Epicurus, Anaxagoras, Empedocles and Parmenides). The secretion of the vulvo-vaginal glands during coitus could mislead in this respect. One could easily take for genitals a secretion, which was only sexual, cf., *infra*, p. 190.

3 Grassmann, *Worterbuch,* see *rasa,* cf. also the passages such as the *Taitt.—s,* II, 2, 10, 4, where it is said . . . "*somaṃ* . . . *raso* . . . *gachaty* . . .", "the *rasa* goes to *soma*", this *rasa* being of one who has been ill for a long time.

4 Suśr., *Sūtr.*, XIV-1. Passage ending in what is quoted in p. 165, f.n. 2. Besides the fire Agni is normally associated with Soma in the Veda and there Soma is sometimes considered as liquid fire, cf., above p. 60.

5 cf., Benveniste—Renou, *Vṛtra et Vrthragna*, pp. 131. 158.

Avesta as *aojah*, associated with *vərəthra*, and in the sense of "force that is naturally infused in the limbs".[1] In medical texts it is "vital juice", a substance whose presence in the body is necessary for active life: "*ojas* is of the nature of Soma, unctuous, white, fresh, substantial, fluid, pure and sweet; it is the principal seat of life".[2] This substance appears only during the eighth month of the life of the embryo and it is its absence which renders the young premature babies unviable.[3] It is essentially that which contributes vigour to the organism, whose nourishing substance is the *rasa*. It is near *rasa* because it has the nature of soma and because, at the same time, it is *tejas*, a calorific radiation of activity, whereas the *rasa* is also, though belonging to the category of liquids such as the soma, impregnated with activity by an internal fire. "The *tejas* accompanying the bodily elements from the *rasa* up to the sperm[4], is certainly the *ojas*. This is what is called "force", according to the decision of our own text. Because of the force inherent in it the flesh becomes firm and develops, there is easiness in all the movements, clearness of voice and of the skin, the internal and external organs fulfil their respective functions".[5] It can be seen that it is not only because of the name that the *ojas* of the medical texts is identified with that whose possession was attributed by the Veda to the warrior Indra.

There have, however, been claims to identify the *ojas* as it is described by Suśruta with albumin. Kunja Lal Bhishagratna has defended this theory[6] on the ground that albumin is precisely an essential element of the constitution of

---

1 ibid, p. 7.

2 *ojaḥ somātmakam snigdham śuklam śītam sthiram rasam| viviktam mṛdu mṛtsnam ca prāṇāyatanamuttamam.*—Suśr., *Sūtr.*, XV, 14, (23 in the Jadavji Trikamji ed. quoted in the *Kumāratantra*, p. 29, f.n. 2). Dalhaṇa explains *somātmakam* by *saumyam* on which see *supra;* cf. also *supra*, p. 27.

3 cf. *Kumāratantra*, p. 29.

4 cf. *supra*, p. 27.

5 . . . *rasādīnām śukrāntānām dhātūnām yat param tejas tat khalv ojas, tad eva balam ity ucyate sva-śāstra-siddhāntāt | tatra balena sthiropacita-māṁsatā sarvaceṣṭāsu apratighātaḥ svaravarṇaprasādo bāhyānām abhyanatarāṇām ca kāraṇānām ātmakāryapratipattir bhavati*—Suśr., *Sūtr.*, XV, 13.

6 *An English Translation of Suśruta—saṁhitā*, Calcutta, Vol. I, 1907 pp. LIII ff and pp. 130 ff.

tissues and that *Caraka-saṁhitā* shows the presence of *ojas* in the urine in case of the disease of *madhumeha*. But it is clear that *madhumeha* is the disease where urine has sugar, the diabetes. The loss of vigour in this disease, where an unusual element appears in the urine and where diuresis is extremely increased, could easily lead to the supposition that *ojas* escaped in the form of this element. But it does not follow that the doctors had discovered albumin or glycogen; what is true is only that they have recognised the presence of an element which they supposed to be *ojas* and which we study in chemistry under the name of glucose. But Kunja Lal confuses glucose with glycogen and supposes a correlation of the latter with albumin and thereby links albumin and *ojas*. He thus brings to Āyurveda the honour of the discovery of albumin without noticing that it implies the attribution of an absurd theory, whereby albumin enters the composition of the tissues of the foetus only in the eighth month of gestation.

It is better to say simply that the Ayurvedic notion of *ojas* is the theoretical concretisation of the Vedic concept of bodily vigour.

One last liquid of the body still remains. The bile has the same name, *pitta*, in both the Veda and Āyurveda. In the theory of the latter, it has an intimate connection with fire, representing in liquid form the fiery element of the organism. This concept could not have resulted from an observation of pathological facts. Undoubtedly the morbid manifestations, in which bile appears to play a rôle, can themselves be febrile, but they are not necessarily so. The bilious vomitings, accidents wherein the participation of bile is particularly evident, can be produced outside all hyperthermia. A theoretical speculation is necessary to make bile into a form of fire, and the existence of some similar speculation in the Vedic period is guaranteed by the *Atharvaveda* and the *Yajurveda*. The same passage in these two texts says to the Fire, "O Agni, thou art the bile of the waters".[1]

The mythology of the fire hidden in the waters or of the fire in aquatic form is Indo-Iranian, as already seen by us

[1] *ágne pittám apām asi, AV.*, XVIII, 3, 5: *Vāj.—s.*, XVII 6; *Kāṭh.—s*, XVII, 17.

(pp. 58 ff). What is new and characteristic here is the identification of the fire with bile. We do not understand how this identification is made, how the fire hidden in the waters, the fire whose prototype is the thunder about to burst, has been assimilated to the fire but the fact that the assimilation is made in the Vedic texts is valuable for its date. The medical concept of the fiery quality of bile goes back to antiquity.

The wind which could be considered as pertaining to anatomy in Indian thought, must be, first of all, studied with regard to its physiological action. The phlegm, the watery element of the organism, is not named in the Vedic Saṁhitās. One of the terms designating it in the classical text is *balāsa* and figures in the Veda but only as the name of a disease and in that capacity we have studied it (pp. 117 ff). It appears, therefore, that to the Vedic Saṁhitās only a part, though an important one, of the anatomical elements having an essential rôle in medicine, is known. The study of the data of Physiology will lead us to an analogous conclusion.

CHAPTER V

THE DATA OF THE VEDIC SAMHITAS ON PHYSIOLOGY

THE INFORMATION that we can obtain from the hymns and from sacrificial formulae relating to the ideas the Vedic authors could have had concerning the play of organic functions, is obviously scanty. Numerous allusions have yielded us the names of diseases, of organs, of parts and elements of the body, but they cannot replace the enunciations of theories. However, people have tried to find in the Veda proofs to show that the fundamental theory of Ayurvedic physiology, that of the three active elements—wind, bile and phlegm—was already known at the time of the composition of hymns.

A hymn addressed to the Aśvins, after saying that they give thrice the remedies of the Sky, of the Earth and of the Waters, calls on them to carry (*vahatam*) to the son of the reciter the *tridhātu śárma* (*RV.*, I-34-6). *Śarman* denotes "protection" or "well-being", but the latter sense has come in only classical Sanskrit. The commentator Sāyaṇa has understood it to refer to the well-being of the three bodily elements of classical medicine. However, *tridhātu* means literally "consisting of three objects", therefore "triple", and it refers to the triple protection of three sorts of remedies which are mentioned here. Moreover, the following verse also contains the word *tridhātu,* and there the sense of triple is unchallenged. The translators have, at a very early date, recognised that the interpretation of Sāyaṇa had been abusive. Langlois who published in 1848 the first complete translation of the *Ṛgveda*, although, generally speaking, he has not been a faithful translator, has rightly recognised and pointed out in a note that *tridhātu śárma vahatam* simply signified "triplex auxilium ferte", although, in translation, he has followed the sense of the commentary. The majority of other translators have not even taken note of the interpretation of Sāyaṇa, except Wilson[1] who has accepted it without reserve because he had

---

1 *Ṛgveda Saṁhitā*, Vol. 1, p. 95, and the French adaptation of this translation by Pauthier and Brunet in the *Livres sacrés de tous les peuples* . . ., Migne ed., Vol. II, p. 39, Col. 2.

made it a rule to follow the commentary, and has thus led the historians of medicine to believe that the fundamental theory of Indian pathology was to be found in the *Ṛgveda*. Reinhold Müller has done well to refute this view once again.[1]

The question has been raised again *á propos* the *Atharva-veda* by Dasgupta.[2] In an article in the *Hastings Encyclopaedia*,[3] Bolling had quite rightly said that the theory of the *tri-doṣas* or *tri-dhātus* did not appear in the early Vedic texts and was found for the first time only in the *Atharvaveda-pariśiṣṭa* (68), a later appendix of the Veda itself. He had also maintained that the expression *vātīkṛtanāśanī* (*AV*, VI, 44-3) does not prove that the wind was already conceived as a bodily element and a cause of diseases; this expression signified "which destroys what is transformed into wind" and not "which destroys that which is made by the wind". Moreover this compound qualifies a remedy which in the preceding verse is called "remedy of the flux (diarrhical, probably)" *āsrāvabheṣajam*, and the wind in question is undoubtedly that of the intestines.[4] But Dasgupta thinks that another passage shows clearly that diseases were divided into three categories caused by the wind, the water and the fire. In the *AV*., I, 12, 3 the words, *yó abhrajā vātajā yáś ca śuṣmo . . .*, seem to signify "(the disease) which is born of the cloud (of the humid), one that is born of the wind and the one which is dry . . . " At least this is the type of translation which results from the explanations of Dasgupta who derives *śuṣma* from the root *śuṣ*, "to dry". But Reinhold Müller[5] has justly remarked that the words *abhrajā* and *vātajā* merely qualify *śuṣma*. One must understand these words to mean, as translators have done so far: ". . . the *śuṣma* which is born of the

---

1 *Die Medizin in Ṛgvéda*, in *Asia Major*, Vol. VI, p. 335. Cordier, although he quotes only the translations of Langlois and Grassmann, had, like Wilson, admitted on the basis of Sāyaṇa that the theory of the *tridhātu* was already found in the *Ṛgveda* (in his first work on Indian Medicine: *Etude sur la médicine hindoue*, Paris, 1894, p. 27).

2 *A History of Indian Philosophy*, Vol. II, Cambridge, 1932, p. 299.

3 *Encyclopaedia of Religion and Ethics*, 1911, Diseases and Medicine (Vedic).

4 Moreover *Vātikāra* (*AV*., IX, 8,20, cf., above, p. 101, n. 1) which appears to be another form of *Vātīkṛta*—can denote only "that which is produced by the wind". On the interpretation of Sāyaṇa, see Dasgupta, *loc. cit.*

5 *Uber pitta oder galle unter Bezug zur Tridoṣa—Lehere der Altindischen Medizin* in *Janus*, 1934, pp. 77 ff.

cloud and the one that is born of the wind . . . . " Besides the sense of *śuṣma* in this passage is uncertain. The root *śuṣ* in Vedic can also denote "to whistle"; in the *AV.* this word has even the sense of "vigour". In any case Bloomfield translates it here[1] by "lightning" and Whitney as "blast" (with doubt). One should, therefore, renounce all attempts at finding the formal proof of the existence of the theory of the *tridhātu* or *tridoṣa* in the *Atharvaveda.* Dasgupta also gives another argument; he observes that in *AV.*, VI, 109, *pippalī*, the long pepper, is at the same time called "the remedy of the *vātīkṛta*" and "the remedy of the *kṣipta*". He interprets *vātīkṛta* as denoting "that which is produced by the wind" and *kṣipta* as madness. The classical literature does consider madness as being due to the wind of the organism. But we have just now seen that *vātīkṛta* denotes "that which is transformed into wind" (grammatically no other interpretation is possible), and *kṣipta* cannot denote madness. The root *kṣip* denotes "to throw". In classical Sanskrit it also frequently signifies "to destroy, to wound". In the passage referred to above, *kṣipta* denotes, as in the classical, "wounded" or, what comes to mean the same thing by a roundabout interpretation, "that which is produced by an arrow that is shot" (Roth : Schuss-oder Wurfwunde). In *kṣiptacitta*, *kṣipta* applies to the spirit to signify that the spirit is troubled or distracted and it is least probable that one has to suppose here, in place of the most natural one, some other sense.

But, If the fundamental pathological theory of classical medicine had not assumed shape at the time of the redaction of the Ṛgvedic hymns and even of those of the *Atharvaveda* or, if at least nothing can prove to us that it had assumed shape, it does not seem to be doubtful that right from the time of the *Atharvaveda*, elements had, in part, been prepared for its elaboration. We have seen (p. 117) that *balāsa* designated swellings, the aqueous infiltration of tissues and that it has become a name of the aqueous element of the organism, the *śleṣman*, "phlegm" or "mucus". The fire which has a manifest rôle in affections like fever, was accepted as an important element in physiology, because of the equivalence postulated since the Veda between

---

1 cf., also Bloomfield, *On the Meanings of the Word Śuṣma*, in *ZDMG.* 418, pp. 565 ff. Last of all L. Renou, *Anthologie sanskrite*, Paris, 1947, p. 55: "violence".

the macrocosm and the microcosm and already the bile had been assimilated with the fire as it is in medical theory.

As regards the wind, the Veda shows that it was already conceived simultaneously as an organic and cosmic force and the multiplicity of the organic winds, already distinguished one from the other, shows that pneumatology which dominates the physiology of Āyurveda was already in the course of formation.

We have already examined in the Vedic texts the most characteristic ideas of ancient India concerning the wind, the cosmic and universal force and the prototype of all motor-force in the microcosm and the macrocosm (pp. 61 ff.). Comparison with the Avestic data has shown us that these ideas were largely Indo-Iranian. Here we still have to show the extent to which the Vedic texts already contain, either in germ or in full form, the special concepts of Āyurvedic medicine on the rôle of the wind in the economy of the organism. For this purpose we have to study those principal passages of the Veda which contain the names of the vital winds, the *prāṇas.*

Arthur H. Ewing has patiently collected the references to these breaths in the entire Vedic literature, adding in an appendix some of their definitions found in classical literature.[1] He has frequently compared and reproduced various translations proposed by philologists. All this work of analysis and classification is and will remain extremely useful. The conclusions reached by him are given briefly here:—

1. The point of departure for the series of *prāṇa* is the word *prāṇa*, "breath in general";
2. The division of the respiratory activity into inspiration and expiration is primitive and appears at an early date in the dual compound, *prāṇāpānau;*
3. With his habit of careful observation, the Hindu could have, and in all probability, has observed from an early date the interval between respirations, wherefrom the supposition of a breath remaining even in the absence of

1 *The Hindu Conception of the Functions of Breath—A Study in Early Hindu Psycho-physics*, in *JAOS*, Vol. XXXII, Pt. 2., 1901, pp. 249-308. But he neglects the data of *Yajurveda* (cf., p. 280) in giving (p. 257) a statistical table of the use of the names of breaths in the *White Yajurveda.* On the concept of the breath in the *Upaniṣads*: G. W. Brown, *the Human Body in the Upaniṣads*, Jubbulpore, 1921.

prāṇa and of *apāna*, i.e., *vyāna*, "separate respiration";

4. With a desire to create a more varied play of symbols, terms analgous to *prāṇa*, *apāna* and *vyāna* have been multiplied by grafting the root *an* on to the pre-verbs *sam-* and *ud-*, which gives us *samāna* and *udāna*;
5. *Apāna* in the sense of expiration has been superceded by *udāna*; secondarily *udāna* appears, etymologically more convenient, to denote expiration;
6. Wishing to establish similarities between the different members of the series of *prāṇas* and the bricks of the altar of Agni, one has been led to give to *apāna* a sense other than the original one;
7. In the Upaniṣads efforts have been made to explain secondarily the localisations adopted to meet the ends of sacrificial symbolism for diverse *prāṇas*. For example, the fact that *apāna* had been placed in the tail of the bird-shaped altar has led to its localisation in the intestines and in the urinary canals; *samāna*, having been placed in the middle, could become an agent of digestion ;
8. Deductions of this type on localisations and functions of *prāṇas* are more or less the contributions to Indian ideas of anatomy and physiology but have no value in themselves, as they do not account for the formation of the series of *prāṇas* on an empirical basis. Each attempt at explanation is to be taken, as the expression of an individual opinion insofar as it is not merely traditional;
9. As regards the translation, the results are mostly negative. Where the entire series appears, it is always symbolic and one can do no more than transliterate.
10. However, a positive result of some value is there: *prāṇa* signifies either the double process of respiration or "inspiration" in opposition to "expiration".

The majority of these conclusions are not at all valid as they are implicitly based on the double postulation that the Indians, speculating on breath in the organism, could only have originally, in view the respiratory breath and that they had, later on, given it no thought except those relative to ritual symbolism. The idea that for the mere requirements of this symbolism and because of the mechanical play of the grammatical rules of the formation of nouns, the Indians found themselves in possession of a nomenclature of breaths and that they have been obliged to invent physiological reasons for justifying this nomenclature, is presented as a result. This, however, is only a strange hypothesis.

Ewing has been led here by the method adopted rightly by him but which he has blindly applied. He has studied the mention of the breaths successively in the diverse strata of the Vedic literature and this was necessary. But, when in an earlier stratum, the context would not yield a definite sense, he has seldom tried to enlighten himself about the definite meaning found in a more recent stratum. He does not seem to have envisaged that the sense given in the more recent texts could have been anything but a novelty in these texts; he had believed that it was the result of an attempt at interpreting a more ancient text. In fact, lightly inserting a value guaranteed only by a Brāhmaṇa or an Upaniṣad into a Vedic Saṁhitā could lead to anachronism. But the lack of seriousness is reflected in the belief, without proofs, that a value clearly expressed only from a certain date did not exist earlier. If an obscure or apparently absurd ancient text gets clarified when such a value is brought in there, one may believe that it was in its place there although it had been found there in so explicit a manner only in a text of later date, from where it had been drawn.

Moreover, although having collected in an appendix (p. 307) the definitions of the *prāṇas* given by Suśruta, Ewing has not thought of seeking light from the works of Indian physiologists regarding the physiological concepts of the breaths. Not only has he limited himself to the data of his texts without clarifying the ones by the others, unless they were of the same epoch, but he has also neglected the tradition of the specialists of the question studied by him. It is true that in this respect he was merely following a usage then current among the translators of Vedic texts. Those could have rejected the evidence of Āyurveda as being very late, but they did frequently accept the still more recent interpretations of commentators like Śaṁkara, who were not physiologists. Evidently the question must be taken up again. It must be taken up here specially as regards the most ancient references to the diverse organic breaths.

In the *Ṛgveda* appear only two names which are given to them later on, firstly the one that is used as the generic designation of all of them: *prāṇa*, followed, only once, by *vyāna*. But the root *an*, "to breathe", is also found accompanied by the pre-verbs *apa-* and *sam-*. *Prāṇa* has the general sense of breath, of life. The most important passage wherein it occurs is the one already noted by us (p. 63) where the atmospheric wind is regarded as produced by the breath of the Cosmic Man. The cosmic wind is already clearly conceived as having for its motor this breath or wind, even when it does not show itself in the form of wind itself because in a hymn to the Sun it is said, "Inside it circulates the brilliant, breathing by its own breath."[1] The passage is obscure, inasmuch as the female being designated by the "brilliant" cannot be surely identified[2] and hence it is not possible to affirm whether *apa* denotes here the "downward" direction or more generally "outside", "keeping itself away", which is imparted to the breath. With the pre-verb *sam-*, *an* is once used in "today he is dead, Yesterday he has gathered his breath".[3] As regards *vyāna*, it is assimilated in the spring of the chariot of *Sūrya* in verse 12 of the epithalamium of Sūrya and Soma (X, 85) a large part of which is found again in the *Atharvaveda* (XIV, 1).[4]

These passages are not very significant and it should be noted that all the uses of *prāṇa*, that of *vyāna* and those of the root *an* with the prefixes *apa-* and *sam-* are found, except one, in the Ist and the Xth Books of the *Ṛgveda* which are the latest. The only exception is in the IIIrd Book. Evidently, it does not follow that breath was not still well-known at the time of the composition of the most ancient hymns. The subjects of these gave no opportunity to its mention. But the references become more numerous in the Xth Book and in the *Atharvaveda* where relations between the Cosmos and the human or animal body are referred to more often, which leads to a mention of breath and the breaths; at the same time the limbs of the body are

---

1 *antáś carati rocanāsyá prāṇād apānatī—RV.*, X, 189. 2 . . . "Sound" is in the masculine; it can, therefore, stand for the breath of the Sun, because of whom the brilliant one (the Dawn) progresses while breathing.

2 cf., Oldenberg, *Ṛgveda, ad. loc.* (p. 366). It is difficult to understand why Ewing says here, "It is clear that *prāṇa* is here viewed simply as physical breath" (p. 251), whereas *prāṇa* belongs precisely to a luminous celestial being.

3 *adyā mamāra sá hyáḥ sám āna—RV.*, X, 55, 5.

4 cf., *infra*, p. 180.

referred to more frequently and there is speculation on the whole subject.

Prāṇa, alone, has the same meanings as in the *Ṛgveda*, meanings which have become fixed elsewhere. It denotes the vital breath, hence life, and hence the cosmic soul. But in the *Atharvaveda*, *prāṇa* is sometimes used in the plural number; upto seven *prāṇas* are counted[1] and the names of seven of them are given. These figures suffice to establish that the breaths in question are not, all of them, respiratory. Thereafter one must ask oneself if they do not correspond to the breaths which are mentioned in classical medicine under the same names, explicitly defining them the while.[2] Even when profound differences in nature could be discerned between the known breaths of the Veda and those whose existence is taught by medicine, it will be evident, solely because of the plurality of the breaths and the identity of their names, that medicine, for its pneumatology, depends on the ancient ideas of the Veda.

Two breaths are most frequently named, *prāṇa* and *apāna*, mentioned separately or in a dual compound. Making a pair in this manner, they seem, at first view, to represent inspiration and expiration and the contexts generally go well with this natural interpretation. The texts of classical medicine sometimes use the compound *prāṇāpānau* in the same sense,[3] when they refer to vital breaths in general and do not limit themselves to mention only *prāṇa*. As these texts interest themselves in the *apāna* chiefly insofar as it circulates downwards in the body, they can group under this name the totality of organic breaths opposed to *prāṇa*. That is why *prāṇāpānau*, even though nominally denoting only two breaths, can represent the complete series of five recognised by medical theory. One may be led to believe that here lies a later extension of the sense of *apāna*, at first limited to that of inspiration,[4] but, if in the *Atharvaveda*

---

1 There are seven *prāṇas*, seven *apānas* and seven *vyānas* (*AV*. XV., 15, 1). The three hymns XV, XVI and XVII of Book XV are devoted to an enumeration of these breaths identified with the astronomical elements of the Universe and some other connected entities.

2 Regarding the medical definition of the *prāṇas*, cf., *supra*, p. 28.

3 cf., for example Caraka, *Śar.*, I, 98. Cakradatta explains here by *ucchvāsanihśvāsa*, "inspiration and expiration", III, 16.

4 For a long time the translators have indifferently given the sense of "inspiration and expiration" to *prāṇa* and *apāna*. Caland has maintained

the interpretation of *apāna* as inspiration fits in generally well with the contexts, it is not always so. Some of them are explicable only if the words *prāṇa* and *apāna* have already meanings approaching those attributed to them by the doctor and also by the Upaniṣads which frequently understand *prāṇa* in the sense of thoracic breath and *apāna* or the abdominal breath as has been very well demonstrated by G. W. Brown.[1]

The hymn XI, 4 applies to the cosmic breath, it exalts the functions of the breath in the universe and mentions twice together, but otherwise separately, *prāṇa* and *apāna* or the corresponding functions, "The *prāṇa* and the *apāna* are rice and barley: The (Cosmic) Bull is called *prāṇa*. *Prāṇa* consists of barley and *apāna* is called rice".[2]

The identification of *prāṇa* with barley and of *apāna* with rice has not been explained. Henry[3] and Deussen[4] have contented themselves by noting that rice and barley were the chief bases of nourishment, but this does not show in the least how the idea of identifying barley with expiration and rice with inspiration could arise if *prāṇa* and *apāna* had denoted nothing but these two phases of breath. Now in hymn XIII, 3, there is the question of an all-powerful god "who, with *prāṇa*, fills up the Sky and the Earth, who with *apāna* fills up the stomach of the Ocean".[5] This shows the idea of a connection between *prāṇa* and nourishment and also of a connection between *apāna* and the waters. These connections will be purely absurd if *prāṇa* here denotes inspiration and *apāna* expiration. But in the classical tradition of physiology, *prāṇa* sits in the mouth and is the agent of digestion of the aliments; *apāna* sits in the lower part of the body where it pushes the liquids to excretion. If it is

(*Zur exegese und Kritik der rituellen Sūtras XXXIV.*, *Prāṇa und apāna* in *ZDMG*, Vol. LV, 1901, pp. 261 ff. and vol. LVI, 1902, p. 556) that originally *prāṇa* was expiration and *apāna* inspiration.

1 *Prāṇa and Apāna*, *JAOS*, XXXIX, p. 104.

2 *prāṇāpānáu vrīhi-yaváu anaḍvān prāṇā ucyate.*
yáve ha prāṇá āhito' pānó vrīhir ucyate//13//AV., XI, 4, 13.
The assimilation of *prāṇa* and of the Cosmic Bull is apparently explicable by the fact that both of them are in turns the centre of the pantheistic speculations, familar in the *Ṛgveda*.

3 *Les Livres*, X, XI, XII . . . p. 148.

4 *Allgemeine Einleitung und Philosophie des Veda*, 4th ed., Leipzig, 1920, p. 302.

5 *yáḥ prāṇéna dyāvā-pṛthivī tarpáyaty apānéna samudrásya jaṭháram yáḥ pṛpati—AV.*, XIII, 3, 4.

admitted that their rôles could have been already envisaged in this manner at the time of the *Atharvaveda*, one can understand the relation established between *prāṇa* and nourishment and *apāna* and the waters. Morever, as barley is a cereal of high terrain and rice is a plant of flooded terrain, in a theoretical repartition of the two aliments between two types of breaths, barley naturally had to be assigned to *prāṇa* and rice to *apāna*. Besides it is not only in the physiological traditions of Suśruta and Caraka that *prāṇa* and *apāna* are conceived under forms other than those of breath. The *Chāndogya-upaniṣad* says of the *prāṇa*, "of the mouth" (*mukhya*), which is the principal one at the same time[1]: "Because therewith one eats, one drinks, one supports the other breaths".[2] In the *Atharvaveda* the epithet of *bhuridhāyas*[3] is given to *prāṇa*. The localisation of *apāna* in the lower part of the body is current in later Vedic literature.

The verse of the *Atharvaveda* which follows the one identifying *prāṇa* and *apāna* with barley and rice, contains yet another inexplicable proposition if *prāṇa* and *apāna* are understood as respiratory breaths: "He puts to play *apāna*, he puts to play *prāṇa*, the Man, inside the matrix. When thou, *prāṇa*, thou, pushest, then he is born again".[4] This refers to the Cosmic Man compared in his development with the embryo and probably to that of the Sun which can concretely represent the Cosmic Man and which is reborn every morning. In any case we understand that the embryo was conceived as having, inside the matrix, pneumatic activity and as being born under the sush of the breath. Now, of all the conceivable organic breaths, the only ones which can have no rôle in the embryo are inspiration and expiration. The others, the animal spirits, which circulate in all parts of the body in formation are according to the classical physiological doctrine the agents of its growth and it is the breaths which determine the delivery. If, following this, we translate, "He put in play his inferior breath, he puts in play his superior breath the Man, inside the matrix . . . ", we can avoid

1 Also in *Bṛh.-up*. I, 3, 7 ff.

2 *tena yad aśnāti yat pibati tena itarān prāṇān avati—Chānd.-up*. 1, 2, 9.

3 *AV*., VI, 41, 2: cf., *infra* p. 181, n. 1.

4 *ápānati prāṇati púruṣo gárbhe antarā|*
yadā tvám prāṇa jínvasi átha sá jāyate púnaḥ||—AV., XI, 4, 14.

the necessity of making the embryo breathe in a full space.[1]

Moreover, one would except that *prāṇa* and *apāna* would not, in the *Atharvaveda*, always designate exhaled air and the inhaled air. As the *prāṇa* or the breath in general of the Cosmic Man is the wind, it is an internal wind because the wind circulates inside the Universe, the body of the Cosmic Giant.

The examination of the data on breaths other than *prāṇa* and *apāna* in the *Atharvaveda* confirms the existence of speculations concerning organic breaths during the period of its composition. These speculations were already quite close to Āyurvedic theories.

Translators have often recognised *vyāna* as a wind diffused all over the body. Ewing has, in this case[2], taken recourse to the reference in the *Chāndogya-upaniṣad* (I, 3, 3) which says that *vyāna* is the "joint" (*sandhi*) of *prāṇa* and *apāna*. He saw therein respiratory air retained between two movements and then circulating inside the body. Elsewhere, the passage of the *Ṛgveda*, where *vyāna* figures as the spring of the symbolic car, had already indicated that this *vyāna* was conceived as the element of junction. But if *prāṇa* is the breath of the upper part and *apāna* that of the lower one or of the back part, then *vyāna* circulating in the middle of the body is exactly the one that unites them.

It is their permanent intermediary in somatic spaces rather than being the occasional interval between expiration and inspiration. The simultaneous mention of the three is more complete as the enumeration of organic breaths than that of *prāṇa* and *apāna* and less equivocal, as the latter two answer also to the two phases of respiration.

This is how, undoubtedly, should be interpreted the passages where the three breaths are mentioned in the *Atharvaveda*.

---

1 It may be objected that if the assertion is absurd, it can in any case be thought to have been made by the author of the hymn. An example may be found in the Chinese Taoist, Ko-hung (Pao-pou-tseu), referring precisely to an intra-uterine respiration (*t'ai-si*). This is pointed out by P. Wieger and he expresses his surprise about it in European medicine (*Histoire des croyances . . .*, 3rd ed., Hien-Hien, 1927, p. 391). But with Ko-hong it does definitely refer to ideas borrowed from India, as underlined by Wieger himself and the respiration in question is, in reality, a *garbha-prāṇa*, a play of animal spirits in the matrix and in the foetus.

2 *loc. cit.*, pp. 277 and 280.

For example, XI, 5, 24, where the pair *prāṇāpānau* and *vyāna* are declared to have been engendered by the Brahmanic student, mythically transposed into a sort of Cosmic Man. For example, once again and chiefly, VI, 41, which is an ordinary charm for health "for the spirit, the thoughts . . . the *apāna*, the *vyāna*, the *prāṇa* giving much of nourishment[1] . . . where evidently *prāṇa* so qualified is not at all the expiration but, as we have seen, the nourishing breath localised by the *Chāndogya-upaniṣad* in the mouth and which will be known to classical physiology.

Samāna is mentioned once in a verse of the *Atharvaveda* where the other three are also named. This is in the hymn X, 2, which asks as to who has made all the things in the cosmic body: "who has woven therein *prāṇa*? Who has woven *apāna* and *vyāna*? Which god has founded the *samāna* in the Man?"[2] This is one of the hymns which enumerate most carefully all that is found in the man; it is natural that its list of organic breaths is more complete than in any other passage of the same collection. The expression *avayat*, "has woven", recalls by pun, as noted by Henry, *avayat*, "has breathed", but it also evokes the idea of the network of the *dhamanis* and of the *sirās* stretched all over the body. One may ask oneself if the author has consciously desired to evoke it as being the one where the *prāṇas* circulate in the body. In any case nothing allows us to specify the special value of *samāna* in this passage.

Udāna, the fifth breath of the classical list, is mentioned twice (XI, 8, 4 and 26) in a hymn which like the preceding one gives us an "inventory of the man". With him are named *prāṇa* and *apāna* in a pair in dual number and it is itself associated in the pair *vyānodānau* with *vyāna*. *Samāna* does not figure in this series. The context does not help us understand the correct sense of *udāna* but its mention does at least show that the *Atharvaveda* already knows all the breaths of the classical series.

Before leaving the data of the *Atharvaveda*, it should be observed that the hymn to the breath (XI, 4), wherein are found very clear passages preventing us from translating *prāṇa* and *apāna* as "expiration" and "inspiration", occupies a separate

---

1 *mánase cétasea...pānāya vyānāya prāṇāya bhūridhāyase*/—*AV*, VI, 41, 1-2.

2 *ko asmin prāṇām avayat kó apānám vyānám u*/
samānám asmin kó devó dhi śiśrāyapūruṣe/—*AV*., X, 2, 13.

place in the rituals prescribed in the Atharvanic Sūtras.[1] This could induce us to suppose that it is a case of aberration or has been introduced specially in the Veda and that it reflected opinions alien to the rest of the collection. But nothing of the kind can be supposed as the interpretations which are valid there, are also valid in the hymns beyond suspicion. The absence of use in the ritual, which, moreover, is not total, does not bear the least significance and, even if it were proved that the doctrine of this hymn was an aberration from the rest at the time of its appearance, it will no less remain a proof of the Vedic sources of classical physiology.

The data of the Saṁhitā of the *Yajurveda* on the *prāṇas* lend itself, like that of the *Atharvaveda*, to an interpretation of the series of breaths made in the light of the physiological theories, expounded later on. Wherever more than two breaths are mentioned, it is not possible to identify these breaths with inspiration and expiration. Even where only two breaths appear, this identification is not always satisfactory.

The formulae wherein *prāṇas* are referred to are mostly limited to a call for prosperity. All the five *prāṇas* are mentioned together a number of times. In the *Vājasaneyī-saṁhitā*, XXII, 33, it is said "That, thanks to the sacrifice, life may succeed, *svāhā* ! That, thanks to the sacrifice, the *prāṇa* . . . *apāna* . . . *vyāna* . . . *udāna* . . . *samāna* . . . the eye . . . the ear . . . the speech . . the spirit, . . . the *ātman* . . . Brahman . . . light . . . the sky . . . . the celestial vault (literally : the back) . . . the sacrifice, thanks to the sacrifice, may succeed, *svāhā !*"[2] The *Kāṭhaka* contains a series of homages to different breaths enumerated in an order a little different, *prāṇa*, *vyāna*, *apāna*, *samāna* and *udāna*.[3] Thus the following formula is twice repeated : "Protect my *prāṇa* and *apāna*, protect my *samāna* and *vyāna*, protect the two forms of my *udāna*".[4] The *Maitrā-*

[1] cf., V. Henry, *Livres X, XI et, XII* . . . p. 147.

[2] *āyur yajñéna kalpatām svāhā prāṇó yajñéna . . . apānó vyānó . . . udānó . . . samānó . . . cákṣur . . . śrótram . . . vāg . . . máno . . . ātmā . . . brahmā . . jyótir . . . svár . . . pṛṣṭhám . . . yajñó . . . yajñéna kalpatām svāhā||*—*VS.*, XXII, 33.

[3] . . . *prāṇāya námo . . . vyānāya . . . námo* in the midst of similar other formulae of homages addressed to numerous entities and diverse divinities—*Aśvamedha*, II, 1-5.

[4] *prāṇāpānau me pāhi samāna-vyānau me pāhi udānarūpe me pāhi.*—*Kāth.*, V, 5; VIII, 12.

yaṇī-saṁhitā also makes an invocation of each of the five *prāṇas* which recalls the one of the *Vājasaneyī-saṁhitā*: "For life *svāhā*! For *prāṇa* . . . . *apāna* . . . *vyāna*, *samāna*, *udāna* . . . the eye . . . the ear . . . the spirit . . . the speech . . . *svāhā*!"[1]

These litanies do not furnish any indications on the precise sense attached to each name. They present the series of five breaths with changes in the order of enumeration proving that the enumeration does not have an essential importance. The one of *Kāṭhaka* asking for protection for the breaths has for its pendent a similar formula but therein figure only *prāṇa*, *apāna* and *vyāna* and this formula is common to the *Vājasaneyī-saṁhitā* and the *Maitrāyaṇī-saṁhltā*[2] Similarly the formula of this latter Saṁhitā beginning with "For life . . ." is also found in a shorter form in the *Vājasaneyī-saṁhitā* : "For *prāṇa*, *svāhā*! For *apāna* . . . *vyāna* . . . the eye . . . the ear . . . the speech . . . the spirit, *svāhā*!"[3] This proves that the enumerations of three or five breaths are absolutely equivalent and that there is no ground for seeking to identify the three breaths with the phases of respiration, which one should not be tempted to establish when there are five of them. Besides *prāṇa* which itself alone designate the totality of organic breaths, the series also designate the same ensemble irrespective of the particular forms that are given and the five particular forms are quite clearly the same as the ones whose notion is preserved in classical medicine while developing the theory thereof.

We should also take note of the nature of entities arranged besides the breaths in the preceding litanies ; these are the organs or the psychic faculties or they refer to psychic activity. Now according to the physiology of the Āyurveda, the breaths are the agents or the motors of these faculties and of these organs in the body. It is not by accident that they are put side by side in the litanies of the *Yajurveda*. Moreover the speculation of the

---

1 *āyuṣe svāhā prāṇāya . . . cákṣuṣe . . . śrótrāya . . . mánase . . . vāćé svāhā*, —*Maitr.* —*s.*, III, 12, 9.

2 *prāṇám mé pāhi/apānám mé pāhi vyānám mé pāhi* . . . —*Vāj. S.* XIV, 8; *Maitr.*—*s.*, II, 8, 2.

3 *prāṇāya svāhāpānāya vyānāya svāhā cákṣuṣe svāhā* . . . , etc.—*Vāj.*—*s.*, XXII, 23. It can be seen that the suppression is preferably of the *udāna* and the *samāna*. When there are four breaths, it is *samāna* which is omitted, cf.; *Kāṭh.*, XXXIX, 3: XL, 5, where it is omitted. But others are also omitted, for example in *Vāj.*—*s* , I, 20 are mentioned only *prāṇa*, *udāna* and *vyāna*.

authors of the Brāhmaṇas and the Upaniṣads has given rise to numerous texts which give us an insight into relations conceived in ancient times between organic breaths and psychic phenomena, particularly sensorial ones. The "prāṇic", "pneumatic" nature of the *ātman*, of the soul is a major principle of Vedic philosophy. It is not, therefore, surprising that from the epoch of the *Yajurveda*, the organic breaths have been placed beside the elements of psychic activity. The medicine of Suśruta and Caraka, in explaining the psychic activity in terms of the interplay of the *prāṇas*, was once again following the organic tradition of Vedic antiquity.

One should therefore not be surpised in having to suppose, at an ancient date, a pneumatic concept of life, carrying the notion that breaths are found in the entire body and command the actions of the same. This is not attributing extremely advanced ideas to the Vedic times. The air coming out of the lungs during expiration is not the only breath of the body, it appertains to the upper part of the front part of the body, which contains others in the abdomen. The pains and the involuntary movements of the entrails are felt as being in evident relationship with the flatuosities which are independent of respiration. Many centuries were not needed, nor as Ewing believed, mystic speculations as intermediaries were necessary so that, knowing and naming inspiration and expiration, one should have noticed the existence of other breaths in the body. And from the time the breath in general had been, since an early date, assimilated with the wind, which latter had from the time of Indo-Iranian pre-history been conceived as the principle of activity, it was easy to conceive a system of pneumatic cosmo-physiology or to feel its existence. If the Vedic Saṁhitās do not themselves offer us a systematic explanation, which they need not have offered, they at least give us, in an already constituted form, the technical vocabulary which was, later on, to accompany the pneumatic theory in its period of full development. Under these conditions, when the intelligibility of Vedic formulae postulates the existence of at least a start of this pneumatic theory during the period of their composition, it is perfectly normal to accept the same.

One can, then, come back to the desperate conclusions of the exegetes who, envisaging only the speculations regarding inspiration and expiration, have declared that the interpretation of the lists of multiple *prāṇas* in ancient Vedic texts is impossible.[1] These exegetes had the tendency to see, in the use of the names of breaths which could not be brought back to those of respiration, a purely verbal and mechanical amplification, wherein primitively only the names of the air coming out of the lungs during expiration had figured as a matter of right. It will be more correct to see therein the first traces of physiological conceptions, very simple besides, but which have later dominated Indian medicine and also the mystical technique of the Yoga, based in part on the control of breaths.[2]

---

1 Ewing already quoted and Deussen on whom Macdonell and Keith (*Vedic Index*, see *prāṇa*) base themselves for saying: "The exact sense of each of these breaths when all are mentioned cannot be determined". Keith, in particular, is sure that the Brahmins understood nothing of what they themselves said of the five *prāṇas*: "The term *prāṇa* is subdivided into five elements among other divisions, and these five are obviously incapable of presenting any intelligble picture to the mind of the priests." (*The Religion and Philosophy of the Veda and Upaniṣads*, Cambridge, Mass., 1925, p. 484). Oldenberg has justly recognised the correlation existing between the nomenclature of the breaths in the Brāhmaṇas and in Medicine (*Die Weltanschauung der Brāhmana-text*, Gottingen, 1919, p. 66), but he has, on that occasion, gone back to the data of the Saṁhitās and has not directed his reflections to that subject, not having recognised the importance of the physiological concepts in the "pre-scientific science" (*Vorwissenschaftliche Wissenschaft*) which he was studying (cf., p. 67).

2 cf., *Les origines d'une technique mystique indienne*, in *Revue Philosophique*, April-June, 1946.

CHAPTER VI

VEDA AND ĀYURVEDA

We have, at first, summarised the data of classical Āyurveda as it is found in the form of already constituted classical doctrines in the schools of Caraka and Suśruta. We have thereafter analysed the medical notions found in the Vedic saṁhitās. We should now try to have a short estimate of these Vedic notions. We can, at the same time, seek to determine the exact position of the Āyurveda in relation to the Veda.

The comparison of the data of ancient Iran with that of the Veda has enabled us to recognise the antiquity of the speculations which were prevalent on both the sides and which were, later, to find a place at the base of the theories of classical Indian physiology. In fact cosmological speculations go back to the period of Indo-Iranian pre-history as they are found in the ancient texts of both India and Iran. They relate to the rôle of elements such as fire and water and to that of wind considered as one of the chief forces of nature. But the details of medical knowledge had, still, not been fixed in this period. The nosological nomenclatures of the Veda and of the *Avesta* are independent and do not share a common heritage.

During the period of the most ancient Vedic texts, between 1500 and 1000 B.C., appear numerous allusions to diseases, to remedies and to limbs of the body or to its constitutive elements. There is already a number of terms which will be found later in the medical texts, and the sense they have therein most of the time helps us to understand the ancient passages where they occur. But the names of explicable diseases refer to affections with evident manifestations and not to doctrinally individualised syndromes. This shows that during the Vedic period pathology, although possessing a rich nomenclature, was not yet scientifically developed. The therapeutics is magical or rudimentary and does not yet prescribe treatments conceived and applied following scientific theories, as will be the case with classical medical texts. These later texts have preserved, only in an extremely reduced measure, the heritage of this Vedic therapeutics.

Anatomy possesses an extremely ample vocabulary in the Veda, but quite a large number of terms in use are only metaphorical designations and all of them have not survived. Many of the internal organs are named, notably in the texts referring to the sacrifice of the horse. But the principal lists of anatomy are found in the hymns which establish similarities between the human or the animal body and the various parts of the universe, considered as the immense body of man or animal. A certain number of notions concerning the constitutive elements of the organism, which have been preserved in classical medicine, come from the Vedic tradition: that of organic sap, the *rasa;* that of the vital sap, seat of vigour, the *ojas;* that of bile conceived as liquid fire.

Vedic physiology is essentially based on the belief that multiple breaths circulate inside the organism. The concept of this circulation is associated with the existence of a system of internal canals. Both this concept and this notion will become fundamental in classical medicine. Already in the Veda the breaths have names which they will constantly have later on. When only two of them are named, they correspond either to inspiration and expiration or to the breath of the antiro-superior part of the body and to that of the postero-inferior part. When three, four or five breaths and sometimes more are named, they correspond to specialised diverse animal spirits whose functions have been specified by classical medicine.

Therefore Āyurveda has chiefly inherited from the physiological speculations and from the anatomical notions of the Veda. It has preserved a part of the nosological nomenclature but has almost entirely abandoned ancient therapeutics. It has thus drawn chiefly for doctrinal elements on Vedic speculations to establish its physiological theories, the one concerning the primordial rôle in the body of the wind of nature, and also the one concerning the rôle of water and fire, the latter being represented by bile. But the theory of three active elements of the organism which, on their equilibrium being disturbed or because of functional anomalies, become its three elements of trouble (*tridoṣa*), the wind, the phlegm and the bile, had not been constituted at the times of the Vedas themselves. In fact the notion of phlegm hardly prefigures in the *Atharvaveda* which limits itself to mentioning an oedomatous affection whose name will be, later on, used to designate occasionally the phlegm itself. It is only in a Brahmanic text, really ancient and going as far back as the first centuries after 1000 B.C., the *Śatapatha-Brāhmaṇa*, that the phlegm is named under one of its principal names, the *śleṣman*. But even here phlegm is not presented as an essential element of the organism.

Indian medicine has, therefore, drawn on the Veda even for the principal elements of its general doctrines. Thereby Āyurveda is the legitimate heir to the Veda, but it has developed to a large extent the patrimony thus received. It has coordinated and systematised ancient ideas and it has constituted an immense treasure of observations and experience, both concerning the diseases and the means of curing them. When we come across it for the first time in classical texts, it seems to us as if there is a chasm between the knowledge accumulated by it and the scanty medical notions which can be found in the ancient Vedic texts. The intermediary works, those where we could have seen the gradual constitution of the vast edifice which, all of a sudden, appears before us in an already achieved form, have not reached us. It is, therefore, all the more precious to measure the considerable depth of the Vedic soil to which go the basic roots of Āyurveda. It is also because of the necessity of a continuity between Vedic speculations and the classical doctrines of Āyurveda that we can affirm with certainty the existence of an intermediary tradition.

The legends of the origins of Āyurveda could not have, in this respect, fixed our judgement. They may take back its origins to the farthest antiquity and attribute the transmission of its teaching to Vedic personalities with known names, but we cannot follow them therein. They do not, as we have seen, inspire confidence. They cannot be taken to be based on authentic facts. Above all, they invoke arbitrary and tendentious geneologies whereby obscure families claim descent from illustrious stocks. They form a part of a system of similar legends concerning the origin of other sciences; therein they resemble more the products of a competition in a sort of nobiliary pride than the souvenirs of schools concerning their real history. At present we see, however, that these legends have not deceived us, at least concerning the essential fact emerging therefrom, namely, the existence of a continuous intermediary tradition between the speculations of Vedic times and the teachings of medicine in the specialised manuals.

It is true that one may ask oneself, whether their data, artificially combined, do not prove that a solution of continuity has been produced in this tradition. In fact, one may suppose that if medical ideas had been regularly transmitted since the Veda, the memory of the actual transmission could have been as well preserved as that of the teachings and could not have been replaced by legends. One may put forward the hypothesis that at first the medical ideas of Veda got fixed without giving rise to evolutionary developments and that the authors of medical systems that arose later, for example, under the Greek medicine, desiring to refer their new science to its antique traditions, have covered this science with Vedic reminiscences and have cooked up the history of a tradition fictive in reality. But such an hypothesis cannot be maintained and we will see that it is essential to look for other explanations because legends have replaced the real history of tradition.

It should be observed first of all that it is not only in the domain of medicine and of other sciences that India has legends in place of history. The desire for perpetuating lists of masters and disciples is attested frequently and in quite ancient times in Indian literatures. Sometimes even the circumstances of the transmission are indicated with a wealth of detail but not in a systematic manner. Evidently more constant attention has been paid to basic things than to the manner in which the ancestors had learnt them and every time it has been desired to establish the continuity of tradition it has been found necessary to reconstitute, with the aid of probability, the chain, all of whose links had not been preserved. This can be undoubtedly explained by the facts that the notions concerning the instruction received, being considered as accessory, were not put to heart with as much of care as the tenor of this instruction. Orally transmitted without the rigour observed in the study of fundamental texts which were, however, exactly learnt by rote, the traditions concerning instruction have got altered and sometimes got lost so as to be later restored by conjectures or by imitation of the parallel traditions claimed by other schools.

In any case, it is impossible that the legendary character of the teaching concerning the origins and the transmissions of instruction implies the non-existence of real transmissions or of long breaks in the traditions, because we see everywhere a legendary character and we cannot suppose everywhere the irreality of or the break in traditions; that means supposing a chasm between the entire culture of ancient India and the entire one of classical India.

In fact, whether we study the Brahmanic, Buddhist or Jaina texts or the scientific treatises, the *Dharmaśāstras* or the technical manuals, we always find legends replacing history we have been looking for. In the most favourable cases the legends are at least mixed with historical data. One should also note that it is in Brahminism, where the continuity of tradition is most certain, that the obscurity regarding the transmission of teachings is at its worst, whether because of the absence of information or because of the effect of legends. However, the old texts are available to us in their authentic form and in their archaic language. They could not have come to us without a continuous and uninterrupted tradition although this itself may have been forgotten. In the presence of this important fact, we must recognise that the legendary character of the data concerning the origins and the transmission of medicine is in conformity with Indian practice and in no way implies that the antiquity claimed for the origins is false and that the existence of a continuous transmission of teaching since antiquity is fictitious.

We have, besides, positive indices concerning the real existence of this continuous transmission and the progressive development of doctrines. A number of allusions and important pieces of evidence, in fact, cover the considerable space of time which separates the Vedic saṁhitās from the manuals of classical medicine.

First of all, there is at least one theory whose permanence can be observed by us and it is an essential theory, namely that of breaths. It appears constantly across the entire literature of Upaniṣads which goes in its origins to the Brāhmaṇas and comes right into the classical period. We have already seen references to breaths in the principal and the oldest Upaniṣads.

notably in the *Bṛhadāraṇyaka* which forms a part of the *Śatapathabrāhmaṇa*. In the more recent upaniṣads these references become more and more clear, and come nearer the final data of classical medicine.

In the *Bṛhadāraṇyaka*-and in the *Chāndogya*-the distinction of five breaths is clear (*Bṛh.*, III, 9, 26; *Chānd.*, III, 13, 1-5; V, 19-23) but it is not found alone, chiefly in the *Bṛhadāraṇyaka*. Sometimes three breaths are considered (*Bṛh.*, III, 1, 10; V, 14, 3; *Chānd.*, I, 3, 3), or four (*Bṛh.*, IV, 4, 1), or six (*Bṛh.*, I, 5, 4) or seven (*Bṛh.*, II, 2, 3); indeed ten (*Bṛh.*, III, 9, 4). Moreover, the precise doctrine of the localisation of five breaths is not formally enunciated therein. Several passages can be understood better on admitting that these localisations were already conceived as indicated in the classical doctrine but they are not described. On the contrary, later Upaniṣads clearly formulate the theory of five essential breaths with indications of their physiological rôle.

The *Maitrī*-, (II, 6) defines *prāṇa* as the breath which goes up *(ya ūrdhvam utkrāmati)*, *apāna* as the one which goes down *(yo'yam avāṅ saṁkrāmati)*, *vyāṇa* as the one which favours other breaths *(yena vā etā anugṛhītā)*, *samāna* as the one which sends the thickest element of nourishment into the *apāna*[1] and brings the minutest in each member *(yo'yam sthaviṣṭho dhātur annasyāpāne prāpayati aniṣṭho vānge'nge samānayati)* and *udāna* as the one which disgorges and swallows the drunk and the eaten *(yo'yam pītāśitam udgirati nigarati)*. These definitions denote a theory which differs in certain details from the classical theory, *vyāna* being simply given as the adjutant of the totality of other breaths and not as a principle of the movement of the body and the function of swallowing being attributed to *udāna*, whereas in the classical doctrine it has become *prāṇa*. This last difference, moreover, does not in the least indicate that classical theory had not been conceived at the time of the *Maitrī* because the *Chāndogya*, (I, 2, 9) had already taught that one ate and drank thanks to the *prāṇa* of the mouth *(mukhya)*. Therefore, it shows simply the existence of a view different from one that has become classical.

---

[1] *Apāna*, therefore, is not, in this text, the inhaled breath but the internal wind of the body, that of the excretion of the refuse of digestion, digestion rendered effective by *samāna*.

The *Praśna* (III, 5 ff) situates *apāna* in the anus and in the organs of generation, *prāṇa* in the eyes, ears, mouth and the nostrils, *samāna* having a digestive function, in the centre (of the body), *vyāna* in the canals and in one of them, *udāna* which loses here its physiological rôle to assume that of conducting the Self of man to its destinies after death.

In later Upaniṣads, particularly in those of the Yoga, references to the doctrine of five breaths are very frequent but are often later than in the texts of classical medicine; they do not have, therefore, as opposed to the earlier ones, much of interest to show this doctrine in an already constituted form between the period of the Veda and that of Āyurveda.

A chance reference in a grammatical text, which was pointed out to me by my *guru*, Jules Bloch, gives us another decisive proof for the history of the Ayurvedic doctrines in this very period. A *vārttika* of Kātyāyana on Pāṇini (V, 1, 38) mentions, in fact, in a number of examples concerning suffixes indicative of cause, the appeasement *(śamana)* and the excitement *(kopana)* of wind, bile, and phlegm *(vāta-pitta-śleṣman)* and their morbific coming together.[1]

This simple reference fully assures us that the pathological doctrine of the *tridoṣa*, whose elements, as we have seen, had not been gathered together in the period of the Vedic *saṁhitās*, as the mention of the phlegm does not appear before the *Śatapatha-brāmaṇa*, had been fully constituted in Kātyāyana's time. Kātyāyana is traditionally said to have lived under the Nandas, overthrown in 313 B.C. by Candragupta, and was therefore an author of the time of Alexander; this is in accord with the chronologies of other well-known grammarians, his predecessor, Pāṇini and his successor, Patañjali[2], although somewhat lower dates could also have been proposed.[3]

Under these conditions and although we do not possess the real medical texts of the period which elapsed between the *Śatapatha-brāhmaṇa* and Kātyāyana, we have to place in this period the definitive formation of the general doctrine of the

[1] Thus *vātika* designates that which appeases or excites the wind, *vāta*; *sannipātika* that which is caused by the reunion of the wind, bile and phlegm.

[2] cf., Max Müller, *A History of Ancient Literature*, repub. Allahabad, 1962, pp. 126-27.

[3] cf., L. Renou, *La Durghaṭavṛtti, Vol.* I, pt. 1, Paris, 1940, p. 23.

pathology of Āyurveda which we have later found to be common to all the great manuals of classical period.

A detailed study of the later Upaniṣads and the Vedic Sūtras will yield still more indirect proofs of the existence of great activity in the field of physiological speculations anterior to these great manuals and on which they have clearly drawn. We have, already, had the occasion to show elsewhere as to how the theories of Suśruta and Caraka on sleep and dreams and on the relation of the spirit with the heart could be related in part to concepts taught in this respect by older Upaniṣads like the *Bṛhadāraṇyaka* and comparable for most of the time to those of the Greeks.[1]

Lastly, another type of evidence comes from without to assure us the continuity and the activity of the Indian medical researches before their literary blossoming. The Greeks who were the contemporaries of Alexander have left this evidence for us.

It is true that their opinions are divided. Nearchos says that medicine has very little use in India, except against snake-bites, the sobriety of the inhabitants ensuring them freedom from disease and that the Sophists cure the diseases that are eventually caused by some divine help (Nearchos in Strabo, XV, 1, 45; Arrian, *Ind.*, XV, 12). Others say that the *Śramaṇas* call themselves doctors but are only magicians (Strabo, XV, 1, 70, where the *Śramaṇas* are 'Pramnai'). On the other hand Megasthenes talking of these very *Śramaṇas* indicates that the second rung in esteem after that of the ascetics who have retired to the forest is given to doctors by the population. Of these doctors he says that they make use more of diet-control than of medicines and that among the latter liniments and cataplasms are made use of more often; the rest appears to them to be more or less suspect of bad effects (Strabo, XV, 1, 60, where they are called 'Garmanes'). The same Megasthenes also talks in the same passage of the existence of the speculations on man and elsewhere of the existence of ideas analogous to those of Greeks relating to cosmology, to elements and attenuates the reproach made of Indians, of mixing too much of

[1] *Le sommeil et les rêves selon les médicins indiens et les physiologues grecs* in *Journ. de psychologie*, July-Sept. 1947, pp. 326 ff., specially pp. 329, 332, 337 and 342.

fiction with philosophy, by saying that Plato had done the same thing. On his side Onesicritos says that the Gymnosophists undertake much research concerning natural phenomena, the presages, the diseases (Strabo, XV, I, 65) and among the Musicanos, where he observes that the sciences are not cultivated, he notes that in this respect medicine is an exception.

We have certainly to reject opinions similar to those of Nearchos, the belief in the perpetual health of Indians being a proof of the insufficience of information. The evidence of Megasthenes who had lived for a long time in India as ambassador and not for a short period as a conqueror is necessarily more competent and is to be accepted as it is in full accord with all the Indian data.

In other points of information furnished by Megasthenes we have got an indirect proof of the activity of medical research in India from the end of the 4th century B.C., because Megasthenes tells us how the diseases of elephants were treated and we see thereby that a secondary branch of medicine, that of the veterinary art of elephants had already assumed a physiognomy which we find it to possess in later texts of elephantology, particularly in the *Āyurveda of Elephants, the Hastyāyurveda* attributed to Muni Pālakāpya. In fact we have already had an occasion to show that the prescriptions indicated by Megasthenes were in conformity with those of this Āyurveda.[1]

We are, therefore, very well assured by the data of the Indian texts corroborated by foreign sources, that Indian medicine, during the seven or eight centuries preceding the Christian era, had never ceased to be actively cultivated and directed towards the definitive constitution of its doctrines; this is when the great classical texts have appeared. The loss of earlier works should be attributed to the exclusive authority acquired by these latter and possibly as we have seen, due to the contempt felt by certain Vedic circles concerning the doctors, in spite of the general opinion which had been favourable to them.

We thus reach the conclusion that classical Indian medicine which is found in a fully constituted form in the didactic

---

[1] *Les gajaśāstra et les auteurs grecs, JA*, 1933, pp. 163 ff.

manuals belonging to the environs of the Christian era, has its essential bases (doctrines of wind and of the breaths, of the fiery nature of bile, etc.) in the ancient Vedic texts, anterior to the formation of the Greek science, but that it has been elaborated and constituted as a system during the period of the efflorescence of Greek science and parallel to it. We have now to examine the analogies and the eventual relationship the two could have had.

CHAPTER SEVEN

THE AYURVEDIC THEORY OF THE WIND AND GREEK PNEUMATISM

THE texts whereby the three oldest Indian manuals of medicine teach that all motor activity inside the organism comes from an internal organic breath identical to the atmospherical wind are in close accord amongst themselves. On this point the doctrine of Āyurveda is particularly clear and definite. A similar physiological concept of the wind also exists in Greek medicine, although it is not equally clearly admitted there. A. Götze has observed that the Hippocratic text *Peri Phuson* (The Winds), makes one think of the great rôle played by the concept of breath in Indian thought of the period of the Brāhmaṇas and he had no doubt that the Greek work had been under oriental influence.[1] The question of this influence can be definitely decided by a simple *rapprochement* but the analogy noted by Götze is evident[1] and the *Peri Phuson* concords even with those of the texts of classical medicine, particularly with those which are said to belong to the school of Ātreya Punarvasu.

Of the two texts which claim to report the very words of Ātreya concerning the wind, the more important is of the *Caraka-saṁhitā*. The one of the *Bhela-saṁhitā* which has reached us in a single manuscript is, at places, considerably altered. This comparison, nevertheless, suffices to show that the ideas presented on either side go back to a common source older than both the texts. The *Suśruta-saṁhitā* usefully completes in details the enunciations of Caraka and Bhela.

CARAKA, SUTRASTHANA, XII[2]

[1] "We are now going to explain the chapter relating to

---

1 *Persische Weisheit in griechischem Gewande*, in *Zeit. fur. Ind. und Ir.*, II, 1903, pp. 84-5. Similarly, although more doubtfully, A.B. Keith, *The Religion and Philosophy of the Veda and Upaniṣads*, in *Harvard Or. Ser.*, Vol. XXXII, Cambridge (Mass.) 1925, p. 602

The editions referred to are abbreviated as follows:

functions and disorders[1] of the Wind". [2], says the blessed Ātreya. [3] *Conference of Ṛṣis:* Desirous of knowing the opinions of one another regarding the knowledge of the functions and disorders of the wind, the great *ṛṣis* sat together and asked one another, "Which property has the wind? What excites

N.=Narendranath Śāstrin, Lahore, 1929, with Vyākhyā (*Ayurveda-dīpikā*) of Cakrapāṇidatta (Cakr.);

J.=Jivananda Vidyasagara, Calcutta, 1896;

Ś.=Śaṁkara Sāstrin, Bombay, no date;

K.=Khemraj Srīkṛṣṇadāsa, Bombay, 1898, with Hindi translation by Pandit Mihiracandra;

H.=Harinath Sarkar, Calcutta, no date(*towards* 1880),with the Vyākhyā of Cakrapāṇidatta almost rigourously identical with that of N. of which it can be the model;

G1.=Gaṅgādhara with the Vyākhyā (*Jalpa-kalpataru*) of the same, Calcutta, 1868-1871, or G2; re-edited by Narendranath Sengupta and Balaicandra Sengupta, Calcutta, 1928; the text of Gaṅgādhara and that of more or less similar editions is without any authority with regard to the text commented by Cakrapāṇidatta, in view of arbitrary corrections and modifications, cf., Hoernle, *Osteology*, p. 21 (which wrongly indicates the edition of 1879 as the first edn. of Gaṅgādhara, but the one of 1868-71, indicated above does not seem to have been complete; in my copy it has 1,200 pages and ends in course of the XVIIIth Adhyāya of the *Sūtrasthāna*). Hoernle is mistaken in affirming that Ś. is a mere reproduction of G., but it follows G. quite closely.

Manuscript: *M. Bibl. Nat. Sanskrit*, 1304, copy of a manuscript in Śārada script kept in the Deccan College written by Cordier on a copy of J. The indications in italics are added by us. Cakr. stands for Cakrapāṇidatta's commentary.

1 According to Cakr., *Kalā-guṇa*' "property, chiefly favourable, quality", or *aṁśa* "portion". The second sense cannot be accepted; it cannot refer to "portions and non-portions of the wind", although Gaṅgādhara has understood it in this manner *(vātasyāṁśāmyorjñānaṁ)* unless it be said to refer to the minute details concerning the wind or the diverse points of the doctrine of the wind. The former sense is found elsewhere in Caraka and is derived from that of portion, Sūtr., X. 3: *catuṣpadaṁ ṣoḍaṣakalaṁ bheṣajamiti bhiṣajo bhāṣante/yaduktaṁ pūrvādhyāye ṣoḍaṣaguṇamiti tadbheṣajaṁ*, "Medicine has four feet and sixteen parts", say the doctors; that which has been said in the preceding Chapter (XI, 9): "possessing sixteen qualities, that is medicine". Wherefrom *kalā-guṇa* (Cakr.), in the sense that the parts referred to here are qualities; four of medicine (instruction, etc.), four of drugs (efficacity, etc.) four of the compounder (ability of preparing the drugs, etc.) and four of the patient (memory, obedience for prescriptions, etc.) One can, therefore, translate "qualities and defects of the wind", or "that which the wind has or does not have as qualities". But *kalā* also denotes the arts and techniques (ordinarily said to number 64, which is 4^3 when 16 is 4^2; *kalā* is habitually in relation with the number 16, the *kalā* or the divisions of the lunar disc are 16 in number, the year has 16 parts, *Bṛh.-up.*, I, 5, 14; similarly the man, *Chānd.-up.* VI, 7, 1; *Praśnopa.*, VI, 1, 6). It can also refer to that which is done by the wind or that which is not done by the wind, or does the wrong way, of its normal and abnormal functions, therefore the translation given above, which fits better than the other ones is possible in the real context of the chapter.

it? or which are the objects that calm it? And how, without having got it, that which lacks both consistency and stability, is it excited by the exciters or calmed by the sedatives? And which are its own actions that it, excited or not, circulates or does not circulate in the body, at the moment when it circulates in the body or outside the body?" [4] *Characteristics of the Wind:* Thereupon Kuśa, of the family of Sāṅkṛtya, said: light, cold, violent, sharp, inconsistent to touch, these are the six properties of the wind.[1] [5] *Exciters of the Wind:* As soon as he heard these words, Kumāraśiras Bharadvāja said: "It is just as the gentleman has observed. These are the properties of the wind; now, the wind is made excited by actions having similar properties and exercised by the drugs of the same type and the virtues of the same kind, because the means of reinforcing the elements are the putting into play of corresponding properties." [6] *Sedatives of Wind:* As soon as he heard these words, the doctor from Bactria, Kāṅkāyana[2] said: "It is just as has been observed by the gentleman. These are the things that excite the wind. Thereafter, the contrary ones are the sedatives of the wind, because the antagonist of the exciter is the means of calming the elements". [7] *Mode of Action of the Exciters and the Sedatives:* As soon as he heard these words, Badiśa Dhāmārgava said: "It is exactly as has been described by the gentleman. These are the sedatives of the excitation of the wind. Also, we are going to explain the way, in which attaining the wind[3], which lacks both consistency and stability, the exciters and the sedatives, excite it or calm it. The exciters of the wind are, in truth, things which produce for the organism the bitter, the light, the cold, the violent, the sharp, the inconsistent and the hollow. The wind, having taken up residence in such and such an organism, growing, gets excited.

---

1 cf., below, (7) where another *ṛṣi* enumerates seven of them. cf. Suśr., *Nid.*, 1, 6, *infra*.

2 That is to say, "of the line of the Sogdians", cf., *supra*, p. 38.

3 Gaṅgādhara and others who have followed him, have changed "in reaching it" into "without reaching it" to reproduce the expression used in [3]. The correction is useless as one feels that at the beginning of the conference [3] one might have supposed that the wind could not be reached, because of its inconsistent character, but once the action on similar or opposite properties having been admitted [6] it might have been thought that it could be reached, wherefrom the change of expression.

The sedatives of the wind are things which produce for the organisms the unctuous, the heavy, the hot, the smooth, the slimy and the sticky. The wind installing itself, circulating in such and such an organism, he is made calm". [8a] *Functions of the Wind:* As soon as he had heard the right statement of Badiśa, approved by all the *ṛṣis*, the royal sage Vāryovida[1] said: "Without any doubt it is exactly as has been stated by the gentleman and, in truth, after having adored the wind, we will explain, to the best of our ability, proving by means of observation, inference and comparison[2], the functions of the wind, excited or not, which circulates or does not circulate in the body, at the moment when it circulates in the body or outside the same. *Nature of the Wind:* The wind is the support of that which retains the chain[3], it consists of the breath of the front, of the upward breath, of concentrated breath, of diffused breath, and of low breath. *Physiological Functions:* It promotes movements of all types, it puts brakes on the wind and also guides it[4], this puts in action all the faculties, it is the conveyor of objects of all the faculties, the distributor of all the elements of the organism, which brings about the coherence of the body, it is the promoter of speech, is the matter[5] of contact and of sound, the basis of the power of hearing and of touch, the source of joy and of liveliness, the kindler of fire, the drier of the elements of trouble[6], the expulser of impurities, the

---

1 Or Vāyorvida, "One knowing the wind", *lectio facilior* which differs from the preceding one by the displacement of only the *repha* written over the syllable *yo* to the syllable *vi*. The aberrant reading of M denotes "knower of that which has reference to the three properties" (of Nature according to the Sāṁkhya philosophy).

2 The three measures-criteria *(pramāṇas)* enumerated are those which are habitually recognised in the Nyāya philosophy, minus the revealed word *(śabda)*, not considered here, except in Ś, which adds its equivalent, the teaching *(upadeśa)*. The reading of M and that of the variant indicated by H, which comprise observation, inference and teaching correspond to the theory of Sāṁkhya. The text has, therefore, been modified respectively by the advocates of Nyāya and Sāṁkhya.

3 The chain (of weaving) is the body (Cakr.: *tantram śarīram*), that which supports the chain corresponds to the joints (Cakr.: *sandhi*). One may, thus, understand *tantrayantra* as the "machine of the body".

4 Cakr. explains: "the one which puts brakes on the mind, which puts itself movement when the object is not desired and is the guide of the mind when the object is desired."

5 Cakr.: *prakṛti kāraṇaṁ*, "*prakṛti*—instrumental cause."

6 Cakr.: *doṣasaṁśoṣaṇaḥ—śarīrakleda-saṁśoṣaṇaḥ*, "drier of the *doṣas*—drier of the humours of the body".

border of the thick and fine canals, the maker of embryos.[1] It becomes the determining cause of the prolongation of life when it is not excited. [8b] *Pathological Functions:* But when, in truth, it is excited in the body, it inflicts on the body all sorts of derangements to the detriment of the forces of colour, of well-being and longevity. It puts in tumult[2] the mind, attacks all the faculties, throws down the embryos, provokes malformation, makes it go on for too long a time, engenders fright, chagrin, bewilderment, sadness, loquacity and blocks the breaths. [8c] *Normal Cosmic Functions:* Of the one which is in its natural state, the functions, when it circulates in the world, are, in truth, the following, i.e., the support of the earth[3], the flaming up of the fire[4], the regulation of the continuous course of the sun, of the moon and of the totality of the stars and the planets, the formation of clouds[5], the emission of waters, the putting into movement of the course of water, the production of flowers and fruits, the piercing of that which pierces, the division of the seasons, of the elements, the determination of the quantity and the aspect of elements[6], the elaboration of grain[7], the growth of cereals, the dryness and the secondary drying up[8] and the tranformation of that which is not transformed. [8d] *Perturbing Cosmic Functions:* Of the one that is excited, the functions, when it circulates in the

---

[1] Cakr.: *bhettā karttaitacca śarīrotpatti-kāle,* "borer, maker and that at the moment of body-formation".

[2] Or variant, *vyāvarttayati,* "it throws upside down".

[3] *lit.,* "of the one that supports". The use of expressions of this type is the mark of a certain *finesse.*

[4] *lit.,* "of the flaming one".

[5] K.: "of the intelligences", bad reading due to the easy confusion between *gha* and *dha* in Nāgarī.

[6] Cakr.: *mānaṁ parimāṇaṁ saṁsthānaṁ ākṛtis tayor vyaktir abhivyaktiḥ kāraṇamiti yāvat,* "*mānam* is the quantity; *saṁsthānam,* the aspect; of these two it is the *vyakti,* the manifestation, i.e., the instrumental cause."

[7] Cakr.: *abhisaṁskāro'ṅkura-jananaśaktiḥ,* "*abhisaṁskāra,* the germinative power".

[8] Ś. K:, the drying of humidity; M.G.: the drying of the dry one (commentary of G.: drying of things which are a little humid, *vikledahīnānāṁ upaśoṣaṇaṁ*). Cakr.: *avikledaḥ pākakālādarvāg aviklinnatvaṁ upaśoṣaṇaṁ ca pākena yavādīnām, ārdrānām eva vikledopaśoṣaṇam,* "*avikleda,* absence of humidity before the movement of maturity and *upaśoṣaṇam,* secondary drying up because of the maturity of the humidity of unripe barley, etc." One should thus understand that it is the cause of the general drying up and of the drying up of the ripening cereals.

worlds, are, in sooth, the following, i.e., the levelling up of the summits of the mountains, the uprooting of trees, the overflowing of the oceans, the rising of the lakes, the pushing back of the courses of water, the trembling of the earth, the swelling of the clouds, the production of the mist, of thunder, of dust, of sand, of fish, of frogs, of serpents, of caustics, of blood, of stones, and of lightning[1], the destruction of six seasons, the clearing[2] of cereals, the calamities[3] for beings, the complete destruction of existences, the production of clouds, of the sun, of fire and of the wind which bring to an end the four *yugas* of the world. [8e] *Divine Nature of the Wind:* It is the blessed and the imperishable source of beings[4], the author of the existence and non-existence, the ordinator of well-being and of troubles, the death, Yama[5], the tamer, the Lord of creatures, Aditi[6], the one which does everything, the one that has all the forms, the one that goes everywhere, the director of all the concatenatious, the atom between existences, penetrating Viṣṇu, who trsaverses the worlds; yes, the wind is the Blessed one". [9] *Objection:* Having heard Vāryovida, Mārīci said: "Even though it is so, what is the relationship of this notion, either for the expression or for the doctrine, with the science of the medical man or whether this doctrine, which has just now been stated, does really concern the science of the medical-man".[7] [10] *The Medical and General Interest of the Doctrine:* Vāryovida replied, "The medical-man, does not consider that the wind possesses an extreme force, has an extreme violence, that it acts very promptly and brooks no delay when it is forcefully excited, what precautions he will

1 Cakr. does not comment upon the expressions between "thunder" and "lightning", probably because he did not think them to be subject to confusion but, since they constitute an hetroclite enumeration inserted accidentally between "thunder" and "lightning" they appear to have been interpolated after the editing of the commentary of Cakr., M. adds "thunder".

2 Cakr.: *asaṅghāto 'nutpādo 'nupacayo vā, "assaṁghāta*, non-production and non-abundance". *Saṁghāta* is, properly speaking, density.

3 Cakr.: *upasargo mārakādiprādurbhāvaḥ, "upasarga*, appearance of pests, etc".

4 Or, "of the elements"; cf., Gayadāsa on Suśr., *Nid.*, 1, 6, *infra.*

5 The god of death.

6 The Vedic goddess "without links".

7 M., Ś., G.: "Is it made in consideration of the science of the medical man?"

take, having prepared himself thoroughly, to protect from the very beginning, to forestall, fearing loss of time. The praise of the wind made in this sense is, besides, worthwhile for health, for increasing the forces and for good mien, for the acme of extreme longevity. [11] *Physiological Rôle of the Fire*: Mārīci said: "It is fire which, inside the organism, incorporated into bile[1], excited or not, renders things good or bad, i.e., digestion, absence of digestion, vision, absence of vision, measure of and its lack as regards warmth, and colour of the normal state and that of the abnormal one, heroism and pusillanimity, anger, joy, aberration, serenity and other pairs (of the opposite) beginning with these ones." [12] *Physiological Role of the Aqueous Element:* Having heard the words of Mārīci, Kāpya said, "It is Soma which, in the organism, incorporated into phlegm, excited or not, renders things good or bad, i.e., firmness, laxity, plethora, thinness, softness, virility, powerlessness, knowledge, ignorance, consciousness, aberration and other pairs (of the opposites) beginning with these ones." [13] *Synthetical Conclusion of Ātreya:* Having heard the remarks of Kāpya, the blessed Punarvasu Ātreya said, "All of you, gentlemen, have said the right thing except that your remarks have been exclusive. All, in sooth, the wind, the bile and phlegm, in normal state, make man, with his faculties intact, full of vigour, good mien and in

1 Cakr.: *pittāntaragata iti vacanena śārīre jvālādi yuktavahniniṣedhena pittoṣmarūpasya vahneḥ sadbhāvaṁ darṣayati na tu pittādabhedaṁ pittenāgnimāndyasya grahaṇyādhyaye vakṣyamāṇatvāt tathā pitta-harasya sarpiṣo'gni-vardhanatvenoktavāt.* "By the expression, 'incorporated in the bile', is specified the real nature of fire in the body in the form of bile and heat, as it is impossible that fire in the body may have flames, etc., but it is distinguished from bile by the fact that in the chapter on chronic diarrhoea mention is made of a reduction of fire by bile and also following what is said about [medicine with the base of] ghee which destroys bile by increasing the fire". The first passage which thus puts fire and bile in antagonism is *Cik.*, XV, 63 (in Ś.: XIX, 63): *pittaṁ...agnim āplāvayat hanti jalaṁ taptam ivānalam*, "the bile... inundating the (digestive) fire destroys it as hot water destroys fire". But this implies that if bile is not fire, it is like hot water and therefore it contains an igneous element. The second passage is *Cik.*, XV, 196: *parīkṣyāmaṃ śarīrasya dīpanaṁ snehasaṁyutaṁ/dīpanaṁ bahupittasya tiktaṁ madhura-saṁyutam*, "Having observed the crudeness (absence of digestion by cooking) of the body, an enflaming (medicine) containing (some) fat (is beneficial), if the body has much of bile, the (beneficial) enflaming (medicine) is one having the pungent along with the sweet one." The two passages belong to the latter part of *Caraka-saṁhitā*, added by Dṛḍhabala.

good health; thus he manages to live a long life, just as morals, interests and pleasures, rightly practised make man attain the utmost happiness in this world. But rendered abnormal, they take him into the abyss of adversity, just as three seasons, rendered abnormal, lead the world to calamity during their respective periods." [14] *Conclusion:* All the *ṛṣis* approved this discourse of the blessed Ātreya, and were glad thereof.[1] [15] And there is (a verse) on this subject: "Hearing this discourse of Ātreya, all approved (it), and the *ṛṣis* were glad like gods hearing the words of Indra". [16] Verse on the above: *Résumé:* The six properties, the cause of two types[2], the multiple function, that which also appertains to the wind, the quadruple[3] function respectively that of phlegm and of bile, [17] the opinion which is of the great *ṛṣis* and that of Punarvasu all this, a propos of the functions and disorders of the wind, has been presented.

COLOPHON:—In the manual of Agniveśa, re-edited by Caraka, in the section of verses[4], the twelfth chapter, entitled, "Functions and Disorders of the Wind", is finished.

The discussion of the *ṛṣis* gathered together shows clearly the various tendencies which have dominated the ancient physio-cosmological speculations of Indians and whose classical theory is the synthesis summarised by Ātreya. He attributed the main rôle in the organism to an unique element, wind, fire or water, the last one of these, water, is represented here by soma, the cosmic liquid *par excellence.* This inevitably recalls the attitude of the Ionian Physiologists seeking the primordial element and finding the same, Thales in water, Anaximenes in air or Heraclitus in fire. In all the cases, the effort aims at supplying a purely physical explanation of the universe and of

---

1 This final formula reminds us of the one which regularly ends the Buddhist Sūtras, "Thus spake the Blessed one; satisfied the... (listeners) were glad of the Blessed one":

idam avocad bhagavān āttamanāḥ te
...bhagavato bhāṣitaṁ abhinandanniti;
in Pāli; idaṁ avoca bhagavā, attamanā te
...bhagavato bhāsitaṁ abhinandun ti.

2 Cakr.: *dvividho heturiti vātaprakopahetur vātapraśamahetuḥ*, "Cause of two types, cause of the excitation of the wind, cause of the calming down of the wind".

3 Quadruple, because it differs according as it is in the body or in the world and whether it is excited or not.

4 Or *Sūtrasthāna*, "section of the sūtras" (*lit.*, place of the Sūtras).

the organism, both conceived as having the same nature. In the opinion of Vāryovida, where wind is assimilated to an entire series of gods, indeed to the Blessed One, to the supreme God, the point of view cannot be held to be mystic, in spite of the protests of Mārīci who feels that the assimilation of the wind to the gods comes out of the framework of speculations that are really medical. The Indian gods in question are not really supernatural beings, powers which freely govern Nature by placing themselves above it. They are included in it; they are eminent therein, but only as participants. Besides, the wind, as it is described by Vāryovida, is nothing but the material element known as such, and when Vāryovida identifies it with the gods, he does not substitute the natural notion of the wind with a mystic representation but, on the contrary, he furnishes a materialistic interpretation of the being of the gods and aims to be fully rational, but not entirely concrete. Our text does not describe in detail the physical action of the breath inside the organism. The *ṛṣis* who discuss the wind or breath judge that it is, in each movement or change, the activating force, but do not see in each case the mode of action of this force. Their conceptions were too vague to be able to concretise themselves as physical representations and a deepened observation would have destroyed them immediately instead of making them more precise. In any case, the consideration of the properties enabled them to materially render the account of the action of wind in the organism without any necessity of having to make it physically precise. From the fact that breath entered the organism, it followed that it introduced therein its properties. When calm it put them to work in normal manner: excited, it disurbed the organism by means of their excesses as also by its own mechanical action. One could, therefore, without having to specify the concrete process of the latter, understand its normal or disturbing functions by referring them to the play of its properties in an abstract manner.

The corresponding text of Suśruta will give us more details on the pneumatic pathology of Āyurveda. But beforehand, the comparison of the text of Bhela, thought to have integrally reproduced the teaching of Ātreya, like that of Caraka, will enable us to go back to the doctrine in the state which constituted the common fund of the teachings of Bhela and Caraka.

BHELA, SUTRASTHANA, XVI[1]

[1] "We will now explain all that relates to the functions and the disorders of the wind," says the blessed Ātreya.[2] [2] "Which is the chief element of trouble, and the least important one?[3]", one asks. Having saluted Ātreya the black, the great *ṛṣis* gave a discourse. [3] *Physiological Functions of the Wind:* Someone has said concerning the same, the main effect: As long as the wind subsists which decomposes[4] nourishment, man lives. [4] It is the wind which, in sooth, causes the semen to fall in the woman. The wind decomposes the menstrual blood of the woman. Because of the wind woman becomes sterile. [5] Neither men nor women are sterile (by nature): either, in the receptacle, the wind is cold and has dried the sperm, [6] or the wind has diminished the sperm and the sperm is suppressed by the wind. All that is seen, blinked and moved, [7] and the diseases of the black (?), in women, it is assuredly thus that they occur. It is because of the wind that the hunchbacked, the crippled, the lame and persons suffering from lumbago, [8] as also those having atrophied limbs or having limbs in excess exist, along with others of the same type. *Cosmic Functions of the Wind:* The inertia of animated beings and the silences of the rivers[5], [9] the quaking of the earth also, is due to the

[1] This text is known through an unique manuscript (Tanjore, No. 10773 of Burnell, become No. 11085 of the catalogue of P.P.L. Sastri, Srirangam, 1933, p. 7410). The transcription of this manuscript has been edited by Asutosh Mukerjee, University of Calcutta, *Journal of the Department of Letters*, Vol. VI, Calcutta, 1921, pp. 26-8 (for this passage). This edition is called E, it gives within brackets the conjectural readings to restore the text, proposed by Ananta Krishna Shastri. They are reproduced here with the sign, *conj.* or *E. conj.* A certain number among them accords with the readings of N. (below) but are less suitable. Three other transcriptions of the same are found in the Cordier collection of the Bibliotheque Nationale: Sanskrit 1183, copy in Nāgarī of Pt. C. Krishnayya, p. 19., l. 1. to 20, l. 1, 6 (N.) *Sanskrit* 1183, copy Telinga; p. 43, l. 5 to 46, l. 8 (T); *Sanskrit*, 1184, Latin transcription in the hand of Cordier not used here because copied from the preceding two.

[2] Reproduces 1 and 2 of Caraka.

[3] E : this is an element of trouble which [in its] least [state] surpasses a hundred.

[4] Literally, "destroyed", that is to say, decomposed, which is a way of representing digestion.

[5] E.: "The inertia of animated beings, sudden and fixed", The conjuncture causing to disappear the mention of rivers is not necessary, because

wind. Steam is produced under the influence of the wind, from steam is born the cloud, [10] from the cloud escapes water from where are born the germs; or the thunder issues therefrom(?). One must know that the force of the group of stars and that of lightning comes from the wind. Thanks to wind, the fire, the husband of the holy oblations, burns. [12] Because of the wind the rivers flow and reach the earth. *Divine Nature of the Wind:* The semen spread in the matrix is affected by the wind of properties. It can destroy bile[1] and phlegm. With[2] one of them, the wind, excited, disperses itself in the body. *Varieties of Organic Breath:* Thus are distinguished the diffused breath, the breath on high, the concentrated breath, [15] the breath below and the breath of the front, according to its multiple specialisations in corporeal beings. The diffused breath, which ensures its own horizontal extension, regularises the breath on high, [16] the breath of the front ensures the placement of the breath below but starts, among corporeal beings[3], the raising of the concentrated breath. It holds also under its dependence, [17] the faculties, the spirit and the soul of the beings, of the corporeal beings. Considered as special, another wind is called "breath below".[4] [18] Drying and marching, and also thought to be without feet, the wind is said to be the principal element among the five elements. [19] These four are linked with the wind; the wind is everywhere, always. From the wind results the emission of the wind, of the sperm and of the excrements, [20] and it is from the cooking of that which

the action of the wind on the rivers is mentioned a little farther (12) and in Caraka, 8d. The silent rivers are a sort of pendant to inert beings. The wind, the force producing noise and movement, stops them when it suspends its action.

1 E.: empoisoned bile.

2 *ādāya* of the following verse, replaced in E. according to an unlikely conjecture, by *āhāra*, "nourishment", which will oblige us to understand that the wind is excited by nourishment. This interpretation is possible but it will oblige us to make *anyataram* as a complement of *hanyād* and to supply "or" after "bile and phlegm". The case envisaged by the text as it is presented here is the one where the wind is associated with bile or phlegm, a frequent case according to the classical doctrine.

3 According to the reading in E.; "puts the corporeal being into action".

4 Following another theory one should, undoubtedly, understand that *apāna* (moreover often opposed alone to *prāṇa* in Vedic texts) is considered as a type of wind distinct from *prāṇa* and possessing an autonomy equal to that of *prāṇa*.

is eaten that results the function of the breath below[1]; this is what is taught. The breath of the front comforts the elements; it is considered that the breath of the front is life. [21] The diffused breath is, in the body[2], the movement and the closing and opening of eyelids. That which, besides, in a creature, goes on high is that which is moved by the breath on high [22] [which produces[3]] sneezing, hiccough, cough, sigh and speech.[4] That which swells the rectum and the body in all the ways, [23] the wind which is held therein is called "breath below". For such reasons and for others which make us see the reality, we will characterize in the corporeal being the wind to be the main element." Thus spake the blessed Āterya.

COLOPHON:—In Bhela, sixteenth chapter.

This passage of Bhela differs externally, in so far as length and presentation are concerned, from the corresponding chapter of Caraka as the latter is in the form of a dialogue in prose and the former a much briefer enunciation in verse. These differences, however, cannot suffice to weaken the tradition which says that both Bhela and Agniveśa have preserved in their texts the teachings received from Ātreya. These differences could be due to the intervention of Caraka who revised the book of Agniveśa. Moreover two versions of the same course by different listeners can considerably differ from each other. The fact that the names of the traditional masters of Āyurveda, such as Ātreya, Agniveśa and Caraka are suspected of being more legendary than historical, does not prevent the two texts from agreeing as regards the basic part of the pneumatic doctrine presented by them as having been taught or approved by Ātreya. If it is not at all sure but only possible that the inven-

1 According to the graphically plausible correction of E. conj.: "it is the cooking of that which is eaten, that is the function of the breath below". This sense, in any case, will not be in accord with the ordinary doctrine according to which it is *samāna* which kindles the digestive fire cooking the aliments, whereas *apāna* ensures the expulsion of the excreta as has exactly been said here. It will, therefore, be better to translate the text without correcting it and to understand that it is the cooking of the aliments which gives rise to excretary function of the *apāna*, because it is the cooking which produces the excreta, thus furnishing the matter on which *apāna* exerts itself.

2 E.: the movement of the body.

3 A verb is supposed by the accusatives, or they should be corrected as nominatives.

4 E. conj.: the syncope.

tor of this doctrine should have been really called Ātreya, is it not at least doubtful that it had existed at a time before the composition of the Saṁhitās of Bhela and Caraka? The considerable differences in editing which appear when the two texts are compared prove precisely that neither of them can be considered as an imitation of the other and that the general concordance between their teachings must be due to a common source of inspiration. We find definitely in both Bhela and Caraka, the notion of the identity of the atmospheric wind as also of the organic breath which, whether in nature or in the body, is the cause of all the activities, the divine cause, but whose divinity consists in its material power of being the element of nature.

The text of Suśruta which follows, again develops and with more details, the same theory although according to tradition, it does not belong to the same school. This pertains to the origin, according to the common appearance, of the two great schools of Āyurveda and guarantees thereby the antiquity of the theory which necessarily pre-existed in its diverse but concordant expressions.

SUSRUTA, NIDANASTHANA, I[1]

[1] We will now explain the etiology of the diseases of the wind.[2] [2] Suśruta questioned Dhanvantari, the best of those

[1] This text has been established following the texts mentioned hereunder: Madhusūdangupta, Calcutta, 1835 (M.).

Jivananda Vidyāsāgara, 3rd. edn. Calcutta, 1889 (J.).

Kālīprasanna Kaviśekhara, Calcutta, 1898, in Bengali script (K.) with the commentary of Dalhaṇa (DK.) and Bengali translation; Yādavaśarman (Jadavji Trikamji), 2nd. edn. Bombay, 1931 (Y.) with the commentary of Dalhaṇa (DY.).

The commentary of Dalhaṇa (D.), the *Nibandhasaṁgraha*, is quoted following the preceding editions as also the separate edition of Jivananda Vidyasagara. 3rd. edn., Calcutta, 1891 (DJ.).

The Nyāyacandrikā of Gayadāsa has been preferred and for the same the MSS. of the Cordier Collection, copied from the MSS. of Bikaner Library '(No. 1762) by Umeshcandra Gupta, *Bibl. Nat. Sanskrit,* 1177, p. 1-37.(G.)

G. gives variations noted here as G. var. A number of the explanations of Dalhaṇa are taken from Gayadāsa; that is why the latter, an early commentator, has been followed before Dalhaṇa. The verses are numbered only in J. and Y., Y. adding a second phrase after the first one of introduction, his numbering thus differs by one from that of J. In K. the numbering is by group of the verses of the beginning.

[2] Y. adds: thus says the blessed Dhanvantari.

who supported the Order, born with ambrosia[1], after having saluted his feet. [3] "O, the best among those who talk, tell me the localisation, the function and the ills of the wind in a natural state and disturbed by excitants". [4] Having heard his discourse, the best of the doctors replied: *General Theory of the Wind:* "The Being existing by himself, that Blessed one is, it is said, the wind. [5] Since it depends only on itself, existed perpetually and also because it goes everywhere, it is for all the objects the universal soul to whom the entire world renders homage.[2] [6] It is he, the efficient cause of the beings[3], in their conservation, their birth and their destruction. Not manifest but with its action manifest[4], it is sharp, cold, bitter.[5] [7] It goes horizontally, has two properties[6], and lots of passion.[7] Its power is inconceivable, it is the conductor of the elements of trouble[8], it shines among the multitude of ills.[9] [8] It acts promptly, circulates constantly. It has its seat in the intestines and in the rectum. Teach me its characteristics when it circu-

1 Reference to the legend which places the birth of Dhanvantari incarnated here in the king Divodāsa, in the churning of the ocean which also produced ambrosia.

2 J., Var. of Cordier . . . the ancients have rendered homage.

3 Or "of the elements". G. justifiably makes a *rapprochement* between Car., *Sūtr.*, XII, 8e (above) and leaves the choice between the two interpretations of—*bhūta*, "beings" or "elements" (p. 8, 1.13: *bhūtānāṃ prāṇināṁ mahābhūtānāṁ vā caturṇāṁ*).

4 D. *avyakto' dṛśyamūrtiḥ / vyaktakarmā prakaṭakriyaḥ*: "*avyakta*, of invisible form, *vyaktakarmā*, of manifest action".

5 cf. Car., *Sūtr.*, XII, 4 and 7, which is reproduced by G., by reading; —*rūkṣah śīto laghuḥ sūkṣma calo viśadaḥ karaiti*, "bitter, cold, light, subtle, mobile, inconsistent, sharp".

6 G., p. 10, 1.4, DY.: *dviguṇa iti śabdasparṣaguṇah*, "has two properties"=has as properties sound and touch (that is to say, those of being heard and felt). DJ. and DK.: *śītasparśa*, "the cold and the touch" (bad reading).

7 This refers to the property "passion" (*rajoguṇa*) which the Sāṁkhya recognises in Nature as a specially active property. The expression amounts to saying. "it has lots of activity", cf., *Śatapatha-brāh.*, VIII, 7,2,10: *dviguṇo bahulataraḥ* (in an entirely different context).

8 Of the impurities of the body or of the three elements of trouble, but in this last case it should be admitted with those who stand for this interpretation, that it is its own conductor because it is one of those three (G. and D.).

9 One could simply translate: "it is the king of the multitude of ills" in accordance with the Bengali version (*vyādhigaṇera rājā*) but G. and D. do not accept that *rāt* be taken here as a synomym of *rājan*. (G., p. 11, 1. 1: *nāyaṁ rāṭśabdo rāja* [Corr.—*'ja*] *paryāyaḥ*;—DY.: *na tu* [DJ. & and DK. have by mistake *nanu*] *rāṭśabdo rājaparyāyah*; G. explains: *rogasamūhe rājati*, D.: *rājate śobhate*.

lates in the body. [9] *Normal Functions of the Wind in the Body:* When it is not excited, the wind ensures the equilibrium of impurities, of the organic elements and of fire, the entering into contact (the sensation) in the domains (of the faculties)[1] and the normal occurrence of various activities. [10] Just as fire is divided into five as regards names, as regards seats and its own functions, similarly is the wind divided, which has only one denomination, one localisation and one activity.[3] [11] The breath of the front and the breath on high, the concentrated breath, the diffused breath and the breath below are the five winds which, when they keep their places, keep the corporeal being going. [12] The wind which circulates in the body is called the breath of the front, *prāṇa*[4], it sustains the body, makes nourishment enter inside and supports the breaths.[5]

---

1 G.: "the entering into contact with the objects of faculties, the disorganisation of faculties, of the organic elements and of fire", that is to say, on one side it closes the circuit on sensation, makes the feeling subject attain the objects falling under the control of sensorial faculties and on the other that it is the antagonist or the regulator of the disturbing elements of the organism.

2 G. and D. specify that it refers to five forms of the fire in the body and enumerate them. They add that it does not refer, as desire some, to five ritual fires.

3 The suffix *maya* here possesses an abstractive value, cf., *vāṅmaya*, "oratorial art", exactly "that which consists of words" (L. Renou, *Grammaire Sanskrite*, Sect. 201). However G. and D. understand: *kriyā—āmayaiḥ kriyayānnapācanādikayā āmayenāmlapākādinā*, "as regards function, i.e., the cooking of nourishment, etc.; as regards disease, that is to say, the acidity, the maturing (excessive combustion), etc." The Bengali translation, seems justifiably, not to follow them (*sei prakāra eka vāyuī nāma sthāna o kriyā*, "similarly the wind, one, as regards names, seats and actions"). The English translation of K.L. Bhishagratna, Calcutta, 1911, Vol. II, p. 3, is too free to judge the interpretation on which it is based. The Latin translator, Fr. Hessler, Erlangen, 1844, Vol. I, p. 169, has understood it as G. and D.

4 G. p. 13, l. 11, notes that "in another book, the breath of the front is said to be seated in the heart; the breath of the front is in the heart, the breath below in the rectum, the concentrated breath goes in the centre of the umbilic, the breath on high is situated in the region of the throat, the diffused breath goes in all the limbs and the articulations. cf., in fact, *Yogacūḍāmaṇyuapaniṣad*, 23-24, with some difference.

5 Others than him or simply "Life" which is a usual sense of *prāṇaḥ*. G. p. 13, l. 14: *prāṇāvalambana-vacanena tu hṛdayāvalambanamuktaṁ / prāṇānāṁ viśeṣeṇa hṛdayamarmasthititvāt*, "by the expression, support of the heart, because the breaths have their seat principally in the vulnerable point of the heart". G. developes thereafter this interpretation, D. takes up a part of this development. Both of them add a quotation *yathā saindhavo'śvaḥ śaṅkumutpāṭya dhāvati tadvat prāṇo* (G. adds *anilo*). "Just as a horse of Sind runs off having uprooted its peg, similarly the breath (G. the breath of the front) arrested, escapes at the time of death tearing off all the winds". In D. this quotation is introduced

[13] Troubled, it produced principally affections such as hiccough and panting. The one called the breath on high, superior wind, goes upwards. [14] By means thereof opens out that which has the characteristic of being said, sung, etc...[1] It produces specially the ills which come above the clavicles. [15] The one that circulates in the receptacles of the uncooked and of the cooked[2], the concentrated breath *(samāna)*, in concert with the fire[3], cooks the nourishment and separates the particular substances which are found to be produced thereby. [16] It produces ills such as the tumours, the weakening of the (digestive) fire[4], diarrhoeas, etc. The one which circulates in the entire body, the diffused breath *(vyāna)* acts to bring in its wake the organic sap, [17] and makes perspiration and blood flow and causes the occurring of the gestures of five types[5] and excited, it provokes chiefly the ills which traverse the entire body. [18] The one that has for seat the receptacle of the cooked (the intestines), the breath below *(apāna)*, it is this wind which, at a convenient moment, brings in its wake the excreta, the urines, the sperm, the embryos and the menses downwards. [19] Excited, it provokes the terrible ills which stay in the bladder and the rectum; but the troubles of the sperm and the urinary ills are produced by the excitation of the diffused breath and of the breath below (associated). [20-21] And, all together, excited, they (the five winds) tear the body undoubtedly.

I am going to explain below the disturbances provoked by the wind when strongly excited, seated in different places. The wind excited in the receptacles of the uncooked (the stomach) provokes ills such as vomitings, etc.

---

by *yaduktaṁ śrutau*, "it is said in the Veda"; in G. by *yaduktaṁ suśrute*, "it is said in Suśruta". Cordier in a note in his hand on the MSS. of G. supposes it to refer to an older edition of Suśruta because it is not the practice of the commentator to thus denote the text commented upon by him. But the good reading must be *śrutau* as the quotation is an approximative reproduction of the *Bṛh.-up.*, VI, 1,13.

1 G., D. variant: the domain of that which is said, sung, etc.

2 The stomach and the intestines.

3 Var.: with the help of the fire.

4 Var.: the tumours, the diarrhoeas where there is association with fire.

5 G. and D.: extension, contraction, flexion, recovery, lateropulsion or according to others reported by D.: march, extension, recovery, opening of the eyes and closing of the eyes.

[22] Bewilderment, swoonings, thirst, the gripping of the heart, the point of the side. The one that has its seat in the receptacle of the cooked (the intestines) provokes the noise of the entrails and the sharp pain (colic) in the nombril.[1] [23] Dysuria and constipation, the intestinal occlusion, the suffering at the trifurcation (of the trunk and of the hips). Excited, the wind can produce the death of faculties (sensorial and active) in the ear, etc. [24] That which is found in the skin can provoke bad tint, the quivering, abruptness, sleep (tegumentary insensibility), cooking, pricking, chapping, desquamation. [25] That which has arrived in the blood can provoke ulcers, that which has its seat in the flesh can provoke painful nodosities,—similarly the one that has its seat in the fat can provoke new ulcerous indolent nodosities. [26] That which has attained the vessels can produce lancinating pain, contraction and the plenitude of vessels. That which has attained the tendons can provoke paralysis and shaking, lancinating pain as also convulsion. [27] That which has reached the joints renders them painful and swollen and can provoke the drying of the bones and their fissuration as also lancinating pain, the one that has its seat in them. [28] And when it has attained the marrow, the illness never gets calm; when the wind has attained the sperm, there is an absence of production or there is troubled production. [29] The wind which goes everywhere, covers successively the constitutive elements of the hands, the feet, the head and can attack the entire body of men. [30] The one that goes everywhere provokes paralysis, convulsions, sleep (anaesthesia), swelling and lancinating pains and mixed (with other elements causing trouble) in the seats that are said to be those of complex ills. [31] The wind that has reached the limbs can provoke innumerable ills. There can be inflammation, heating and swooning when the wind is associated with bile. [32] Cold, swelling and heaviness, when it is enveloped in phlegm.

Pricking as by needles, horror of touch (hyperaesthesia) [33] and other disturbances of the bile can occur when the wind is associated with blood. When the breath of the front is enveloped in bile, vomiting takes place and inflammation

[1] Var.: the sharp pain and the intestinal occlusion.

appears. [34] When it is enveloped in phlegm, there appear weakness, depression, lassitude and bad mien. When the wind of high is associated with bile: swooning, inflammation, dizziness, lassitude. [35] Absence of transpiration and horripilation, diminished (internal) fire, cold and impotence, when it is enveloped in phlegm.

[36] When the concentrated breath is associated with bile, sudation, inflation, burning and swooning. And when it is enveloped in phlegm, excess of phlegm, excreta and urines, horripilation. When the breath of below is associated with bile, there can occur inflammation and burning and (in women) flux of the blood.

[37] When it is enveloped in phlegm, heaviness in the lower part of the body. When the diffused blood is enveloped in bile, convulsions, lassitude. [38] All the limbs are heavy and there is the stiffness of the points of bones, (such is) the symptomatology *(liṅga)* when the diffused breath is enveloped in phlegm and there is also the paralysis of movements. [39][1] Generally, in delicate persons, in those who take undue amounts of nourishment and live beyond measure, because of excessive fatigue due to women, due to spirituous drinks and exercises which are the paths of ills[2], [40] following a deviation in the regimen of the seasons and irregular use of fatty bodies, etc., the windy blood gets excited in those who are chaste as also in the corpulent ones. [41] The one who goes with elephants, horses, camels and others, has his wind excited because of the habitual causes (of excitation), because of nourishment of vegetables, etc. pungent, hot, acid and caustic edibles as also because of heatings, etc. (becoming) too habitual. [42] Rapidly the blood gets corrupted and blocks the path of the wind. This wind, immediately rendered violently excited by the blocking of its route, can immediately trouble the blood a great deal. [43] The latter, mixed with the wind, disturbed by its predominance, is called "Windy Blood". Similarly bile mixed with disturbed blood, disturbed phlegm mixed with disturbed blood. [44] Fearing the touch, suffering from pricking pain and drying up, from

---

1 39 and 40 probably interpolated.

2 Var.: following the affliction.

sleep (anaesthesia), are the feet because of the windy blood. Because of bile and blood they have a violent inflammation, are extremely hot, have red swelling and are smooth. [45] They are pruriginous, white and cold, swollen, inflated and impotent when the blood is disturbed by phlegm. And the ailments, when the blood is disturbed by all, make manifest in the feet, their individual aspects. [46] As premonitary symptoms, they are soft, perspiring, cold (or) possess opposite characteristics, have a bad colour, a pricking pain, sleep (anaesthesia), heaviness, heat. [47] When it (the blood) has reached the sole of the feet, sometimes also the palm of the hands, like rat-poison[1], it infiltrates the body. [48] When it has spread up to the knees, and when it is an effusion, being fragmented (that is to say, in the form of spread-out spots, petechiae) and when it is accompanied by complications like those of the weakening of the breath and of the flesh, [49] blood can become incurable (or) curable after several years. But when excited wind invades all the vessels, [50] then by a sudden attack it causes lively convulsions all over the body occurring at all moments, and as this convulsion is caused at all times, it is traditionally called "convulsor" *(ākṣepaka)*, [51] is called "tension-producer" *(apatānaka)*[2], the one which makes descend *(pātayati)*, by intervals, if the wind associated with phlegm violently occupies the (vessels). [52] The one which makes it hard like a stick is serious, that is the "tension-producer like a stick" *(daṇḍapātanaka*, upright tetanus*)*. When it seizes the jaws very strongly

[1] D.: poison of *Ficus glomerata* which is in reality the name of a skin-disease (*audumbara*, Suśr., *Nid.*, V, 3), but the rat-poison, thought to be contained in its sperm, is well-known to Suśruta as giving rise to extended accidents, *Kalp.*, VI, 5-7, which describes exactly the swellings, eruptions, fevers, panting, weakness, etc. caused by the corruption of blood.

[2] This word depends on *tan*, "to extend", and not on *pat*, "to fall"; hence the etymology proposed here is fallacious. The diseases in question are the different forms of tetanus whose "convulsion-causing" wind provokes spasms. The names of *ākṣepaka, apatānaka* are the epithets of the wind as tetanus-causing functions but easily become names with morbid forms provoked by the latter; in that case these words are used for *ākeṣpaka-roga, apatānaka-roga*, etc. It has been believed that *apatānaka* denoted epilepsy (Suśr., trnsln. of K.L. Bhishagratna) undoubtedly because of the indication that there is a fall but epilepsy is well-known and is described elsewhere as *apasmāra* and the mention of falls, which are not the characteristics of tetanus (whose access, in any case, is incompatible with the standing position), seem to be due to the care shown for etymology; the rest of the piece refers clearly to tetanus and to the diverse forms of tetanic accidents.

(trismus) use of nourishment becomes difficult. [53] The one that makes the body bend like a bow draws its name from the hardness of the bow *(dhanuḥstambha)*. It has its seat in the fingers, in ankles, abdomen, heart, chest and throat. [54] When the wind, impetuous, causes the convulsive expansion of the tendons, (the patient) has his eyes fixed, the jaw rigid, the side twisted (pleurothotonos), and (he) vomits phlegm. [55] When the man is bent like a bow inwards, then the wind, powerful, provokes its "contraction inwards" (emprosthotonos), [56] and if the tendons of outside[1] are found in the expansions it provokes the "outward contraction" (opisthotonos). The experts call incurable the one that causes the chest, the hips and the thighs to incurvate.

[57] The wind associated with phlegm and bile and even the wind alone can produce the "convulsion-producer" *(ākṣepaka)* and another, the fourth is born of the traumatisms.[2] [58] The "tension-producer" which has abortion for its cause, or which occurs because of haemorrhage, or which has the traumatisms as cause, is not cured. [59] When the wind, excessively excited, attains the vessels going downwards along with those going horizontally and those which go high in the body, [60] then, releasing the links of articulations on one side, it injures the side and the best of practitioners call him "affected on the side" (hemiplegia). [61] The one who is tormented by the wind and whose entire half-body is paralysed and insensible, (he) falls[3] and even loses life. [62] It is known that the side injured by pure wind[4] is the most difficult to cure, the curable is that which is in relation with another (element of trouble), and the incurable is that which brings atrophy in its wake. [63] The wind

---

1 D.: "the tendons of outside are those which have their seat in the soles of the feet, in fleshy mass (calf of leg, etc.), in the posterior parts of hips, of the back and of the neck". These are the muscles whose contraction causes opisthotoṇos.

2 There are three types of "convulsion-producers" due respectively to wind, to wind associated with phlegm and with wind associated with bile, a fourth type is of traumatic origin. This last form, where the coming in of the disease is apparently due to traumatism, is distinguished from tetanus seeming to be spontaneous, which were considered as pertaining to medical pathology, even in modern times before it was known that D. lists various classifications of tetanus in four types.

3 Var.: following the same.

4 Alone, without the intervention of the phlegm and of bile.

excited can climb from its seat to the heart and the head, it torments the temples and can cause convulsions in limbs and can also bend them. [64] With eyes closed, without any movement, or with eyes fixed, one whimpers, without breath, or one can breathe with difficulty, with consciousness abolished. [65] One can be in one's normal state when the heart is freed and one swoons when it is enveloped (in the wind) by the wind accompanied by phlegm, one should know it to be *apatantraka*.[1] [66] As against sleeping during daytime, in one posture[2], in one position, of one look in an abnormal sense[3] the one that is enveloped in phlegm provokes torticolis *(manyāstambha)*. [67] In pregnant women, in parturition, in children, old men and the weak[4], in the case of the diminution of blood, the one who cries aloud and masticates hard objects too much, [68] laughs, yawns, and due to weight, due even to an unequal level[5], going to the head, the nose, the lips, the chin, the forehead, the junctions of the eyes[6], [69] the wind torments the visage and engenders thereafter facial paralysis *(ardita)*. Half of the face becomes twisted and even the neck gets twisted, [70] the head deviates, there is liming of speech (Aphasia) derangement of the eyes, etc. and suffering on the same side of the neck in the chin and in the teeth. [71] The one who has horripilation in the beginning, trembling, eye-trouble, wind going up, sleep (anaesthesia) and pain in the skin, seizing of the muscular mass of the neck and of the jaws, the experts in diseases call his (trouble) the disease "*ardita*".[7] [72] The one who is weakened, whose eyes do not blink, whose

1 According to Y. (note): "hysteria". The design suits well enough the convulsions and the "hysterical" coma, but also the manifestations with an organic substratum such as can provoke a number of neurological affections, meningeal haemorrhages, etc.

2 Specially of a posture in sitting position. Var.: of an irregular position.

3 Var.: of an upward glance.

4 The first half of the verse is rejected by Jejjhata and others.

5 Var.: of unequal respiration.

6 Lines of junction between the brows and the lids, the eye-lids and the white, etc. (Suśr., *Utt.*, I, 14). In fact, in facial paralysis there is a complete displacement of the eye-lids in relation to the eye.

7 Here it does not refer merely to facial paralysis, but rather to facial neuralgia with trophic troubles (troubles of the eye), or to serious facial paralysis with lagophthalmia (absence of blinking indicated in verse 72), secondary contractions and neurological troubles associated together (paralysis with hemiplegia and aphasia).

speech is continually limy[1], his *ardita* is not cured assuredly as also if he is three years old and of the one who trembles. [73] The tendon of the heel and that of the toe which is tormented by the wind can retain the extension of the thigh; this is what is called "sciatica" *(gṛdhrasī)*. [74] The tendon of the palm and of the fingers, in the back in the region of the arm, diminishes the function of the arms; this is what is known as "brachial paralysis" *(viśvācī)*. [75] The swelling in the centre of knee, due to the wind and to the blood, very painful is the "jackal's head"[2], massive like the shout of the jackal. [76] When the wind happens to sit in the hips and causes the tendon of the thigh to convulse[3], then the man can become lame and, following the death of the two thighs, become paraplegical *(paṅgu)*. [77] The one whose legs shake while walking and who walks like a lame person, one should know him as the "lame because of sinewy fasciculia" *(kalaya-khañja)*, whose ligaments of articulations are loose. [78] When the foot is placed in an irregular manner, the wind can produce pains; it should be known that it is the "thorn of the wind" *(vātakaṇṭaka)* which has its seat in the ankle.

[79] The wind associated with bile and blood provokes inflammation in the feet and specially following a walk: it is called "inflammation of the feet" *(pādadāha*, acrodyny*)*. [80] The one whose feet have horripilation and are as if asleep[4], it should be known that he has the horripilation of the feet *(pādaharṣa)* born of the excitation of the phlegm and of the wind. [81] The wind which, having its seat in the region of the shoulder, after having dried up the articulation[5] and bent the tendons, stays there, engenders the "arm below" *(avabāhuka)*. [82] Where the wind stays filling the vectorial canal of speech[6], whether pure or associated with phlegm, deafness *(bādhirya)*, is produced because of it. [83] The one

---

1 Var.: whose speech is limy and indistinct.

2 Literally: "head" but preceded by jackal, that is to say that its name is formed of *śiraḥ*, "head", preceded by *kroṣṭhuka*, "jackal", therefore, *kroṣṭhukáśiraḥ*, "head of the jackal".

3 According to G.: "convulses a little". Here it refers in fact not to violent contractions but to paraplegia or spasmodic monoplegia.

4 Var.: and can be put to sleep.

5 Literally: "that which has a link". Var.: the link of the shoulder.

6 Literally: "of the words".

in whom the wind provokes a shooting pain in the ears as if cutting the jaws, temples, head and the neck, he is said to have the "shooting pain of the ears" *(karṇaśūla)*. [84] The wind with phlegm having filled the vectorial canals of speech, renders men inactive, dumb, speaking through the nose, or makes them stammerers. [85] The suffering that goes downwards, arriving in the receptacles of the faeces and of the urines, as if cutting the rectum and the genital organs, is known as the "quiver"[1] *(tūnī)*. [86] The suffering which, arrived in the rectum and in the genital organs, winding the wrong way, occurs with paroxysms in the receptacle of the cooked (in the intestines) is called "contrary quiver" *(pratitūnī)*. [87] The abdomen with rumbling, the seat of extremely violent pains, strongly swollen: one should know that to be "distension" *(ādhmāna)*, terrible due to the stoppage of the wind. [88] When the side and the heart are untrammeled and when it reaches the receptacle of the undigested (stomach) it should be known as the "contrary distension", where the wind is filled with phlegm.

[89] One should know that a nodule, firm like seed-stone, enlarged upwards, elevated, is a "seed-stone of the wind" *(vātāṣṭhīlā)*, blocking the external outlets. [90] One should say that the one accompanied by pains, blocking the winds, the faeces and the urines, developed horizontally in the abdomen is the "seed-stone in the contrary direction" *(pratyaṣṭhīlā)*.

The Hippocratic Manual "On Breaths"

The three great Indian texts of medicine are thus unanimous in making the wind as the soul of the world and of the body, in the concrete sense of the word "soul". The various winds, organic breaths or "animal spirits" are the principles of the entire manifestation of life in the body. The differences between Suśruta and the texts of the tradition of Ātreya do not go to the basis of the doctrine; they are, above all, a result of the fact that Suśruta does not insist on the cosmic rôle of the wind and, on the contrary, gives details of its action in the body. Suśruta makes a concordant enunciation, though technically

[1] Pain as if due to a quiver full of arrows. Similarly the "shooting pain", *śūla*, is the pain caused by a blow of the lance.

much more medical, referring to a later development of medicine. The Hippocratic manual *On Breaths* teaches the same general doctrine as taught by the three Indian texts, being nearer the first two texts, because of the much less technical nature of its enunciation and, in any case, offering concordances in detail with those of Suśruta.

For a long time the Hellenists have been struck by the literary character of the manual, *On Breaths,* composed, it is said, like a discourse meant for a large audience.[1] E. Maass has thought that his author had imitated Gorgias[2] and the most trustworthy opinion today seems to desire it to be the discourse of a sophist. This will explain its much less technical character —which, in any case, is a fact—and will imply that its attribution to Hippocrates is false.

On this last point, it is difficult to reach a definite judgement. The critics have never been unanimous on the manuals that are to be accepted as authentic[3], the proposed criteria of authenticity being hypothetical and a thousand hypotheses being possible according to the manner in which are conceived the spirit of the Master and his preoccupations. But it is probably certain that the manual *On Breaths* is, in its form and doctrine, different from the majority of the most important pieces of the collection. Yet, the peripatetician Menon thought this text to be a work of Hippocrates and this implies, as has been shown by Diels, that Aristotle had considered it as such.[4] Diels and Wilamowitz have thus come to the conclusion that Aristotle had seriously deceived himself and this opinion of theirs has generally been accepted.[5] One must, however, observe that it is not only the form of the text which militates, in the eyes of modern critics, against its authenticity but also the mediocre esteem they have for it and which makes them think it to be

---

1 cf., Axel Nelson, *Die Hippocratische Schrift,* PERI PHUSON; *Text und Studien,* Uppsala, 1909. p. 98.

2 Hermes, XXII, 1887, pp. 566 ff., Nelson, p. 99.

3 cf., A. Diés, *Autour de Platon,* Paris, 1927, pp. 14 ff., and review of the Congrés de l'Association Guillaume Budé, (Nice, 1935), in A Rey, *La maturité de la pensée scientifique in Gréce,* Paris, 1939, p. 433.

4 *Hermes,* XXVIII, 1893, p. 432.

5 cf., Nelson, *loc. cit.,* pp. 106-7. Nelson ends with a quotation of Wilamovitz whose conclusion he accepts. "*Aristoteles hat im ihm* (Hippocrate) *den Sophisten von. P- Ph. gesehen: das ist schlimm fü die Medicin, die er in Stagiros gelernt hatte*".

unworthy of Hippocrates.[1] Yet, the manual *On Breaths* (14) describes a natural pathogeny of the sacred disease closely resembling the one described in the special manual *On the Sacred Disease* which is generally thought to be one of the chief claims to glory of the "Father of Medicine". However it may be, the manual *On Breaths* did not appear to be quite denuded of value to Aristotle and we will see, after having summarised it, and in part reproduced in the translation of Littré[2], that it had been in accord with the generally trustworthy doctrines of Greek medicine at least since the epoch of Hippocrates. It belongs definitely to the Hippocratic tradition as it had been constituted before the epoch of Aristotle and Alexander

SUMMARY AND EXTRACTS OF THE MANUAL "ON BREATHS".[3]

(1) *Greatness and Difficulties of Medicine. Necessity of recognising the general cause of diseases.* (2) *The Cause of Diseases is one:* All the diseases have one single mode of being; they differ only in their location. Firstly, they have among themselves no similarity, because of the diversity and the dissimilarity of places they affect. However, for all of them there is only one form and one cause, always the same. That which it is, I will try to explain it in the following part of my discourse.

(3) *Of Air considered as an agent in the world*[4]: The body of men is nourished by three types of aliments; they are called food, drink and breaths. The breath[5], is known as wind *(anemos)* in the body, air *(air)* outside the body. The air is the most powerful agent of all and in all[6]; it is worthwhile to consider its force. The wind *(anemos)* is a flux and a current of air; when, therefore, accumulated air becomes a violent current,

[1] Blass, *Hermes*, XXXVI, p. 405, has supposed that the manual *On Breaths* attributed to Hippocrates by Aristotle and Ménon was not the one that has reached us but a text of greater value on which the existing one was composed. This hypothesis has been approved by Th. Gomperz, *Les Penseurs de la Grèce*, French trnsln., Paris, 1928, Vol. I, p. 321, note: it remains, nonetheless, a simple hypothesis.

[2] The summarised portions are in italics.

[3] E. Littré, *Oeuvres complétes d'Hippocrate*, Paris, Vol. VI, 1849, pp. 90. ff.

[4] cf., Car., above, 8 c-d; Bhela, 8-12.; Suśr., 4-8.

[5] Littré: *pneumata*, Nelson: *pneuma*.

[6] cf., Car., 8e; Bhela, 12; Suśr., 5.

the trees fall, being uprooted by the impetuosity of breath, the sea raises itself[1], and the ships of large dimensions are thrown on high. Such is the power it possesses. Invisible, in truth, to the eye, it is visible to thought; because which effect would be produced without it ?[2] From where is it absent or where is it not present ? The entire interval between the earth and the sky is filled by breath. This breath is the cause of winter and of summer[3]: dense and cold in winter, in summer soft and tranquil. Even the march of the sun, of the moon and of stars takes place by breath[4]; because for the fire the breath is nourishment, and the fire deprived of breath could not live[5], so much so that the eternal course of the sun is maintained by air, which itself is light and eternal. Evidently the sea also has a part of the breath[6]; because the swimming animals cannot live when deprived of this breath, and how can they live except by drawing the air through water and from water ? The earth is the base where the air rests[7], the air is the vehicle of the earth, and there is nothing that be devoid thereof. (4) *Of Air considered in the body of the animals:* Such is, therefore, the reason of its force in every other thing; as regards mortal beings, it is the cause of life in them and of the diseases in patients[8], and so great is the need of breath for all the bodies that man, who deprived of all solid and liquid nourishment can live two or three days and even longer, would perish if the outlets of the breath in the body were to be intercepted, even for a brief part of the day. So very predominant is the need of breath ! Moreover, in man, all the actions are subject to intermissions, as life is full of mutations, this action alone is never interrupted in mortal animals, all busy in inhaling and exhaling air. (5) *The Air is the cause of diseases:* Therefore it is said that all the animals participate largely in the air; now

1 cf., Car., 8d.

2 cf., Car., 8e; Bhela, 12; Suśr., 6.

3 cf., Car., 8c.

4 cf., Car., 8c; Bhela, 10.

5 cf., Bhela, 11.

6 *To pelagos metekhei pneumatos*: Littré translates less clearly, "the sea is in communication with the breath."

7 Other reading: "and, for the moon, its base is on it" (*khai ti minī epi touteou to bathrion*).

8 cf., Car., 8a and b; Suśr., 6.

one should explain immediately, that according to all probability, the source of diseases should not be placed elsewhere, so that when it enters the body, whether in excess or in lesser quantities, or too much at a time, or dirty with morbific miasma. These remarks do not suffice for the thing in general; now coming to the facts themselves in the following part of this discourse, I am going to show, that all the diseases are produced thereof and proceed therefrom. (6) *Air is the cause of fevers and first of all of epidemic fevers and of epizooty. When air is infected with miasma which are the enemies of human nature, men fall ill; when it becomes improper to another animal species, it is the latter which is struck.* (7) Air is the first cause of sporadic fevers *determined by aerophagy:* When the body is filled with aliments, it is also filled with air, abundantly if the aliments rest; now, if they rest, their quantity preventing them from going on; the lower part of the abdomen thus obstructed, the winds spread themselves in the entire body, and, falling on the most sanguine parts, they cool them off; following this cooling off of these parts which are the sources and the roots of blood, shivering runs in the entire body, and the blood being entirely cooled, the entire body shivers. (8) *Air is the cause of the principal phenomena which accompany the fevers, shivering, trembling, yawning, resolution of articulations, transpirations, cephalalgy:* This is why shiverings precede fevers. Depending on the quantity and on the coldness of the winds which irrupt, shivering is as much stronger as they are more abundant and colder, as much weaker as they are reduced and less cold. In shiverings the tremblings of the body are produced in this manner: the blood, flowing back before the cold which pursues it, agitates across the whole body to run to the hottest parts of the body. Such is its vagabond course. The blood having thrown itself far from the extremities, the viscera and the fleshes tremble; because certain parts of the body become hyperemic and others anaemic, now the anaemic parts, under the influence of the cold, far from keeping their immobility, are seized by spasmodic movements as heat has left them; and the hyperemic parts, due to the accumlation of the blood, tremble and cause inflammations, as there can be no immobility where there is superabundance of this liquid. Yawns precede fevers, when lots of accumulated air, coming out of the upper side at the same time, opens forcibly the mouth as is done by a lever; there is, in fact, the easiest exit . . . when the largest part of the blood has thus been gathered, the air that had cooled it, gets heated in turn, being dominated by the heat: having thus become an incandescent mass, it communicates its heating to the entire body. And the blood cooperates with it; because put on this *brasero*, it evaporates; and it shuts itself from the breath; this breath arriving at the pores of the body, perspiration is produced because the condensed breath falls into water, and, traversing the pores, shows itself outside . . . The cephalalgy accompanying the fever is explained as follows: the paths of the blood get narrow in the head; because the veins are filled with air; thus filled and burnt, they cause cephalalgy; in fact, the blood, forcibly pushed in one path, being hot, cannot flow rapidly, as it encounters lots of obstacles. Therefrom the throbbings which are produced in the temples. (9) *Air is the cause of Ileus and of colic pain:* The breath when it falls on soft parts, unhabituated and intact, it pushes itself in like an arrow, and penetrates the flesh, throwing itself sometimes into hypochondrium, sometimes into sides, sometimes into both.[1]

(10) *Air is the cause of fluxions and of Hemoptyses:. . .* when the veins of the head are filled with air, firstly the head becomes heavy because of winds that oppress it; then the blood whirls, which the winds cannot make flow because of the narrowness of the paths; but the thinnest part is shown across the veins; this liquid, when it has been accumulated, flows out by other exits, and the point of the body where it flows becomes the seat of disease . . . Because phlegm mixed with acrid humours, wherever it goes, causes ulcers in parts of the body not used to its presence . . . The inhaled air arrives by the throat in the chest, and goes out by the same path; so when the breath which comes from below, encounters the flux going downwards, cough occurs and phlegm *(phlégma)* is thrown upwards. Things being so, ulcer is caused in the throat . . . because necessarily a painful part retains the breath . . . (11) *Air causes the ruptures, Rigmata:* The ruptures *(Coan Prognoses*, 418) have the following cause: when different parts of the flesh, by some violence, get detached from one another, and the breath insinuates itself in

1 cf., Suśr., 20-22.

the interstice, this excites suffering *(On Diseases,* I, 20*)*[1]. (12) *Air is a cause of Hydropsy:* If the winds spread themselves in the fleshes, dilating the pores of the body, these winds are followed by humidity for which the path has been made by air; the body having thus become imbibed, on the one hand the fleshes melt, and, on the other, the legs get tumefied . . . *(proofs drawn from what occurs when the ascites is punctured)*. (13) *Air is the cause of Apoplexies:* When the winds, abundant and cold, penetrate the fleshes, the penetrated parts become insensible[2]: abundant winds run across the entire body? The entire body is struck with apoplexy; do they get fixed in a certain part? it is this part; do they get dissipated? the disease gets dissipated; do they persist, the disease persists. The continual yawnings of these patients prove that it is so. (14) *Air is the cause of Epilepsy:* I attribute the same cause again to the disease called sacred. (*It is the blood*) *which in the body, unites most with intelligence (phronisis)*. When it is in its normal state the intelligence remains intact, otherwise it gets altered. This is the case in sleep where the blood gets cooled and in drunkenness where it gets suddenly increased in quantity. Much of the breath being mixed in the entire body with all the blood, it creates several obstacles in several places in the veins *(phleps)*. When much air charges the thick veins full of blood and charging them, stays there, the blood is prevented from flowing; here it stops, there it goes slowly, elsewhere more quickly. In such a way that the flow of the blood across the body becomes irregular, and all sorts of irregularities are the result; the whole body is drawn on all sides; the parts get contracted under the action of the trouble and the derangement of the blood; perversions of all types manifest themselves in every way; during this time the patients are struck with anaesthesia, (they are) deaf to what is said, blind to what is done (and) insensible to suffering: so much has the air by its trouble troubled the blood and dirtied it! It is also not without reason that froth comes to the mouth, air, penetrating by jugular veins *(sphagitidan phleban)* passes, it is true, but while passing, draws

---

[1] Suśr., 20, 26, 27.
[2] Suśr., 24, 30, 32.

along the thinnest part of the blood, the liquid thus mixed with air gets white, because the air appears in its purity across the subtle membranes; this is why all the froths are white. So, when do persons who are victims of this disease get free from the access and the tempest which assails them? This is what I am going to say. The body, because of the exercise it receives from suffering, gets heated, and the blood with it; the blood, heated communicates its heat to the winds; under this influence, the latter get dissolved and dissolve the coagulation of the blood; they come out in part with exhalation, in part with the phlegm. The ebullition of the froth ceases, the blood comes back to normal, the tempest roused in the body gets pacified and the attack is over. (15) *Conclusion:* In definitive, the winds are, in all the diseases, the principal agents, all the rest are only concomitant and accessory causes; this alone is the effective cause; I have shown it. I had promised to show the origin of diseases, and I have established that the breath, sovereign of the rest, is the same in the body of the animals. I have applied the reasoning on known diseases, where the hypothesis is seen to be veritable. If I were to enter into details of all the affections, my discourse on the same would become too long, but it would be neither more exact nor more convincing.

The general concordance of the doctrine of this text with that of Indian pneumatism is evident. The similarities in detail of the pathogenic representations are equally so. But there are also differences. The manual *On Breaths* (5, 6) talks of spots introduced in the body by the inhaled air and explains the epidemics. Our Indian texts contain nothing similar. The Greek discourse explains a pathogeny by the association of blood and wind which recalls the totality of the theories of Suśruta (42). But in his theories corrupted blood blocks the wind, from where the excitation of the wind, which in its turn troubles the blood. In the former, it is the wind which cools the blood and then gets heated by contact and pushes it violently, even though its heat obstructs its circulation. The final result is the same: there is an obstacle in the normal course of the breath and of the blood, but somewhat different on both sides, there had been speculations on the mechanism of this accident. It should, therefore, be recognised that there is a profound analogy between the doctrine of the manual *On*

Breaths and Indian pneumatism but not a close correlation. It seems excluded that there was textual borrowing. On the Indian side the doctrine propounded is too ancient, because of its Vedic attachments and because of its Indo-Iranian pre-history, to have been born under Greek influence; at the most it could have been influenced in certain details. On the Greek side, only a free imitation of an Indian model could be admitted as there is no literal concordance. It is true that the eventual Indian model could have been a text other than the ones that have reached us. But, besides the fact that it will be a gratuitous hypothesis to put forward and defend, the Greek puts forward a doctrine which appears, on enquiry, to have been very well attested in the Hellenic world. If there has been a borrowing from India, it has been in the shape of general ideas and it has been of an entire part of the Greek medical text rather than that of the author of the manual *On Breaths* acting alone. The problem posed by the concordances between this manual and the Sanskrit works is not one of borrowing a text but that of cultural relations.

Nelson has already justly noted (p. 101) that the rôle of the essential element of the cosmos attributed to the air goes back at least to Anaximenes, that Diogenes of Appollonia and others have exalted the all powerfulness of the air, considering it as the principle of life and of thought, and lastly that in the Hippocratic manuals *On the Sacred Disease* and *On the Nature of Man*, also appears a doctrine of pneumatic physiology.

It is easy to find in the Pre-Socratics[1] and in the Hippocratic Collection many other concordances with the manual *On Breaths* which show the extent to which the latter is linked with several theories current among the Greeks and at the same time quite analogous to those of India. Just then, in the Pre-Socratics, are found teachings on the rôle of the air or of the breath in the world, and in the Hippocratic Collection are found the data concerning its action in the body. Nevertheless the pre-occupations of anatomy and of physiology are frequent in the pre-Socratics.

1 H. Diels, *Doxographi graeci*, Berlin, 1879. (quoted hereafter as Dox and by number), trnsln. in P. Tannery, *Pour l'histoire de la science helléne*, second edn. by A Diés, Paris 1930, (quoted as T. and by page-number); J. Voilquin, *Les penseurs grecs avant Socrate*, Paris, 1941 (quoted as V and by page-number).

Diogenes of Appollonia, who died towards 428 B.C. recognised numerous vessels in the body; he believed that the soul entered the child after birth with the cold air attracted by the heat of the body and that death came when the air quitted the veins. The blood during sleep pushed the air towards the chest and towards the abdomen (Dox., 426, 436; T., 334,; V., 149-159). But a little earlier undoubtedly, Empedocles (who died towards 430 B.C.) had defended the existence of canals traversing the fleshes and ending in the nostrils where alternatively, by the flux and the reflux of the blood, air entered and went out. According to him, sleep would correspond to a moderate cooling of the blood (Dox., 435; T., 336; V., 126) and this last doctrine is found in our manual (14) with the one saying that intelligence depends on the blood; an opinion which also belongs to Empedocles (T., 345, V., 116; frag. 105). Empedocles did not admit breathing in the embryo before birth (Dox., 425; T., 335).

On this last point, Empedocles and Diogenes of Appollonia have been contradicted by the Hippocratic manuals which, like the Indian books, taught the existence in the embryo of the circulation of the breath coming from the mother: *On the Embryo of eight months* (12) *On the Nature of the Child* (12) [wherein are recognised, as in India, a feminine and a masculine semen[1], with which the breath gets united, this breath organises all the parts of the embryo (17)] and *On Flesh* (6). As opposed to this, the school of Sicily, which had very strong links with Empedocles, has given a great deal of importance to the theory of pneuma[2] which was to become much later, after Celsus, the characteristic doctrine of the "pneumatic" school[3] and which was to play, in Hellenic and Hellenistic philosophy and mysticism, a rôle comparable and parallel to that of *prāṇa* in India.

The circulation of air in the vessels is admitted again in the Hippocratic manual *On the Alimentation* (31). The retention of air intercepted in the vessels is considered as the

---

1 cf., *supra*, p. 165-6.

2 cf., M. Welmann, *Fragmente des sikelischen Arzte*, Berlin, 1901 W. Jaeger, *Diokles von Karystos*, Berlin, 1958.

3 cf., M. Wellmann, *Die pneumatische Schule bis auf Archigenes*, Berlin, 1895.

cause of the sudden loss of speech, with dizziness, convulsions, etc. in the manual *On Diet in Acute Diseases* (App., 4 & 5). According to this text the breath and the blood united produce Quincy (App., 6). The manual *On Ancient Medicine* (22) refers on its side, to the action of the internal winds, the pains and even to the abcesses in the region of the liver and of the diaphragm, its exposition reminding us of *On Breaths* (9).

The manual *On Breaths* thus belongs to an entire Greek literature of pneumatic[1] physiology which serves as a pendant to Sanskrit literature concerning the physio-pathological rôle of the wind inside the organism. It is the eventuality of the relations between these two literatures rather than that of the relations between the texts themselves compared by us that we should envisage.

---

1 On the role of the pneuma in stoicism and its dependence on medical theories, cf. G. Verbeke, *L'évolution de la doctrine du pneuma du stoicisme ā saint Augustin*, Paris-Louvain, 1945, pp. 6, 12 et passim.

CHAPTER EIGHT

THE *TIMAEUS* OF PLATO AND INDIAN MEDICINE

ANALOGIES of the same type as those that have been noted between Indian medical texts and the Hippocratic manual *On Breaths*, being expressions of ancient Greek pneumatic conceptions, have already been pointed out between a theory taught in the *Timaeus* and the Indian doctrine of pathology. Armand Delpeuch[1] has been struck on finding in the *Timaeus* in the form of explanation, quite aberrent in comparison with Hippocratic medicine, the classical teaching of Ayurveda, whereby diseases are provoked by the wind, bile and phlegm. But he believed that he could refer this teaching back to the Veda and thought that Plato had received it from the Pythagorean tradition, Pythagoras being reported to have searched for a medical philosophy in India.

It is impossible to accept the idea that the doctrine in question goes back, in its complete form, up to the Veda, but it is certain that its analogy with the thesis of the *Timaeus* is remarkable.

Plato recognises three classes of diseases. The first are due to the alterations of the four constitutive elements of the body similar to that of the universe—earth, fire, water and air (82 a-83 e). Others are related to humours produced by the elements and are susceptible to corruption (83 e-84 c). The third class (84 d) comprises diseases due to pneuma, to phlegm (*phlegma*) and bile (*khole*). This is the thesis which is in accord with the classical Indian doctrine. The exposition of Plato is, unfortunately, extremely rudimentary and very confused.[2]

Summary and Extracts (84 d-86 a):

"When the lung, distributor of air in the body, is obstruct-

---

1 A. Delpeuch, *La goutte et le rhumatisme*, Paris, 1900, pp. 26 ff.

2 The quotations which follow are borrowed from the translation of M.A. Rivaud, Coll. Guillaume Budé, *Platon*, Vol. X, Paris, 1925, pp. 217-219, with very minor changes.

ed by discharges of (*reūma*), the circulation of air in the body is troubled, on the one hand the parts that do not receive their freshening (supplies) get corrupted and, on the other, air does violence to certain vessels (*phleps*), causes them to be distended, twisted and dislocates them. And it shuts itself in that part of the body where the diaphragm is found.[1] Thus are born frequently a number of painful diseases accompanied by abundant perspiration. Often in this way, the flesh gets disjointed inside the body, air gets therein, unable to get out therefrom and (becomes) the cause of suffering identical to that provoked by air come from without.[2] Such suffering is, above all, very great when the air applies itself to the tendons (*neuron*)[3] and to the vessels which are there and causes them to swell. Then it causes the extensor muscles to distend as also the muscles adhering thereto and causes them to contract in the contrary direction. The diseases resulting from this tension have, for this reason, received the name of tetanus and episthosnos. It is difficult to bring any remedy to them and, most often, it is the fevers which, coming in then, resolve them."[4]

The white phlegm (defined in 83 d as mixed with bubbles of air) is dangerous if the air of the bubbles contained by it is retained in the body; it is less dangerous, if the air goes out, but then the skin gets spots of white (85 a). If the phlegm gets mixed up with black bile and troubles the "extremely divine revolutions" which occur in the head, there can be produced the disease called the sacred one because it appertains to

---

1 Rivaud thinks that it refers here to the pathogeny of pulmonary congestions and to bronchitis, but the air which shuts itself in the diaphragmatic region could not determine similar affections. It refers to the air retained in the centre of the body and which provokes the diseases that follow, the latter not being of the respiratory type.

2 cf., *On Breaths,* 11; Suśr., 20, 26, 27.

3 The nerves and the tendons, all the 'cords' are confused in Greek anatomy, the same being the case in Indian anatomy, the 'nerves' in the modern sense of the word are confused with the *snāyus* or tendons.

4 The Hippocratic manual *On Diseases,* III, 14 and 15, describes the tetanus quite well and also admits its curability in certain cases. It omits among the symptoms fever, which is, nevertheless, extreme and which is noted by Plato, who, in accord with other Hippocratic manuals (*Aphor.,* IV, 57; *Coan Prognoses,* 348; *On Diseases,* 1, 7; *On Crises,* 61) makes of it a favourable symptom. On tetanus and on opisthotonus; Suśr., 51-57, who relates them similarly to the wind, but in association with the phlegm.

the sacred substance in us.[1] The sour and salty phlegm produces extremely diverse catarrhal diseases.

"For the ailments called phlegmonous, because they provoke burning and swelling, they are, all of them, caused by bile" (85 b). When the bile goes out, it provokes tumours; retained, it provokes inflammatory diseases, mostly when it gets mixed with the blood. The blood contains fibres which prevent it from being too liquid (it is the observation of the coagulum separating itself from the serum which, apparently, has given rise to this theory of fibres). The bile which belongs to the blood become old, which is "hot and liquid", causes by its heat, if it flows in the blood in abundance, disorder in the fibres. It can penetrate up to the marrow and burn it, provoking death. But if it is in small quantities it can be pushed back by the vessels in the thorax or in the abdomen and from there can be evacuated (85 e).

The passage terminates with an enumeration of fevers. The continuous ones are due to fire; the daily ones are due to air; those occurring every third day to water, slower than fire and air; those occurring every fourth day are due to earth, which is slower still. The sources of this pathology have not been fully elucidated.[2] Mr. Rivaud asks himself if Plato had not accepted from all sides different hypotheses which he had not sought to reconcile. It is certain that one could find, scattered in various texts, the elements of the doctrine of the *Timaeus* and that uptil now no Greek medical text, grouping these elements in the manner in which he has grouped them, has been pointed out. The Hippocratic manuals present different pathological theories but they recognise most often the action of the four elements (which is also done by Plato in his description of the first class of the diseases), or of four properties, the cold and the hot, the dry and the humid (cf., *On Ancient Medicine*, 1, which combats this theory); or of four humours, blood, phlegm, yellow bile and black bile (*On the Nature of Man*, 4) or blood, bile,

[1] This explanation of the name is not, as is known, in accord with the Hippocratic manual *On the Sacred Disease* which says that it should be so called as it is considered to be coming from the gods, but who contests the opinion that it can be provoked by divinity.

[2] cf., A. Rivaud, *loc., cit.*, pp. 114-5. A.E. Taylor, *A Commentary on Plato's Timaeus*, Oxford, 1928, p. 599, is embarrassed; he believes that Plato must have made use of a source which he does not find in what is known of the Greek medical tradition.

water and phlegm (*On Generation*, 3 and *On Diseases,* IV, 32); or of bile and of phlegm (*On Diseases*, II, 2), etc. Only in Indian medicine is found in the form of a received doctrine a pathogeny similar to that of Plato, some details being in concordance on the two sides, some being different.

The pathogeny of troubles due to the wind differs in the Sanskrit texts and in the *Timaeus*, because of the fact that, in the latter, Plato brings in the lung as the distributor of the air in the body whereas the Sanskrit texts do not even mention it on that occasion. Plato has also a theory of breathing which says that something like a trap of fire and of air was introduced by God in the body, where it would go out alternatively.[1] This theory does not appear to be found in India. But the idea that the wind retained in the body provokes therein pains and convulsions, is a part of classical Indian teaching. The text of Suśruta, studied above, links specially tetanus to the wind under its various forms, stressing the predominance of contractions on such and such a group of muscles, extensor or flexor. The concordance with the *Timaeus* in this respect is complete.

The theory of phlegm in Plato is quite similar to that of the *śleṣman* of Indian doctors. Plato has described the phlegm before indicating its rôle in diseases. "Serosity (*ikhor*) when it comes from the blood is sweet, the one that comes from black and acid bile is malignant, above all, when because of the action of heat, it gets mixed with the salted quality. Another type of serosity is formed from new and tender flesh, dissolved in the air . . . we call it white phlegm (*leukhon*)" (83c-d). Suśruta, on his side, teaches: "The phlegm is white, heavy, unctuous, viscous and cold. But, sweet when it is not burnt; when burnt, it can be salty".[2] Although the formation of the phlegm is taught differently in the Greek and Indian texts, and although only the Greek text brings in the black bile, both agree on a theory which is quite strange and to which the observation of real facts does not naturally lead, namely the

[1] 78. Galen had rightly judged this concept to be difficult to follow. He has, nevertheless, explained it in detail, cf., Ch. Daremberg. *Fragments du commentaire du Galien sur le Timeé de Platon*, Paris-Leipzig, 1848, pp. 18 ff.

[2] Suśr., *Sūtr*., XXI, 12: *śleṣmā śveto guruḥ snigdhaḥ picchilaḥ śīta eva ca, madhuras tv avidagdhah syād vidagdho lavaṇah smṛtaḥ.*

passage of the phlegm from sweet to salt under the action of heat.[1]

Concerning the 'hot and liquid' nature of the bile, Plato agrees fully with the old Vedic idea of the igneous nature of bile, an idea inherited by Ayurvedic medicine. He brings in the bile from a liquefaction of extremely old fleshes, getting black under the action of prolonged heating and becoming bitter or acid. The bitter parts plunge themselves in the blood and this results in a green tint. Finally the younger parts of the flesh give the yellow colour along with bitterness (83 a-b). Suśruta cites a verse summarising the Indian ideas concerning the bile: "The bile is bitter, liquid, fetid, black and also yellow, hot and of acrid taste, and when it is burnt, it is acid."[2] Some of the notions which agree on both sides, are of little significance. The amertume of the bile is a commonplace and universal fact but the same is not true of the theory saying that the bile, under the influence of heat, becomes acid.

The explanation of certain diseases by the irruption of bile in blood is common to Plato and to Indian doctors who call this accident *rakta-pitta*, "blood-bile" (Suśruta, *Uttara-tantra*, XIV) and attribute to it the origin of the spontaneous haemmorrhages which occur principally in the course of acute diseases. It is probably because the idea has been conceived in the presence of the forms of grave icterus, relatively frequent in a tropical country and characterised both by jaundice and multiple haemmorrhages. But the Platonic theory of the fibres of the blood does not appear to be found in Indian medicine.

The fevers enumerated by Plato, while finishing his exposition concerning the diseases of the body, are well known in India, not only to doctors, but even to the authors of the magical conjurations of the *Atharvaveda*.[3] In any case their knowledge is necessary in all those countries where they occur within the eastern basin of the Mediterranean as also in India.

---

1 The experience of heating the phlegm and of subsequently testing it after having tasted it before could have been carried out. The manual *On Flesh*, 4, prescribes to cook the tissues to appraise the properties. But the phlegmatic secretions (mucosity for example) are salty before being cooked. It should, therefore, be a theoretical opinion and not an experimental statement.

2 *pittam tīkṣṇam dravam pūti nīlam pītam tathaiva ca,*
uṣṇam kaṭurasañ caiva vidaghan cāmlameva ca.—Suśr., *Sūtr.*, XXI, 8.

3 cf., *supra*, pp. 115-116.

The explanation of their varieties, given by Plato, according to the elements in question, does not agree with the usual pathogenic theories of Indians.

Leaving aside the passages dealing with the pathogeny by air, with phlegm and with bile, and those that concern the very nature of phlegm and bile, other concordances with Indian ideas are also found in the *Timaeus*.

One and the same comparison is proposed in the *Timaeus* and in Suśruta. Plato says that the gods have "dug canals in our body, similar to those established in the gardens, so that it may be watered, as by the course of a stream" (77c-d). Suśruta does not bring in the demiurge but says that by the presence of vessels "the body is like a garden or like a field with water-drains".[1] But it is evident that such a comparison is so natural that it could have come to the minds of both Plato and Suśruta quite independently.

Among the vessels Plato distinguishes two conduits placed on both sides of the vertebral column, and of the generating Medulla and which, near the head, branch out in interconnected form (77d-e). Mr. Rivaud rightly hesitates regarding their identification[2], but it seems to refer in Plato to a theoretical concept, based merely on a vague knowledge of the existence of thick vessels near the vertebral column, because he says: They (the gods) dug two dorsal vessels, as the body was in double, having a right and a left" (77 d). These vessels do not really correspond to any anatomic reality but are, on the other hand, a datum of theoretical anatomy of India which is, this time, not furnished by the Sanskrit medical texts themselves but by the mystical literature o f the *Tantras*. In fact it is a thesis current in this literature as also in the later Upaniṣads which refer to the same ideas. It amounts to saying that two canals called *iḍā* and *piṅgalā* are found on the two sides of the vertebral column and of a central canal called the *suṣumnā*[3],

---

1 Suśr., *Śār.*, VII, 1, cf. *Supra* , p. 163. This comparison is also found in Aristotle (*De part. anim*, 668 a, 10) as has been pointed out by Rivaud, *Timaeus*, p. 207, note.

2 Page 207, note, he identifies them with the Aorta and the veins of the superior and the inferior cave, but, at p. 98, he shows the difficulties in this identification.

cf., *Ahirbudhnya-saṁhitā*, XXXII, 27 and 29; *Kṣurikopaniṣad*, 16. Numerous references are to be found in the index of Mahadeva Sastri, *The Yoga Upanishads*, Adyar, 1920.

the three cross one another in the body. Moreover, the tantric texts vary as regards the question of their crossing one another.[1]

In *Timaeus* is to be found yet another concordance with the doctrines of Tantric mysticism. Plato, while establishing a relationship between the elements of nature and geometrical forms (55e-56b), gives the figure of the cube to earth, that of the triangular pyramid to fire, that of the octahedral to air and that of the icosahedral to water. Now the *tantras* also represent the elements symbolically in various diagrams (*maṇḍalas*) by means of analogous geometrical figures, although plane ones; earth by the square, fire by the triangle, air by a figure of six points (two equilateral triangles superposed one on the other), water by a figure resembling the crescent Moon and ether by the circle.[2] This is a case of the encounters of symbolism whose history is quite complex; because in Egypt on the Zodiac of Denderah, a monument later than Plato (of the epoch of Ptolemy) is found a representation of the solar light by several chains of triangles.[3] The Tantric texts containing these several points of agreement with the ideas of *Timaeus* are also much later than this last work.

One should also count the belief of Plato in metempsychosis and his theory of the vision among the concordances of his ideas with that of India. This is not the place to examine the former but the latter conforms to the medical concepts of India in so far as Plato admits the existence of a fire inside the eye, the fire which, on meeting the external light, links up, by the union of the similar with the similar, the object with the perceiving soul (45 b-d). Similarly Suśruta describes a fire which is a form of bile called *ālocaka* and which, localised in the eye, is the agent of vision.[4] The Platonic theory of the visual fire

---

1 The idea of a similar crossing of thick vessels in the body is found in the Hippocratic collection (*On the Nature of Man*, 11, where several "veins" forming the third pair of the system described, go from the temples to the lungs, the one from the right side coming to the left side and vice versa).

2 cf., Avalon, *Tantric Texts*, Vol. III, Calcutta, London, 1944, p.7 (Introduction to the edition of the *Prapañca-sāra-tantra* by Tārānātha Vidyāratna).

3 cf., Antoniadi, *L'astronomie égyptienne*, Paris, 1934, fig. 25 and p. 88.

4 Suśr., *Sūtr.*, XXI, 7.

is, moreover, far from being isolated in the Hellenic world[1] and Bühler had, long ago, drawn the attention of Th. Gomperz on the analogy presented by the theory of the vision of Alcmaeon of Croton (VIth century B.C.) and that of the *Nyāya-Vaiśeṣika* philosophy of India.[2] In Alcmaeon the theory seems to be different from that of Plato but the existence of an intra-ocular fire is put forward in principle.[3] On this point the accord is complete between India on the one hand and Alcmaeon and Plato on the other.

The interpretation of all these concordances between the doctrines of *Timaeus* and those of the physiologists, indeed the mystics, of India is delicate. It seems difficult to relate all of them, at the same time, to the coincidences of hazard. The similarity of subjects studied and the rudimentary means then available, both in India as in Greece, to the human mind for solving the problems of Physiology and of Pathology can explain all of them only with difficulty. Noted at a time when it was readily believed that Plato had reproduced the ideas of the so-called Pythagorean *Timaeus* and that Pythagoras had known the ideas of India, these concordances could have been easily considered as the witnesses of the dependence of Pythagorism and Plato on India. But today, and although the question of the eventual relationship of Pythagoras with India has never been seriously settled, this question cannot be settled with equal ease. The romance of the Pythagorean *Timaeus* is considered as based, for a large part, on the dialogue of Plato[4] himself and the value of the ancient tradition which says that Plato had probably borrowed the clearer part of his Physics and Biology from the Pythagoreans, is contested.[5] From another side, the possible influence of the Orient on Plato has been postulated by several authors[6], without anybody having

---

1 cf, Rivaud, *Timaeus*, p. 105.

2 cf., Th. Gomperz, *Les penseurs de la Grece*, French trans., p. 185, f.n. 1.

3 cf., Theophrastes, *Des Sensations*, 27.

4 Rivaud, *Timaeus*, p. 18.

5 ibid., p. 24.

6 cf., W. Jaeger, *Aristoteles*, Berlin, 1923, pp. 123 ff; H.S. Nyberg, *Questions de Cosmogonie et de cosmologie mazdéennes* in *JA*, July-Sept, 1931, pp. 104 ff. Last of all J. Bidez, *Eos ou Platon et l'Orient*, Brussels, 1945, and A.J. Festugiere, "Platon et l'Orient." in *Revue de Philologie*, XXI, fasc. 1, pp. 5 ff. (the latter is more reserved).

been able to point out any precise data as our sources of information, concerning the Iranian or 'Chaldean' doctrines, which have been almost exclusively considered, are quite precarious. All that we can say today is this: that the concordances of *Timaeus* with Indian doctrines appear to us to be more striking because these Indian doctrines are much more accessible to us.

We have briefly pointed out the resemblances between the *Timaeus* and the Indian ideas found at quite a late date. We have chiefly stopped to look at patent similarities between the medical doctrine of the *Timaeus* and the Ayurvedic pathology whose essential elements, as we know, date from the Vedic epoch and which became a system between the epoch of the *Śatapatha-brāhmaṇa* and that of the grammarian Kātyāyana, i.e., approximately between the VIIth century and the end of the IVth century B.C. Plato lived from 428 or 417 to 347 B.C. and the *Timaeus* belongs to the end of the life of Plato, to the second quarter of the IVth century. On his side, the Hippocratic manual *On Breaths*, whose pneumatism has been found by us to be comparable to that of India, although not dated, belongs to a period quite near that of Plato and, in any case, to a period before that of Aristotle and of Alexander.

Thus the two groups of precise concordances noted by us between Greek and Indian medicine refer to the same period, anterior to the expedition of Alexander in India, an expedition about which it is generally said that it marked the first contact between India and Greece. In order to interpret correctly the concordances noted above, we will, therefore, have to see if the two worlds presenting them were, at that time, in reality, totally strangers to each other.

CHAPTER NINE

COMMUNICATIONS BETWEEN GREECE AND INDIA BEFORE ALEXANDER

It is currently admitted that it is because of the expedition of Alexander to India that India has been put in communication with the Hellenic world. It is quite natural to state that only when the Greek armies entered India and for the first time occupied the basin of the Indus did the Greeks and the Indians start really knowing each other. It suffices to compare the data on India possessed by the Greeks before Alexander, for example at the time of Herodotus, in the middle of the Vth Century B.C. with the data acquired by them during this expedition (an idea of the same can be had by the numerous fragments of Nearchos, of Aristobulos, of Onesicritos or of Megasthenes) to appreciate the immense progress that the direct contact had realised in the knowledge of India in the West. It is also clear that this progress has had no immediate consequences because the direct contact was very soon broken by the expulsion, after the death of Alexander, of the Prefects he had left in India and by the reconquest of the Indus basin by Candragupta.[1] To convince oneself about the same, one has only to note that during the centuries that followed, the majority of Greek and Latin authors who have written on India have borrowed their information from the contemporaries of Alexander and Seleucos. And, in this matter, one should not limit oneself only to noting the facts gathered from what we possess of Greek and Latin writings because the evidence of Strabo gives us the guarantee that even in those writings that have not reached us, but which were available to him when he wrote his *Geography*, about the beginning of the Christian era, little had been added to the data of the epoch of Alexander. Strabo, in fact, strongly deplores that this state of affairs does not enable him to draw a satisfactory picture of

[1] Justin, *Epitoma Historiarum Philippicarum*, XV, 4, 12, ff.

India (XV, 1, 23).

Strabo is even severe on those companions of Alexander who have written on India and on their rare successors. According to him, these men had rushed through India as soldiers, had seen only some parts, had learnt a great deal only by hearsay and did not agree, even among themselves on what they had seen with their own eyes. If, therefore, even those who, in a large number of cases, had been able to learn directly about the Indian world, have such a precarious and such an uncertain knowledge of India, it is difficult not to believe that, for better reasons, during the preceding period, the two worlds of Greece and India have been completely unknown to each other.

If one were to hold to these considerations one could be tempted not to pursue the enquiry and to conclude right now that no intellectual communication could have taken place between India and the Hellenic world before Alexander and that the analogies observed between the medical doctrines of India and Greece of that epoch are purely fortuitous, no matter how numerous and precise they may be. However, it must be observed that intellectual exchanges do not necessarily suppose complete and reciprocal knowledge, not even direct contacts. It will, therefore, not be correct on our part to say that because India and Greece had not known each other very well in antiquity, nothing could have passed from one to the other. To pursue the examination of the question of their relationship, it will suffice to find out if any intermediary had existed between them. We know that the Persian Empire had been this intermediary.

The conquest of a part of India by the Achaemenian Persians or rather the conquest of India in the narrow and original sense of the word, that is to say of the Indus valley, is attributed to Darius I, but it should go back partly to Cyrus, as has been shown by Foucher.[1] In fact Darius, in his inscription of Behistan, declares that he has re-established his authority on the entire domain of Cyrus and mentions amongst

---

[1] *Les satrapies orientales de l'empire achéménide*, in *Comptes rendus de l'Acad. des Inscr. et Belles Lettres*, 1938, pp. 340-341; *La Nicée d'Aghanistan*, ibid., 1939, p. 438. *La vieille route de l'Inde de Bactres á Taxila*, with the collaboration of Mrs. E. Bazin Foucher, in *Mém. Deleg. archeol. franc. en Afghanistan*, Vols. I & II, 1947, pp. 190 ff.

the satrapies forming this domain of Gadara, that is to say Gandhara which, at that time, extended from the Hindukush up to the Hydraotes at least, descending towards the south up to Multan, thus comprising the entire far North-West and the greater part of the Punjab. Moreover, Pliny has reproduced an older piece of information which said that Cyrus had destroyed Cappissa, that is to say, Kāpiśī, to the South of the Hindukush, therefore at the beginning of his conquest of Gandhara.

These facts, in their totality, are corroborated by Arrian (*Ind.*, I, 3) who writes that the people living between the Kophen (Kubha, river of Kabul) and the Indus, had been the subjects of the Assyrians, then of the Medians and then of the Persians and that they had paid tribute to Cyrus. These facts are nowhere contradicted by tradition, which, though contested, said that the same Cyrus had met with a disaster while trying to attack the Indians, because it manifestly relates to an attack on the people of the lower Indus, of Sindh. It seems that this attack was directed through Gedrosia as, according to Strabo who refers to this tradition without giving it much credence, it was for the glory of marching his entire army through a region, where Cyrus had lost his, that Alexandar withdrew from India through Gedrosia (XV, 1, 5).

It was left to Darius to bring Sindh into the Achaemenian Empire but, as Gandhara was a land of Indian culture, a narrow and direct contact of this culture with the Achaemenian civilisation should undoubtedly start before 528 B.C., the date of the death of Cyrus.[1]

Herodotus has recounted how Darius had (apparently in 519 B.C.) deputed the Greek Skylax of Karyanda in Caria, to explore the lower course of the Indus and how Skylax, starting

[1] According to Ktesias (*Persica* 6) Cyrus died of a wound inflicted on him by an Indian soldier belonging to a corps allied against him with the Derbices, people living to the east of the Caspian sea, and who had brought to them the elephants of war. But Ktesias is contradicted by Xenophon (*Cyrop.*, VIII, 7, 3-38) who makes Darius die in his place, by Herodotos (I, 214) who says that he was killed in a battle against the Massagetes and by Berose (*Fr.*, 29, 6-7) who makes him die in a war against the Dahai of Parthia. The incertitude, therefore, is very great, although some parts of this information are irreconciliable. The fact reported by Ktesias can lead only to the inference that the presence of a corps of Indian soldiers with elephants in a region to the east of the Caspian was not considered impossible. It is true that Ktesias has often left the domain of probability in his writings but we will see that at least commerce did regularly bring Indian goods to such regions.

from Kaspapyros or Kaspatyros (now Multan) reached the Indus, took to the sea and arrived, thirty months after his departure, at the Egyptian port, from where, in earlier times the Phoenicians had left for the periplus of Africa. The conquest followed a little later. The inscription of Darius at Persepolis, between 518 and 515, mentions the Hidu, that is to say the Sindh among the satrapies.

The Persian occupation continued up to the conquest of the Achaemenian Empire by Alexander in 331. It was, therefore, kept up, probably with variations in the extent of subject territories, during approximately 185 years. Over this long period, the India of the North-West had been subjected to the deep influences of Persia, and which has, often been noted. One of the most notable ones was the local adoption of the Aramaic alphabet used in the Achaemenian administration confined in the whole empire to the functionaries of Babylonian culture. This alphabet had been completed with new forms and diacritical signs and adapted to the phonetic transcription of the Indian languages, just as had been the case, at a later date, with regard to these languages of the Arabic and European alphabets. It constituted the script called Kharoṣṭhi which should, for the sake of clarity and exactitude, be called Arameo-Indian.[1] Unfortunately, no document in this script and dating from the period of the Achaemanian domination has reached us. The oldest specimens known are the inscriptions of Aśoka which date from the middle of the IIIrd cent. B.C. and are, in consequence, about eighty years later after the end of the Persian administration. We can, consequently, know nothing of the relations between the learned of India and the functionaries of Irano-Babylon. At least we have the proof, in the existence of the Arameo-Indian script itself, that these relations were effective, because the adaptation of the Armaic alphabet to Indian languages is the result of a savant effort and supposes the intervention of competent grammarians.

This fact is pregnant with consequences. In 525, a few years before the conquest of Sindh by Darius, Cambyses had conquered Egypt and there also had been installed the

[1] cf., *Ecritures aramea indienne.*--in Ch. Fossey, *Notices sur les caractères étrangers, ancienstet modernes* Paris, 1948, pp. 203 ff

same administration of the Aramaic language as had been the case in India. By means of this step, the Achaemenians had thrown a bridge of Mesopotamian culture between Egypt and India. The big unit formed by the Persian empire had been sufficiently coherent to enable numerous exchanges between its farthest parts. Historians have not always justly appreciated the organisation of this empire. As has been very well pointed out by Sylvain Lévi, "We have taken up the cause of Greece, espoused, exaggerated its just grudges; the Persians are the vanquished and the Barbarians".[1] It is true that they have not imposed, not even powerfully spread in their territories a civilisation which was specifically and exclusively Iranian. But they have created political unity transcending races and religions. It is to the glory of Cyrus and Darius that they tolerated the beliefs of their subjects and this toleration has favoured the flowering and the exchange of thought. On the side of syncretisms (all of them have not been happy though) this has given rise to a large interchange of ideas where all the tributary people could bring in theirs and obtain those of others.

The Greeks had put in many products of their genius and had been easily able to draw therefrom many new suggestions or precious knowledge. The King of Lydia, Cresus, had conquered the Greek establishments of Asia Minor[2] towards 560 and Lydia fell to Cyrus in 546. Ionia did not remain a peaceful subject of the Persians for long. It revolted from 499 to 494. The Persians sacked the Ionian towns and the bloody battles were not conducive to activating intellectual exchanges. Those which could take place with the Greece of Europe were also undoubtedly compromised by wars. But a large number of Greeks did, at that time, espouse the cause of the Persians and the conflicts between peoples did not hinder the activity of scientific and philosophical speculation. Moreover, the war was not continual. Miletus having taken the oath to Cyrus, stayed for some time, in perfect peace with the Achaemenians (Herodotus, I,169) and some of the most notable of its children, like Hekateus were the partisans of an *entente* with the Persians. Moreover, the war itself was sometimes the occasion of deport-

[1] *L'Inde civilisatrice,* Paris, 1938, p. 40.
[2] Herodotus, I, 26-27.

ing captives who, humanely treated in exile, could take the ideas of their country far. After the occupation of revolted Miletus in 496, a contingent of Milesian prisoners was first led to Susa, and then settled on the Erythrean sea at the mouth of the Tigris (Herodotos, VI, 20). The epoch of these wars is precisely that of the philosophers of Ionia. Thales and Anaximander flourished at the time when Cresus subjected Ionia. Anaximenes died in 525; Heraclitus wrote a little after 478; Anaxagoras, born in Asia Minor, at Clazomenes, lived chiefly at Athens but came back to end his days in Asia Minor, at Lampascus, towards 428. At the boundary of the Persian empire or incorporated therein, Ionia in its essential period of intellectual activity, has remained a part both of the Asian world and the Hellenic world. Its radiance reached both of them. It is difficult for us to believe that the Ionian thinkers have had no influence from the side of orient and that they remained blind and deaf to all that came from that side. India was not unknown to Miletus. One of its illustrious citizens, Hekateus, towards 500 B.C., possessed information concerning the geography and the peoples of India; the little fragments of his work that have been preserved for us show it to us directly. Unceasing relations, chiefly maritime, had put Ionia in contact with all the insular and the riverain people of the Mediterranean, especially with Egypt. Thales whose ancestors, according to Herodotos, were of Phoenician origin[1] and Heraclitus are often considered as having acquired important knowledge in Egypt.[2] As regards Thales, Tannery even thought that he had acquired the means of forecasting eclipses in Egypt and that, as this means was rather Chaldean, possibly the Egyptians had borrowed it from the Chaldeans, before the time of Thales.[3] But Tannery forgot that Lydia, to which the motherland of Thales was then subject, was of Mesopotamian culture. This fact renders useless the hypothesis of an intervention of the Egyptians, at least for

1 I, 170. Modern authors have seldom noticed this fact. Many have sought to combat it. However Th. Gomperz has remarked that their objections only prove that probably Herodotos may have been mistaken, but it is unlikely that the Greeks had, without any motive, given a foreign origin to one of their great men. (*Les penseurs de la Grèce*, French trans., p. 76, f.n. 2).

2 P. Tannery, *Pour l'histoire de la science hellène*, Paris, 1930; *On Thales*, pp. 57 ff.; *On Heraclitus*, pp. 179 ff.

3 ibid., p. 62.

a loan of the Chaldean astronomy. The exchanges take place not only in particularly suitable countries; the political state of the Mediterranean Orient made them possible everywhere and in all directions.

They took place equally with the Greek colonies of Italy, of Sicily and of Cyrenaica. We know the precise circumstances of the historical relations about which we do not know positively whether they ended in intellectual exchanges but which, at least, offered the requisite conditions for the establishment of such exchanges. This is how at the beginning of the reign of Darius, in the same epoch when the Great King was having the lower course of the Indus reconnoitred by the Greek Skylax, a part of the inhabitants of Barka in Cyrenaica[1] was abducted and transported to Bactriana where lands were allotted to them for founding a new Barka (Herodotos, IV, 204). The presence, at the end of the VIth Cent B.C., of Greeks or of men of Greek culture in India or at the gates of India is thus well attested. The deportees of Barka, of course, never came back to the West but they could have brought western ideas to India. Skylax, for his part, came back from his voyage and wrote a report thereof, which has unfortunately not reached us. Herodotos (III, 125-127) has also recounted the story of the doctor of Crotona, Demokedes.[2] This doctor who accompanied Polycrates, the tyrant of Samos, when the latter was drawn towards an ambush at Magnesia by the Persian Oretes, was made a prisoner and sent to Susa in 522 B.C. A little later, Darius, suffering from an ankle-sprain and not finding himself any better after eight days of treatment by the Egyptian doctors, was informed of the presence and of the qualities as doctor of Demokedes; the latter was then forced to treat Darius. The doctor was successful and remained, although against his will,

---

[1] At Cyrene flourished an important medical school but chiefly a little later, in the Vth century, cf., M. Wellmann, 'Alkmaion von Kroton', *Archeion*, XI, 1929, p. 156. Herodotos says that at one time the Crotonians were considered as first among doctors and those of Cyrene as second (I, 131).

[2] Suidas, under the word *dimokhydis*, says that his father had been the priest of Asklepios at Cnida and Jamblique makes a Pythagorean of him (*Vie de Pytha.*, 357), cf. A. Gotze, "Persische Weisheit in Griechischem Gewande", in *Zeit. fur Ind. und. Ir.*, p. 97, who rightly notes the importance of the presence of three doctors in India, for the history of medical communications between Iran and the Hellenic world.

attached to Darius. Having, later on, cured the queen Atossa of a suppurated ailment in the chest, he succeeded in making her to persuade Darius to send him under escort to reconnoitre Greece in view of an invasion. There he succeeded in escaping from the Persians and re-entered Crotona where he married the daughter of the famous athlete Milon. He sent word of this marriage to Darius because, says Herodotos, the name of Milon was, at that time, very well-known in the Persian court. Suidas says that he wrote a book on medicine.

Demokedes was certainly an eminent doctor although his cures at the court of Persia have probably been more fortunate than difficult. The sprain of Darius, painful as it naturally is during the first days, was not very serious, otherwise it could not have been rapidly cured as is said to have been the case by Herodotos. Undoubtedly Demokedes was lucky to have been called in a little before the normal attenuation of painful phenomena, but it is certain that the medical school of Crotona, the town of athletes, had specialised in the treatment of traumatisms and that Demokedes had personally acquired a great renown in the Hellenic world before he got attached to Polycrates. He was, therefore, capable of spreading in Iran Greek medical knowledge of great value as also of learning foreign theories and methods.[1] As he was able to come back to Crotona and was probably able to write there, he could have made known the Oriental data and techniques. The Achaemenian Court was certainly a meeting place for intellectual exchanges as reports from all the satrapies converged there and as the story of Demokedes himself tells us about Egyptian doctors and a Greek one assembled there. Moreover, relations between Susa and Crotona existed independently of the chance captivity of Demokedes at Susa as, according to Herodotos, Milon was well known in the Iranian Court.

Two other Greek doctors have been employed by the Achaemenians. It is known that according to a legend and certain texts, which are very probably apocryphal[2], Hippocrates had refused the parents of Artaxerxes, who had ordered him to

---

[1] On the probable Oriental influences on Demokedes and his own influence on the Greek schools of Italy, cf., P.M. Schuhl, *Essai sur la formation de la pensée grecque,* pp. 307 ff.

[2] Hippocrates, Vol. IX, pp. 308 ff.

come for fighting against an epidemic, but Appollonides of Cos practised in the Court of Artaxerxes from the beginning of the reign of this prince, even if he had not been there before him. In fact, he cured Megabyze, wounded during the troubles which followed the failure of the conspiracy of Artaban against Artaxerxes[1] in 464, seven months after the assassination of Xerxes which took place during the summer of 465. He had more time than Demokedes to propagate Greek medicine in Iran, but did not return to his country. He was shamefully executed in 440 for having seduced Amytis, the widow of Megabyze, under the pretence of curing her of an hysterical disease.[2]

Lastly Ktesias of Cnidus, who has narrated these facts, was for a long time the doctor of Artaxerxes II and is said to have ended his days in his own country. He has remained famous by the fragments of his writings preserved by Photius and one of which was specially devoted to India. This work is of little value, in so far as it has reached us, because it is full of fables, but its existence positively guarantees that which was rendered, *a priori*, probable by the state itself of the Achaemenian empire, that is to say, that information concerning India could reach the Greeks by the intermediary of Iran. If the information of Ktesias is fantastic, it does not follow that nothing serious could have been then brought from India. Ktesias is not a critical author—the fragments of his work on Persia prove this point—he is certainly responsible for having listened to fables. Besides, Photius has been able to choose in his work the most extraordinary allegations and leave aside data which were truer but less striking. It is not doubtful, however, that the functionaries of the satrapies of Gandhara and of Sindh could bring nothing but the marvellous to the Achaemenian Court.

It may be stated that the facilities offered by the great unity of the Achaemenian empire to the cultural exchanges between India and the West have proved to be of little effect. A serious error of Herodotos incidentally proves it. The Father of history was a Greek of Asia, he hailed from Halicarnassus, in Caria

---

1 Ktesias, *Persica*, 30.
2 ibid., 42.

which was under the Persians. He lived from approximately 480 to 425. A great traveller and a man of great learning, he knew things Iranian and Egyptian particularly well. He was therefore seemingly well-placed for having exact information concerning the Mesopotamian sciences then in use in the Persian empire administered by the functionaries of Babylonian culture. He says, nevertheless, that the Babylonians have no doctors, that among them the sick are exhibited in the public place and that the passers-by give them advice according to their experience (I, 197). His information presents on this point an enormous lacuna; we possess a large number of the fragments of the medical literature of Babylonia[1] and the code of Hammurabi had already, towards 2000 B.C., fixed the fees of the doctors and the punishments they incurred in case of default.[2]

Badly informed of the social life and of the state of science at Babylon, Herodotos' knowledge of farther India is, generally speaking, still worse. This leads to the consequence that, in the Greek world of Asia, one was not generally and regularly well-informed on all that touched the peoples of the Persian empire. It does not follow in the least that it was impossible to have occasionally precise information concerning the ideas of their peoples.

Herodotos himself fortuitously gives us the proof that under the Achaemenians Greeks and Indians could meet and know the ideas of each other. He describes (III, 38) how Darius, one day, asked the Greeks, his subjects, if they could force themselves to nourish themselves on the dead bodies of their relations. The reply was, as was to be expected, that they would never do it. Thereupon Darius confronted the Indians called Kalatiai[3],

1 Description and bibliography in G. Contenau, *La médicine en Assyrie et en Babylonie*, Paris, 1938.

2 ibid., pp. 30-45.

3 Hekateus of Miletus also mentions the Kalatiai. The word can refer to some people of the North-West because Megasthenes has, later on, reported that the inhabitants of the Indian Caucasus ate the dead bodies of their relations (Strabo, XV, 1, 56). Herodotos himself attributes an analogous custom to the Padaioi (III, 99). After having summarily described the customs of another category of Indians, he adds that those of whom he has talked are black in colour, farther from the Persians towards the centre and who have never been the subjects of Darius. If these latter details relate to the Padaioi as also to the Indians mentioned after them, these Padaioi have nothing in common with the Kalatiai, except for a similarity of customs. From then onwards it is difficult to recognise, as Lassen has claimed to do after

who had the custom of eating their relations. They showed as much indignation as the Greeks when Darius asked them about the amount of money which could persuade them to burn the dead bodies of their relations. An interpreter, Herodotos specifies, was explaining to the Greeks all that was being said on both sides. Such conferences and conversations with the help of interpreters evidently facilitated the exchange of ideas. Therefore it is not only the voyagers like Skylax who could have learnt something about India and could have carried Hellenic notions of the same. The Greek doctors of Susa could have found themselves in a position to communicate with the Indians, of whom many, at that time, were more cultured than the Kalatiai cannibals. And, in a more general way, to enable the intellectual contacts among the peoples of the Persian empire to be more efficacious, it was sufficient to have suggestions and points of general information to pass from one country to another. It was not in the least necessary that the corpus of entire doctrines had to be carried and taught with a popular repercussion so that the memory of the same could not have failed to reach us.

On the other hand, and above all, it should be observed that precise enquiries which help us to obtain deep knowledge are often those which take place without much noise and we have the proof that such enquiries have been made on India inside the Persian administration. Strabo tells us that one of the rare authors for whom he has great regard among those who have written on India following the expedition of Alexander, namely, Patrocles[1] had said that the companions of Alexander had only an extremely superficial knowledge of India, whereas Alexander himself could have been better informed, as he had got detailed descriptions from people knowing the country well. Patrocles was able to see these reports as an act of special favour by the treasurer Xenocles (II, 1, 6). These exact reports were therefore secret or at least were not written for being circulated and largely known. Their authors being men

---

Bohlan by basing himself on Herodotos (*Ind. Alt.*, I, pp. 465-466; II, p. 639) the word *kāla* "black" in the name of the Kalatiai. One may ask oneself if this name does not cover a form *khalati*, "bald" attested since the *Yajurveda*, not, of course, as the name of any people.

[1] Named also by Pliny (VI, 21) as the admiral of Seleukos and of Antiochos Soter.

who knew the country were not the Greeks brought by Alexander. They were, in all probability, the functionaries of Achaemenians who had passed under the authority of the conqueror, come to take possession of the satrapies administered by them. Their reports must have been devoted more to the geographical, economic and political conditions than to Indian thought but they could not have ignored the latter and they were in a position to give information regarding the same to the Greeks. It is through men of this type that scientific ideas have been easily able to pass through the Achaemenian Empire and reach the Greeks of the Orient. Moreover, it is quite possible that some of these men were Greeks and had been in the service of the Persians in India for a long time, because, before conquering Sindh, Darius had sent Skylax there.

It is certainly through them rather than through the soldiers, or even the philosophers who accompanied them in their march, that theoretical data on science could have been transported. Even a philosopher cannot always collect useful information only by chance encounters during his passage. Onesikritos gives us an example of the same. Sent by Alexander to talk with the gymnosophists, he was able to have a sufficiently important conversation with them, but it became necessary for him to abandon the idea of knowing their thoughts fully because it was necessary to have recourse to three successive interpreters.[1] Men conversant with the country could have informed him more effectively about the ideas of these gymnosophists than the latter themselves encountered in passing.

Besides, it is not excluded that Indians themselves may have sometimes established themselves in Greek lands for a sufficiently long time for having been able to disseminate among the learned some of their ideas. We have, on this subject, a text whose authenticity is not ordinarily admitted but which does deserve to be examined.

[1] Strabo, XV, 1, 64. Onesikritos has nevertheless drawn from this conversation certain data which are interesting even for us today. This is how he has understood a legend according to which the earth was at first covered with food but this food disappeared as a punishment for the insolence of human beings. A similar legend is found much later in texts like the *Mahavastu*, ed. Senart, I, pp. 338 ff. The report of Onesikritos teaches us usefully that this legend existed in the IVth century B.C.

Mr. Bréhier, Mr. Bidez and Father Festugiére have drawn attention to an extract of Aristoxenes of Tarentum, quoted after Aristocles by Eusebes in his *Préparation évangélique* (XI, 3, 8)[1], Aristoxenes, who lived towards 320-300 had narrated how an Indian who used to see Socrates at Athens, made fun of him one day when he learnt that Socrates did research on human life, saying that it was impossible to understand things human as long as things divine were ignored. If Socrates had thus been able to communicate with an Indian philosopher in Athens, it would have been quite natural for Plato to have knowledge of the medical doctrines of India which are evoked in his *Timaeus* by so many characteristic resemblances. But this piece is considered as presenting a purely imaginary anecdote. The possibility of the presence at Athens of an Indian before 399, the date of the death of Socrates, that is to say, more than seventy years before Alexander, had opened the Indian world to the knowledge of the Hellenes, does not seem to have been found worthy of examination. The only effort made has been to find out the reasons as to why such encounters between Greek and Oriental sages have been evoked.

In fact, the dialogues between Greek and Oriental sages were numerous and appear during certain periods in Greek literature; they should be considered together as has been done by the Father Festugiére and there is every reason to think that the majority of them, far from having been composed on the basis of original documents giving an account of real dialogues have been forged, in imitation of one another, during those periods when the vogue of the Orient called for placing the Greek and Oriental sagacity side by side. Similarly the hypothesis of the Father Festugiére (p. 36) that in the Orientalist circles to which he belonged, Aristoxenes thought of India, then better known thanks to the expedition of Alexander, is quite likely. In fact it is quite certain that during the time of Aristoxenes, India was quite in the news, this was approximately the time when Seleukos had sent Megasthenes to the court of Candragupta. But Father Festugiére adds that the anecdote of

[1] E. Bréhier, *La philosophie de Plotin*, 1928, p. 132; *Eos ou Platon et l'Orient*, Brussels, 1945, pp. 122 ff; A.J. Festugiére, Grecs et sages Orientaux, in *Rev. Hist. des Rel.*, Vol. CXXX, July-Dec., 1945, pp. 34 ff.

Socrates and the Indian, the result of the presence of the sage of India and of the sage of Greece "is already in favour of the Oriental wisdom, following a fashion which will prevail later during the Greeko-Roman epoch", and he refers on this subject to his book, *La Révélation d'Hermés Trismégiste*[1], wherein he has studied the vogue of Oriental wisdom during the first centuries of the Christian era following the decline of ancient rationalism. On this point, however, one should hesitate to follow him. A fashion cannot be active several centuries before its existence; in order to link up the invention made by Aristoxenes of a dialogue between Socrates and an Indian with the Orientalist infatuation seen during the Greeko-Roman period, it should be supposed that in reality the fashion reputed to be that of this period had commenced much earlier. But in the attention paid by the Greeks to the Oriental doctrines must one explain everything by simple fashions. There is, in any case, another point of view where the Orientalist finds himself quite naturally placed and we should stop a moment to see what can be discovered through this point of view.

When a Greek text refers to the Orient, the first job of the Orientalist is to find out whether what is alleged is exact. If it is found to be false, it follows automatically that we are dealing with a text of fantasy and the reasons that prompted the author to write it, should be looked for only in the preoccupations of the author himself or those of his circle. Things become altogether different if the indications regarding the Orient found in the text are found to be correct. Then the reasons of the author should not be sought only in his ideas or in those of his nation as the real influence of foreign thought on him is evident. Now on examining the facts regarding the wisdom of Indians found in various works or in the dialogues claiming to present Indians, it is perceived that they are generally exact; therefore, it can be said that the vogue of the Orient among the Greeks has not been solely due, in so far as India is concerned, to a purely internal evolution of ideas but it is due to a real contribution made by true facts. We have already had the occasion to show the same elsewhere *a propos* of the texts of the

---

[1] Vol. I, Paris, 1944.

first centuries of the Christian era.[1] We can today give a new example of the same, concerning the anecdote of Aristoxenes studied here.

In his article quoted above, *Gréce et sages orientaux*, Father Festugiére has made a *rapprochement* between the opinion credited to the Indian in the anecdote of Aristoxenes, that things human cannot be understood without knowing things divine, the theory of the *Ist Alcibiades* that knowing one's soul is to discover God and the assertion put in the mouth of the Brahmin Iarchas, in the Life of Appllionos of Tyana, that all knowledge depends on the knowledge of oneself and that to know oneself is to know God (p.38). These concordant opinions have appeared to him to be inseparable and he asks himself if the remarks ascribed to Iarchas did not derive from the idea expressed in the *Ist Alcibiades*, which could have been well known to Philostratos, the author of the life of Appllonios. This would be quite probable if India had been an imaginary country; in that case, the Greek authors could not but have sought inspiration from one another for talking of India. But the idea reported to have been expressed by the Indian of Aristoxenes and that of Philostratos is in conformity with the chief doctrine of the Upaniṣads according to which supreme knowledge consists in the identity of the *ātman*, the self with *Brahman*, God. The passages of Aristoxenes and Philostratos agree between themselves because they refer to the same truth and if Philostratos lends to a conventional Brahmin a veritable Indian doctrine, it is in no way because he was inspired by the *Ist Alcibiades*. From then on there is no problem of filiation between the three texts put near one another. Two of them echo the true information that came from India. Only the third, the passage of the Platonist dialogue, because of its concordance with others poses a problem, namely, that of finding out how this dialogue contains an idea which is found to be a classical idea of the Brahmanical philosophy elsewhere.

We will not let ourself be led into examining this last problem here, but this example shows that Greek assertions concerning India, even on the most fictitious stage like that of

---

[1] *JA*, 1943-45, pp. 349 ff (Book-review of Festugiére, *op. cit.*); *La doctrine des Brahmanas d'apres saint Hippolyte*, in *Rev. Hist. des Rel.*, July-Dec., 1945, pp. 59, ff.

the *Life of Apollonios* are not necessarily pure fantasy and the opinion ascribed to the Indian interlocutor of Socrates in the anecdote of Aristoxenes is an authentic Indian opinion. One cannot therefore *a priori* reject this anecdote of the Indian and Socrates, as one would have had to do if Aristoxenes had credited his Indian with impossible views. It is, besides, quite natural that Aristoxenes, writing towards the epoch of the expedition of Alexander, was able to have a correct notion of the words that could be ascribed to an Indian philosopher. But the fact remains that he wrote precisely at a time when attention had been drawn towards India and when the conditions, under which knowledge about it was obtained, were well-known. He could not have, at such a time, evoked the presence of an Indian philosopher at Athens a century earlier, if it had been thought that such a presence was impossible before the great events of the conquest which then took place. It is, therefore, not very important whether the anecdote of Socrates and the Indian sage is true or false; even if false, it guarantees that towards the end of the IVth century B.C., it was known in the Hellenic world that Indians knowing the doctrines of their country had been able to visit Greece for a long time, just as the Greeks had been going to India. It is, therefore, in no way impossible that Plato had knowledge of the Indian medical theory before he explained the one which is near it and which he does not seem to have borrowed from the known schools of Greek medicine.

Indices furnished by chance positively tell us on the other hand that Indian data on medicine had been received in the Greek medical circles where an Hippocratic manual namely *On Woman's Diseases* had been elaborated; this manual being quite generally considered as Cnidian.

In this manual (I, 81, Littré, Vol. VIII, p. 203) is prescribed an ingredient used in the composition of a pessary, the "Indian medicine (variant-Median), which is for the eyes and which is called pepper (*peperi*)". The same prescription is found with slight variations in the manual *On the Nature of Woman* (32, Littré, Vol. VII, p. 365). In this latter passage, Littré has adopted *midikhoi* in his text and indicates the variant *endikhoi*; in the other he has adopted *indikhoi* and gives as variants *midikhoi* and *mildikhoi*. It is not doubtful that in the two cases, the correct readings be *indikhoi*, "Indian", because *peperi* is a derived form of the name of the pepper from Sanskrit *pippali* (or *pippalī*) and that pepper is an Indian product and not a Median one. One can even specify that it does not refer to pepper in general but to "long pepper" which is denoted by *pippali*, excluding the "round pepper", because the two Greeks just now quoted by us immediately add the mention of the "round" one (*strongulu*). Moreover, the indication that the medicine in question is meant for the eyes agrees very well with the teaching of the classical Indian medicine which frequently includes *pippali* in its formulae of collyriae.[1] Last of all, two other passages of the book, *On Woman's Diseases*, confirm that one should read "Indian" and not "Median" and one of them enables us to explain the wrong reading while giving a precious indication.

First of all a pessary similar to the preceding ones is prescribed where the "Indian medicine" is included as one of the elements, without being named this time, and for this indication there is no variation (II, 358, Littré, VIII, p. 337). The second passage (ibid., 205, p. 395) again gives a similar formula where the Indian substance re-appears; about this substance, here it is said that "the Persians call it *peperi*" and there is inside it something round called *murtidanon*. The variant Median for "Indian" can come in only after an unhappy effort at correction is made, under the impression that the drug belonged to the Persians from whom its name had been received, but the passage says specifically, without giving any variant, that the drug is Indian, although the name given to it may have been Persian. In fact the name is also Indian but it is true that in the form of *peperi*, it is Persian, as was earlier noted by Lassen, *r* in Iranian standing for *l* in Indian.[2] It follows therefore that this product along with indications concerning its medical usage passed through the Persian empire to reach the Greeks.

The same manual *On Woman's Diseases* also mentions another Indian formula for dentifrice (II, 185, Littré, Vol, VIII

---

1 Suśr., *Uttaratantra*, XI, 11; XV, 29, XVII, 4. 6, 14, 18, 21, 22, etc. In these passages in verse the name of *pippali* is often replaced *metri causa* by various synonyms.

2 *Indische Alterthumskunde*, Vol. I, p. 278, IInd edn., p. 326, f.n. 3.

p. 367), which has the characteristic of having been offered along with a precept of general alimentary hygiene; to eat little and to partake of only substantial things. This characteristic is part of the tradition of Indian medicine, which has always been careful to regulate the use of food as much as the use of drugs.

The presence of Indian data in the *Hippocratic Collection*, consciously received as such proves that at least indirect communication of Greek and Indian medical sciences had been realised during the elaboration of certain elements of this *Collection*. These communications must have commenced before the time of Alexander, to which the basis of the large part of these texts is anterior. However, in view of the state of extreme uncertainty of Hippocratic chronology, it will be imprudent to peremptorily affirm that the passages noted by us as referring to Indian remedies have not been written much later. It remains true, nevertheless, that the certainty of Indian influence on the texts *On Woman's Diseases* and *On the Nature of Woman* brings in the possibility of a similar influence on the other texts such as the one *On Breaths* and that what is said of the Indian medicine *péperi* leads one to think that it has been known to the Greeks through the Persians and therefore this knowledge did not have the need to wait for the expedition of Alexander.

Moreover, we need not limit ourselves to a vague indication when we invoke the passage of an Indian product across the Persian empire, because an old and regular commercial route between India and the West is described for us by Strabo and Pliny and probably, in general, enough attention has not been paid to the consequences arising out of the existence of this path of communication.

In fact, Strabo (II, 1, 15) indicates that Indian goods used to arrive easily after being transported by the Oxus up to Hyrcania, that is to say, in the region of the Caspian, the region where they spread by means of the rivers right up to the Bridge. Pliny gives the details of transit on this route. The goods of the Oxus are routed by the Icare into the Caspian (Now the Oxus flows into the sea of Aral, but its ancient bed has been found), from where they are taken to the Cyrus. Thereafter they are transported by land up to the Phase, a tributary of the Euxine, in, at the most, five days. It is true that

Pliny, while describing this itinerary (VI, 19, 2) says that Varron, from whom he has borrowed this information declares that it has been gathered under Pompei, during the war of Mithridates. The information of Pliny thus goes only upto 66 B.C., but Strabo, whom Pliny has not quoted and who drew from other sources, has specifically indicated these sources in a second reference made to the same route (XI, 7, 3); they are Aristobulos, who participated in the expedition of Alexander and Patrocles, the informant who had access to secret documents established for Alexander and about whom Pliny tells us that, as the admiral of Seleukos and of Antiochos Soter, he made a periplus of the Caspian Sea (VI, 21). As nothing enables us to suppose that the route from India to the Euxine was opened to commerce precisely by the expedition of Alexander, it is clear that it has been established earlier and it became known to the Western people only on this occasion.

One could, therefore, under the Achaemenians, pass from India to Greece not only by reaching Ionia through the south or the centre of Asia Minor, but also by the Euxine and Thrace and it will be convenient to remind oneself of this fact while studying the possible connections between the doctrines of India and those of Orphism, connections held not as improbable by some critics but which they envisage as only across Iran.[1]

However it may be, other ways were also open for the passage from India to the Hellenic world. We know, from the time of Herodotos, that Cinnamon was brought up to there (III, 111), and as it refers, in all probability to cinnamon-bark, it should have been brought from Indian seas. The same text *On Woman's Diseases* which, several times, mentions the Indian pepper also knows the cinnamon (II, 187) and similarly the text *On the Nature of Women* (34, Littré, VII, p. 373). But Herodotos also indicates that it was brought by the Arabs and he did not know from where they drew it. On this point he merely repeats the tales about which Pliny has said that they were fabricated without any basis in order to make the most of the rarity of the commodity. It is therefore improbable that

---

[1] Boulanger, *Orphée*, p. 45; taken up again by P.M. Schuhl, *Essai sur la formation de la pensée grecque*, p. 239; M.J. Lagrange, *Les Mystéres: L'orphisme*, Paris, 1937, p. 81.

information regarding Indian ideas could have reached Greece by the route of the cinnamon, as this route became really known to the Westerners only towards the beginning of the Christian era.[1] Elsewhere again the voyage from India to Egypt which was accomplished by Skylax, starting from the mouth of the Indus, as a prelude to the Achaemenian conquest of Sindh, has been accomplished again, but on this subject we do not possess precise and sure evidence.

In any case, we see that sure paths and intermediaries, i.e., Greeks in the service of the Persians, being the functionaries of the Achaemenians who dominated both the Greek and the Indian lands, and may be Indians also, were there for assuring scientific communication between India and Greece before Alexander. Undoubtedly they did not suffice for making India largely known to the Greek public, nor did they suffice for making Greece known to the Indian public, but they were easily able to carry across the notions on which minds on both sides, whether by conscientious emulation or not, marked. This is the explanation of why there are, between Indian and Greek medicines, so very particular and precise similarities which are not easy to ascribe to chance. This is again why we come across, both in Greece and India, so many similar speculations during the same moments. If the two worlds, while knowing each other only in a vague manner, have brought the level of their science to the same level, it is because they communicated with each other on the under-side.[2]

---

[1] cf., *Les échanges de l'Inde et de l'Empire romain aux premiers siècles de l'ère chretienne*, in *Rev. Hist.*, January-March 1949, pp. 6 ff.

[2] While terminating this work, I have to express my thanks to all those who have been kind enough to take interest in it and to favour it with their criticism and advice, especially Messrs E. Benveniste, J Bloch, A Foucher and L. Renou who know all that I owe them on this occasion as on many others. I also have to thank the Centre national de la recherche scientifique and the Imprimerie Nationale who have been kind enough to undertake the printing and publication of this book. (in French)

APPENDIX

ACCADIAN, GREEK AND INDIAN MEDICAL PROGNOSTICS[1]

A RECENT publication of Mr. René Labat, *Traité akkadien de diangostics et pronostics médicaux*[2] has considerably enriched our knowledge of Mesopotamian medicine. It has a particular significance for the general history of science because of the light it throws on one of the oldest medical traditions and due to the point of comparison furnished by it, as regards other ancient medical traditions, which can be linked with it or which have at least been developed only a little later.

The collection edited and translated by Mr. Labat had a large circulation in Mesopotamia; this is proved by the variety of the sources of fragments constituting the same. This fact alone shows that the work represents a tradition which was recognised everywhere and which was, consequently, quite old. The analogy with other technical collections has enabled Mr. Labat to accept as probable the fact that the composition of the work could possibly go back to the Hamurabbian period and more probably to the end of the Kassite era. But the majority of the tablets, which acquaint us with the manual, were written on the orders of Assurbanipal (668-627 B.C.), an older one going back to the reign of Mardukapaliddin of Babylonia (721-710 B.C.) and a more recent one being dated in the eleventh year of Artaxerxes, that is, in 453 (pages xiv, 212-213, tablet 35). Regardless, therefore, of the original antiquity of the manual, we have to deal with teachings which were in vigour in Mesopotamia from the VIIIth to Vth centuries B.C. This is the period of the beginning of Greek medicine and it is contemporary with that of the Vedic and Brahmanic elaboration of Indian doctrinal medicine. One could, therefore, ask oneself if there is any analogy between such Mesopotamian teaching and the two great

---

1 *JA*, Vol. CCXL, 1952, pp. 299-321.

2 Académie internationale des sciences, Paris; E. J. Brill, Leiden, 1951, pp xlix and 247.

medical traditions of antiquity, of which one was born in the East in India and the other in the West, in the basin of Eastern Mediterranean. Mr. Labat has himself looked for the analogies of the manual in Greek medicine and we are here going to look for the same in Indian medicine.

But before presenting us with analogies with these two medical systems, the Mesopotamian shows up a striking difference. Whereas the former are characterised by an effort at constructing rational theories aiming at an explanation of physiological and pathological states, the Mesopotamian does not show itself under a theoretical form.. It does not, however, follow that it had never known any theory. The absence of theories in documents that have reached us could have been due to the extreme rarity of doctrinal works. Everywhere and in all the periods, the practical medical literature, the collections of usual data for diagnosis, prognostics and treatment are much more numerous and more widespread than dogmatic works; it is, therefore, the former that have more chances of being found when the tradition is dead and is revealed only by the chance-discovery in excavations. Whatever it be, in the particular case of Mesopotamian medicine, we know it only by the collections meant for the use of the practitioner and not for that of the theoretician.

However, the practicai teachings of Accad are methodically arranged; they show a great effort of regular observation and of rational classification and are well-suited for being compared with more elaborate teachings which have reached us more completely, i.e., those of Greece and India.

The Accadian manual published by Mr. Labat consists of five parts. The first gives a series of prognostics drawn from signs observed by the exorcist when he goes to the house of the patient. It refers, therefore, as has been noted by Mr. Labat, more to divination concerning the patient than to medicine. The type of indications is as follows: "If, in the street, he (the exorcist) sees a potsherd planted (in the earth), anxiety will not approach that patient". Or "If he sees a table for offerings (?), the patient in question has been seized by some charm, he will remain ill and then die" (Table I, 2-3). In the latter case a diagnosis concerning the medical origin of the disease precedes the prognostics. This first part, designated according to its commencing words, *When the exorcist goes to the house of the patient*, also carries the enigmatic designation of *Sick Muscles*.

The second part, *When thou approachest a patient*, after reminding the doctor of the necessity, for his personal safety, of performing a prophylactic charm prealably, enumerates the signs presented by the patient at the time of the doctor's approach and which reveal the origin of the disease, most often due to the "hand" of such and such a divinity, which has put itself over the sick person. For example: "If he is 'struck' in the cranium: the 'hand' of Papsukkal . . . If, being 'struck' in the cranium, his ears do not hear: the 'hand of Istar' " (Table III, 9-10). The prognostic often follows or is given alone, without a prealable diagnosis.

This part, written according to a prototype of Babylonia, is, properly speaking, an *aide-mémoire* of semiology, enumerating the symptoms, organwise, going from the head to the feet and indicating their significance. Most of the time, it is a case of isolated symptoms and its medical value is nil. It will be even difficult to believe that the Mesopotamian doctors could have preserved, for a long time, in their traditional lists of significative symptoms indications such as these: "If his nose is cold: he will die" (Table VI, 3) or: "If the tip of his nose is yellow, he will die" (ibid., 25). One should suppose that probably some complementary oral instruction existed or that the indications furnished by parallel manuals specified the conditions in which similar symptoms could become significant. Besides, these conditions are indicated in certain cases: they are constituted by the presence of other symptoms associated with the one referring to the part of the body in question, that is to say, in the existence of clinical entities or syndromes of recognised individuality. Here the manual does assume a really medical character distinguishing it from the collections of divination. For example, certain crises of convulsion are described in these terms: "If the neck of the patient continuously turns towards right, if his hands and his feet are clenched (?), if his eyes are closed and upturned, if slaver flows out of his mouth, if he snores: that is a crisis of high disease *(antasubbū)*" (Table X, 1). There are even indications of differential diagnosis, because the text immediately adds: "If, when seized by the crisis, he remains conscious: it is sure; if (on the contrary), at the time of the seizure by the crisis, he becomes unconscious: that is not sure". This distinction, as has been ably noted by Mr. Labat, appears to refer to the differential diagnosis of epilepsy and other crises of convulsion, the loss of consciousness being characteristic in epilepsy. In any case, the still more characteristic symptom, regarding the absence of the memory of the epileptic accident, is not indicated and the given description nohow constitutes a complete and general *tableau* of the disease. Descriptions of this type prove that certain diseases were the object of efforts for nosological individualisation and not that these efforts had been in an advanced stage among the Mesopotamians as they had been a little later, among the Greeks and the Indians.

In the third part, prognostics are drawn from the observations of symptoms during the first day of sickness and the moments when changes take place in the disease. Moreover, in this part the first efforts at drawing clinical pictures reputedly characteristic of the action of various gods or demons reappear. Diverse prognostics are added thereto in accordance with the psychical state of the subject and, eventually etiological indications also (for example, the fever due to dryness, Table XXIII, 29).

The fourth part, extremely mutilated, depicts the multiple forms of the "malignant attack" *(misittu)*, diseases provoked by various demons, the malignant transformation of certain diseases under a determined influence and the magical therapeutics meant to combat them. Lastly it indicates the prognostics resulting from the nature of the various hallucinations of the patient.

The fifth part, which has reached us in an extremely incomplete state, deals with women and young children, specially with the prognostics concerning the sex of a child to be born and his chances of life. It also discusses the conditions of delivery and the sentiments to be shown in future by the child to his mother; this rather belongs to divination than medicine.

Mr. Labat has then compared the Accadian and Greek prognostics, noting in the *Hippocratic Collection* as also in the Accadian literature, the existence of works specially dealing with prognostics, diagnosis being less mixed up with prognostics among the Greeks. Certain similarities of detail appear, but there are also big differences. Mr. Labat thinks that the personal action of Hippocrates has eliminated from Greek medicine, many teachings which could have borne the traces of Babylonian heritage (p. xlii). [This marked a great step forward.] One may also think that Greek medicine developed entirely out of the important influence of Babylonia. However, in the domain of the veterinary art, not turned upside down by the intervention of a Hippocrates, Mr. Labat notices closer concordances with the Accadian manual, specially in the listing of the enunciation of prognostics, although these latter were not gathered together in special manuals.

It is certain that the chapters on prognostics in the *Hippocratic Collection* show certain gifts of clinicians which are entirely different from those seen in the Accadian manual. The impression that one is in the presence of the results of a personal medical experience and not that of a repertory of traditional data, is confirmed by the eventual reference to the cases of patients who are designated by name and are, in consequence, personally examined or whose observation has, at least, been personally known (*Prorrhétique*, I, 27, 32, 34, 72, 99, 104, 119). In any case, the personal twist thus given to the teaching of prognostics, does not efface the analogy of the general structure of certain Greek manuals with the Accadian text. This is how, as has been remarked by Mr. Labat (p. xxxviii), the *Prénotions de Cos* catalogue organwise the symptoms, having the value of prognostics, in a manner sufficiently similar to the second part of the Accadian manual.

It could be claimed that this analogy does not have much interest, as any doctor desirous of enumerating symptoms could be tempted to do so organwise, beginning from the head. But precisely it is already remarkable that on both sides, in the Accadian medical literature and also in the Greek medical literature, similar enumerations have been constituted. The study of medical data put in such a form, does not form part of a method necessary for medical teaching wherever it be given and the instinct of the clinician not influenced by a mode of explanation which had been traditional before him, would make him understand his observations in a more natural manner, just as he may have gathered them; that is to say that he would describe the entire disease either in each particular patient or in a type summing up the common traits of similar morbid developments observed by him. The pre-determined way of listing the signs establishes a good relationship between the Accadian manual and the *Prénotions de Cos*.

The examination of the *Prénotions de Cos* and of other Greek texts seems to be able to enlighten us even regarding this relationship as also concerning certain other peculiarities of the Accadian manual.

After a list of symptoms, largely fatal and of signs showing themselves chiefly in fevers[1], the *Coan Prognoses* (beginning from 156), concern themselves with local physical signs approximately classified from the head downwards and in association with various other signs. Now certain groups of symptoms are found identically described, almost word by word, in the *Prorrhétique* 1, with additions in this latter text of a reference to a given patient.[2] One may *a priori* suppose either that the author of *Prorrhétique* 1, has borrowed elements from *Prénotions de Cos*, adding thereto the names of the patients where he remembered having seen these symptoms, or that the *Coan Prognoses* or some of them, have been gleaned from the collections of clinical notes like the *Prorrhétique* 1, with clinical references being suppressed, or that the two manuals have drawn from a common source. It is the second hypothesis which is confirmed. It is confirmed by the fact that one of the *Coan Prognoses* (543), coinciding with the propositions of *Prorrhétique* 1 includes the reference to the patient, discussed by the corresponding proposition of *Prorrhétique* 1 (119)[3], whereas others do not include the same. It appears, therefore, that the editor of *Prénotions de Cos,* as we have them, has had recourse to *Prorrhétique* 1, but habitually leaving aside, except once, personal indications; and this helps us observe the compilatory process of the composition of the semiological collection of the *Coan Prognoses*. By a similar process particular or exceptional clinical observations

1 Littré (Vol. V, p. 588), has abusively entitled the series: "Des fievres considerées comme maladies générales."

2 *Pror.* 27-*Coa.* 2 and 69; *Pror.* 32-*Coa.* 194; *Pror.* 34-*Coa.* 76; *Pror.* 99-*Coa.* 606; *Pror.* 104-*Coa.* 257; *Pror.* 119-*Coa.* 343 and 543.

3 Save some orthographic variants the text, on both sides, is identical (cf., Littré, V, pp. 550 and 708) and denotes, following Littré's translation: "In hysterical women, spasms without fever are easy, as among Dorcas".

could have easily found themselves arranged in pair with regular and frequent morbid facts, and one can understand that detached symptoms, and since then without significative values, be on the contrary presented as important signs, beside other really characteristic signs. A recapitulatory registration of clinical data had taken place with a view to a mode of traditional transmission which appears to be quite analogous to the Mesopotamian mode and which, while not naturally imposing itself, could very well have been inspired by the example of the former, extended up to the Persians and which the Oriental Greeks could not have ignored.

The analogy of conditions in which certain propositions of the Accadian manual and certain *Coan Prognoses* are presented serves, in reality, to simultaneously help us seize a similitude of the compilation of this text and of *Prénotions de Cos* and explains to us the apparent futility of analogous propositions found on both the sides.

We have taken note, a little earlier, of the Accadian preposition, "If his nose is cold, he will die", and supposed that such indications of prognostic could be held valid only after they had been completed by the knowledge of the conditions of their validity. Now we read in *Prénotions de Cos:* "Ears cold, transparent and contracted, fatal sign" (188) and exactly like the Accadian manual, here also nothing indicates in the context the clinical table under which this sign can have a value, which evidently it does not have it itself. But Littré in his translation refers to a passage of *Prognostics* (2, t. II, p. 115), which yields us the key to the enigma posed by the presence, among the *Coan Prognoses* of a proposition, which in itself is so insignificant and so false. This proposition detaches, simply for classifying it among the symptoms furnished by the ears, a sign, which in the *Prognostics,* is part of an entire clinical table whose significance is finely discussed over there. It refers to the examination of the face of the patient in serious diseases and not to that of the ears of no matter which subject, as one would have believed on reading only the *Coan Prognoses.* The comparison of the physiognomy of the patient is to be made with that of normal persons and chiefly with the physiognomy habitual to the patient himself. It is also specified that the patient will have to be asked if he had felt various types of fatigue or debilitating causes (prolonged awakening, strong diarrhoea, hunger). It is only when the possibility of these conditions, in themselves capable of producing alarming symptoms, is eliminated that one will relate the symptoms in question to the violence of the trouble and will hold them as really significant of a fatal prognostic. It is only then and when it is associated with the totality of other described signs, that the coldness and the contraction (?) of the ears can take on the value of a fatal sign.

It can thus be seen that studied in isolation and not completed by data as that of *Prognostics*, *Prénotions de Cos* will lead to such gross errors in prognostics, under which no medical practice could survive. They suppose, therefore, and the persistent reputation of the Accadian tradition across entire Mesopotamia equally supposes the existence of a complement of teaching such as that of the *Prognostics*, preserved for us by the *Hippocratic Collection*, whereas the chance discovery of cuneiform tablets has not yielded us so far, for Mesopotamia, anything equivalent.

It is also to be observed that the collections of the lists of symptoms which could not have, in themselves, sufficed as medical manuals, do not constitute a very natural mode for the fixation of the medical tradition and this can lead one to think that this mode having been habitual in Mesopotamia, it is by means of the Mesopotamian example that it got established among the Greeks, leading among them to compilations like *Prénotions de Cos*.

We will see that closer analogies of the Accadian text with the aberrant parts of the Indian medical tradition equally lead us to think that the Mesopotamian mode of divinatory prognostication and of the presentation of signs could have been the example on the Eastern side.

The art of diagnosis and of prognostic presents itself in India as a branch of the medical art, much less detached from others than in Mesopotamia. The medical diagnosis and prognostics constitute a part, as is normal in scientific medicine, of nosology and establish themselves in respect of each trouble described in its totality. It is only at a late date that special manuals of prognostic such as the *Narapatijayacaryā*, A.D. 1232, are met with.[1] But the big classical medical texts

[1] cf., E.G. Kashikar, *Indian Medicine by Dr. J. Jolly*, translated from

devote full chapters[1] to special collections of symptoms having the value of prognostics which remind us of the Accadian manual. As in the latter, which mentions twice more often the signs of the coming death than the favourable symptoms, Indian medicine is chiefly attached to the traits of incurability, the doctor being under the obligation of not taking up the useless treatment of the incurable[2], although according to Caraka, he must also refrain, on humanitarian grounds, from revealing too promptly the gravity of his prognostics (*Indr.*, XII, 61, 64).

The external analogies in the methods of the explanation of this matter, common to Sanskrit texts and to the Accadian manual, are not rare. The headings are put at the end of chapters, the colophons resemble those of the Accadian manual. This first analogy, however, deserves to be noted only for the sake of memory, because this is the general usage in the entire Sanskrit literature. Another analogy is somewhat more remarkable as it refers to a usage, which is not equally widespread in India, though found in the Upaniṣads (*Kena*, *Īśa*), and which is nowise to be found in any Accadian text. This relates to the use of the first words of the text as its title.

In the *Caraka-saṁhitā*, eight out of twelve chapters which constitute the section, *Indriyasthāna*, specially devoted to prognostic, have for titles words which begin them or a part of these words: CHAP. I, *varṇasvarīyam indriyam*, beginning: *iha khalu varṇaś ca svaraś ca* . . . II, *puṣpitakam indr.*, beginning: *puṣpam* . . . IV, *indriyānīkam indr.*, beginning: *indriyāṇi* . . . V, *pūrvarūpīyam indr.*, beginning: *pūrvarupāṇi* . . . VI, *katamāni-śarīriyam indr.*, beginning: *katamāni śarīrāṇi* . . . VIII, *avākśirsīyam indr.*, beginning: *avākśirā* . . . IX, *yasya-śyāvanimittīyam indr.*, beginning: *yasya śyāve* . . . XI, *aṇujyotīyam indr.*, beginning: *aṇujyotir* . . . XII, *gomayacūrṇīyam indr.*, beginning: *yasya gomayacūrṇābhyām*.

The other chapters, without reproducing the initial words in

German and supplemented with Notes, Poona, 1951, p. 207.

1 *Caraka-saṁhitā*, *Indriyasthāna*, XII Chapters; *Bhela-saṁhitā*, *Indriyasthāna*, XII Chapters; *Suśruta-saṁhitā*, *Sūtrasthāna*, XXIX-XXXIII; Vāgbhaṭa, *Aṣṭāṅga-saṁgraha*, *Śār.*, IX-XII.; *Aṣṭāṅgahṛdaya*, *Śār.* V-VI; *Kāśyapa-saṁhitā*, *Sūtr.*, XXVIII and *Indriyasthāna*; *Hārīta-saṁhitā*, 2, II, V and VIII-IX.

cf., J. Filliozat, *Le Kumāratantra de Rāvaṇa*, Paris, 1937, p. 56, n.

their headings, draw them from the words of commencement. But the method is often employed, even in chapters belonging to other parts of the text, having no similarity with the Accadian collection.

The accounts in Sanskrit frequently resemble the Accadian accounts in the formulae. For example, Caraka, *Indriyasthāna*, III, enumerates the symptoms of troublesome prognostic in phrases of the following type, which remind us of the Accadian method of presentation:

> "If the respiration is too long or brief", one should know that "his vital breath will go away".
>
> "When palpated, if the two (lateral) cervical regions do not have the throbbing", one should know that, "his vital breath will go away".
>
> "If his teeth are charged white, with gravel on them", one should know, "that his vital breath will go away."[1]

But these are merely external analogies which, even when grouped, do not have any significance in themselves. Much more important are the concordances in the tenor of teaching, although they appear along with considerable differences. The most detailed explanation of special Indian prognostics is the one which covers the totality of the twelve chapters of the *Indriya-sthāna* of *Caraka-saṁhitā*. Their brief analysis and that of similar principal texts will enable us to take up the comparison of their teaching with that of the Accadian text.

The first chapter enumerates the signs to be considered in a patient or with reference to him to know the time left to him for living. The anomaly (*vikṛti*) of which he is the victim, is of three types: (1) *lakṣaṇa-nimitta*, "assigned by the types", that is to say, signified and caused simultaneously[2] by the congenital structural types of the body; (2) *lakṣya-nimitta*, "assigned by the typifiable, that is to say, by the morbid manifestations, capable of

---

1 *Indr.*, III, 8-10:
tasya ced ucchvāso 'tidīrgho hrasvo vā syāt/
parāsuriti vidyāt//8//
tasya cen manye parimṛśyamāne na spandeyātām/
parāsuriti vidyāt//9//
tasya ced dantāḥ parikīrṇāḥ śvetā jātaśarkarāḥ syuḥ/
parāsuriti vidyāt//10//

2 *Nimitta* is both cause and sign. The chief sense is 'sign', 'presage', but in view of a reasoning current in medicine, both outside and in India, according to which *post hoc ergo propter hoc*, the preceding sign is easily taken as the determining cause; this gives the value of "cause" taken by the word.

being referred to nosological types, to individualised syndromes; (3) *nimittarūpa,* "conforming with the assigned ones", that is to say, with presages which occur and are thought to determine the consecutive trouble.[1] These are, then, more advanced theoretical views than those found in the manuals of the *Hippocratic Collection* concerning the prognostics as also in the Accadian manual. The chapter, thereafter, gives the unfavourable signs observable when the colour (of the skin, *varṇa*) and the voice *(svara)* of the patient are examined. That is the beginning of an explanation of objective symptoms which covers the two following chapters, while the fourth is devoted to a description of subjective symptoms.

The second chapter describes the *ariṣṭas,* symptoms which appear to announce the death as flowers announce the fruit. These *ariṣṭas* are the odours spread by the patient and tastes of his secretions, these secretions not being tasted directly by the doctor, but he infers the savour thereof according to the behaviour of flies, leeches, etc., which suck it or which turn away from it.

The third chapter concerns the information of prognostics furnished by palpating various parts of the body enumerated from the feet to the head (III, 5), the observable symptoms (III, 4) being: inertia *(stambha)* of the parts of the body, normally ever vibrant *(spandamāna)*, the coldness of those which are normally hot, the stiffness *(dāruṇa)* of the supple, the rugosity of the smooth, the absence of the normally existing parts, such as the testicles, the relaxation, the rupture and the dislocation of the articulations, the diminution of flesh and blood, the (general?) stiffness *(dāruṇa)*, the non-interruption of perspiration or its stoppage and all other abnormal symptoms. Thus are described the signs to be recognised by various sensorial faculties *(indriyas,* wherefrom the name of the section) of the doctor, those of sight, hearing, smell, taste and touch.

The fourth chapter commences the examination of the

---

1 The commentary of Cakrapāṇi explains that it "reproduces the significance of assigning (presage), which shows itself as engendering the effect or as taking note of the effect" *(nimittasya yo 'rthaḥ kāryajananarūpaḥ kāryabodhakarūpo vā tam anukaroti)*. Cakrapāṇi, therefore, does not entirely accept the sophism *post hoc ergo propter hoc* and admits that the sign is not necessarily the cause, but can simply be an announcement (*Indr.*, I, 7).

manifestation of signs perceived by the sensorial faculties of the patient: vision, hearing, various sensorial errors regarding odours, tastes, hot and cold, etc. and various hallucinations.

The fifth chapter studies the premonitory symptoms of death in diseases of various types, the objective ones observed by the doctor and the subjective ones reported by the patient. These latter consist chiefly of dreams, only a part thereof being considered as premonitory ones and a rational theory having been elaborated to explain, by means of the influence of the organic elements of trouble on the perceptions, the troubles of premonitory value of some of them.[1]

The sixth chapter describes the groups of the symptoms of incurability during diverse morbid conditions.

The seventh chapter enumerates the forebodings of death, furnished by the anomalies of the shadow or the reflection of the body, as regards their state *(saṁsthāna)*, their dimension *(pramāṇa)*, their colour *(varṇa)* and their luminosity *(prabhā)*. It adds diverse groups of the symptoms of the coming death.

The eighth chapter continues the study of similar groups of symptoms to be specially noticed on the eyelashes, in the hair, on the tongue, in respiration and adds short clinical tables, such as the following, which remind one of exactly the tables of the Accadian manual.

> "Rubbing the knee against the knee, letting fall the feet after having raised them, the patient who often twists his face, does not live. Cutting the tips of his nails with teeth, cutting his hair with his nails, scratching the earth with a baton, he does not get rid of his disease."[2]

The ninth chapter takes up once again the signs of incurability in various sorts of diseases and other groups of symptoms, particularly in relation with the action of the bile (internal fire).

The tenth chapter discusses the signs of imminent death

---

1 cf, J. Filliozat, 'Le sommeil et les rəves selon les médicins indiens et les physiologues grecs', *Journal de psychologie*, 1947, pp. 326 ff., specially pp. 332-34.

2 *Indr.*, VIII, 17-88:

ghaṭṭayan jānunā jānu pādāv udyamya pātayan/
yo 'paśyati muhur vaktram āturo na sa jāvati//
dantais cchindan nakhāgrāṇi nakhais cchindañ cchiroruhān/
kāṣṭhen bhūmim vilikhan na rogāt parimucyate//.

particularly those where the action of internal wind intervenes. The eleventh classifies the signs according to the time, at the end of which death will occur: a year, a month, a shorter period.

Finally, the twelfth chapter, after certain indications of the same type as in the preceding one, studies the forebodings obtained by the doctor by observing the messenger come to fetch him for the patient or of the presages encountered by the doctor on the way to the patient's house and on entering that house. It terminates in a recapitulation of the entire *indriyasthāna* and in new indications concerning the necessity of hiding the fatal prognostic as also the favourable signs.

The *Bhela-saṁhitā* which concurrently with the *Caraka-saṁhitā* presents teachings going back to the same master, Ātreya[1], enables us to go, in comparison with this *Caraka-saṁhitā*, to an older tradition, from which both of them are descended. What is common to both of them has every chance of belonging to an ancient source. Unfortunately the *Bhela-saṁhitā* has reached us only in a single mutilated manuscript.[2] But the *Indriyasthāna*, which corresponds to the section of the same name of the *Caraka-saṁhitā*, is sufficiently well-preserved. It has, like its pair, twelve chapters.

The first chapter, whose title has been lost along with the beginning, relates to the signs of the time left for living, one, two or four months and the signs announcing a short life or one more or less long, up to a hundred years. Only the first part has its analogous one in Caraka (C), in Chapter XI.

The second chapter, *Svastyayana*, "favourable course", describes the symptoms of the coming return to health, as are found at the end of Chapter XII, but differently. The end is lost.

The third chapter, the title and the beginning lost, indicates a series of symptoms of troublesome prognostics—certain sensorial hallucinations of the patient, certain fetid emanations, the considerable alterations of urine, etc. These symptoms, in

1 cf. *supra.*, pp. 2, 196 and 207.

2 Other known manuscripts are mere copies of the former, whose edition has been given by Asutosh Mookerjee, *Cal. Univ., Journ. of the Dep. of Letters*, Vol. VI, Calcutta, 1921. In this edn., the *Indriyasthāna* runs from pp. 97 to 115. The editor (p. 97, n. 1) underlines that in this part there is closer conformity between the *Bhela-* and *Caraka-saṁhitā*.

effect, in most cases, in the actual state of therapeutics leave little hope (here are to be recognised notably the symptoms of grave diabetes).

The fourth chapter, *Sadyomaraṇīya*, "concerning imminent death", with its title identical with that of Chapter X, has the same contents in general in an editing greatly differing in details. It does not begin as Chapter X, with *sadyas*.

The fifth chapter, *Yasyaśāvīya* (correct *Yasyaśyāvīya)*, has an almost identical title with Chapter IX, and similarly starts with *Yasya śyāve*. It gives a teaching similar in its totality but altogether different in detail.

The sixth chapter, *Pūrvarūpīyam*, "concerning the signs", a title similar to that of Chapter V, is altogether different though devoted to the descriptions of the symptoms occurring in various diseases.

The seventh chapter, *Indriyāṇīka*, named after its first word, is identical word for word, except for numerous variants, with Chapter IV, similarly named and which contains only two additional *ślokas* (14 and 20).

Chapter VIII, *Dūtādhyāya*, "chapter of the messenger", corresponds to the part of Chapter XII, devoted to signs furnished by the observation of the messenger but completely differs in explanation.

The ninth chapter, *Gomayacūrṇa*, has an almost identical title with Chapter XII, *Gomayacūrṇīya*, although it starts with *cūrṇam śirasi yasyaiva śuṣkagomayasannibham* . . . and not like Chapter XII with *yasya gomayacūrṇābham cūrṇam mūrdhani jāyate*. Its only *raison d'etre* consists in taking up the first words of the text as is done in Chapter XII; it follows that the editing of Caraka carrying *gomayacūrṇa* immediately after *yasya* is surely more faithful, at least here, to the original account, whose beginning is altered by the *Bhela-saṁhitā* while guarding the sense and keeping intact the old title which retains the traces of the first form of this account. After a common verse, with some variants, the two texts become divergent, that of Bhela merely describes various clinical tables of bad prognostic.

The tenth chapter, *Chāyādhyāya* "chapter of the shadow", is named after its first word *anuchāyā* . . . but only the first two verses refer to the shadow. The remainder describes the symptoms of incurability in the course of the diseases provoking haemorrhage *(raktapitta)*, those of cough *(kāsa)* and those of dyspnoea *(śvāsa)* and other hopeless morbid tables.

The eleventh chapter, entitled *Puṣpīya* corresponds in part with the second chapter of Caraka, called *Puṣpitaka* because it commences with *puṣpam.* But in Bhela, this chapter, which of course describes first of all the *puṣpita*, that is to say, the patient in whom appear the symptoms announcing some result as the flower announces the fruit, does not begin with *puṣpa.* It appears, therefore, that the ancient tradition referred to Ātreya agrees, in both Bhela and Caraka, in ascribing to Ātreya an account commencing with *puṣpa,* but that the text of Bhela has not preserved here as that of Caraka, the old beginning. After five verses devoted to *puṣpita* Bhela continues with an explanation of premonitory signs drawn from the dreams of the patient, identical with those found in the fifth chapter of Caraka but of a different tenor.

Finally, the last chapter, *Avākśirsīya*, is named after its beginning, similar to the eighth chapter, *Avākśirsīya,* of Caraka and also discusses the same subject, particularly related to fatal symptoms seen in eyelashes, in hair, etc.

The two *Indriyasthānas* relating the teaching of Ātreya, i.e., those of Bhela and Caraka, have, therefore, a common stock, with many similar details, but with different classifications and with internal changes in the contents of parts, which at first sight look similar. The spirit and the matter are the same but the latter has been kept similar only to enable one to admit that at the point of departure the tradition already had a definite formulation. This is not surprising. We do not know how the teaching received by Bhela has been transmitted, but we know that in relation to Ātreya, Caraka has come in only later. It is Agniveśa who might have received the teaching of Ātreya. Caraka intervened for revising the work of Agniveśa. Many of the divergences can be ascribed to him. However all should not be put to his account. We have seen that at least once he has been more faithful than Bhela in preserving the text which gave the title to a chapter. Moreover, he deals with subjects, which though missing in Bhela, must not be considered as new additions due to him. The investigation of the messenger is neglected by Bhela but is found in other words, in Suśruta[1], whose tradi-

[1] It is summarily recommended, *Sūtr.*, X, 4, without its name being given,

tion parallel to that of Ātreya, is very close and in Hārīta[1], reputed to be a co-disciple of Bhela under Ātreya.

In the *Suśruta-saṁhitā*, the third among the chief texts of Indian medicine, the teaching corresponding to the *Indriyasthānas* of Bhela and Caraka is incorporated in the *Sūtrasthāna* and is much better systematised. The five chapters XXIX-XXXIII, devoted to the same, respectively deal with the presages, subjective fatal symptoms, the "shadow" of the patient, other objective signs and particularly incurable diseases.

The presages (Chap. XXIX) are drawn from the messenger, from encounters had while rendering oneself to the patient's house, while entering that house or they are drawn from the dreams of the patient or of those of his entourage. The subjective fatal symptoms (Chap. XXX) are the *ariṣṭas*, consisting of sensorial errors and of the hallucinations of the patient. The *chāyā* corresponds in general with what we call the good or bad "looks" (Chap. XXXI), but the chapter deals with it only at its beginning and discusses thereafter the signs drawn from the state of the tongue, of the nose, of the eyes, of hair, of eye-brows, of attitudes, of respiration, of various groups of symptoms shown in the course of certain affections, of the state of the mouth, etc. These are, then, mainly objective signs and their study continues in chapter XXXII. The next chapter enumerates the circumstances wherein appear the hopeless cases of patients who are victims of eight diseases particularly dangerous by their nature itself.

As a whole, the doctrine is the same as that of Caraka and of Bhela. The account of Bhela looks less orderly and that of Suśruta as the best-arranged. It is also Suśruta who most often mixes up the enumerations of prognostic with general considerations regarding morbid causes. It seems that with him, traditional learning, in part divinatory and in part resulting from real medical experience, and which Bhela and Caraka have only half adapted in the theoretical medicine of scientific import, has tended to be integrated more closely into this medicine.

In relation to these Indian documents, the Accadian

---

but described in XI.

1 II, 8, *Hārīta-saṁhitā* actually known is, in any case, largely apocryphal, cf., *IA*, 1934, pp. 127 ff.

manual appears as similar but typologically more archaic, less developed as regards the progress of empirical knowledge and of the collection of the facts of experience, for scientific knowledge and the comprehension of acquired experience. The theoretical Indian classifications of morbid manifestations and Indian attempts at a rational explanation of certain signs, viz., the production of dreams of bad augury by organic perturbations in the canals of the organ of thought, do not have any equivalent in the Accadian manual. But the rest of the teaching has, with this manual, both a general concordance and particular similarities.

The general concordance is due to the principle itself of the grouping of symptoms having the value of prognostic in these lists, wherein they are detached from the concomitant signs, from the morbid atmosphere and from general conditions, which alone could give them fully significant value. The analogy between the Accadian manual and the special portions devoted to the same subject in the Indian manuals here is the same as is the case with this Accadian book and the Hippocratic manuals specialising like the former in the enunciation of prognostics, particularly the *Prénotions de Cos*.

The incorporation among medical symptoms of purely divinatory signs, as those which consist of observations made by the doctor or the exorcist during his passage towards the patient's house, is the first particular analogy between the Accadian manual and our Indian teaching. It is striking for anyone who studies Indian medicine in its totality. Divination in India, at least in the scientific circles, about which we are informed by the principal Sanskrit texts, is in no way a dominant part of its preoccupations. In the *Caraka-saṁhitā* itself, a full chapter *(Sūtrasthāna,* XXIX*)*[1], which is devoted to the description of the qualities of a good doctor and which gives details of the activity of a quack, enumerates in great detail the knowledge which a doctor worthy of that name must have and it makes no reference to an interpretation of divinatory signs. The texts devoted in various manuals to *nidānas*, that is to say, to the conditions in which diseases appear and develop

[1] French translation by J. Filliozat in L. Renou, *Anthologie sanskrite*. Paris, 1947, pp. 394-97.

and which enumerate the symptoms of these diseases and discuss their prognostics, are essentially based on direct clinical observations and on the interpretations of these observations as a function of admitted pathological theories and not, or as a rare exception, on divinatory data. Such data, though present in special sections like the *Indriyasthānas* of Bhela and Caraka or in particular groups of chapters as in Suśruta, and there mixed, as in the Accadian manual, with the enumerations of clinical signs detached from general clinical tables and which are, most of the time, the signs of serious or fatal prognostics, such divinatory data generally remain in the margin of the chief teachings of Indian medicine, which is complete without the same. In short, Sanskrit accounts similar to that of the Accadian manual are admitted in all the principal medical texts of India, but they have therein a place entirely to themselves. They are added to these texts and are not intimately incorporated therein.

Yet another trait which brings the accounts of Sanskrit medical texts near those of the Accadian manual, also separates them, though less completely, from the rest of the teachings of Indian medicine.

The Indian medical texts are well acquainted with the phenomenon of demoniac possession, which gives rise to diseases. In these texts it is called *graha*, "seizure". A belief in such "seizure" belongs to universal folklore. It will therefore be in vain to observe that it is found several times in the Accadian manual, which frequently indicates that if the patient presents such and such a symptom or if such and such a foreboding takes place, then the "hand" of such and such a god "is on him", or that such and such a god or demon "has seized him or her". On the other hand, the data of Sanskrit texts, summarised by us, do not relate to the diagnosis of possession, but other parts of the main texts in Sanskrit give such diagnoses based on symptoms similar to those which establish demoniac possession in the eyes of the Accadian doctors, and these parts, as those which describe forebodings, also have a separate place in the teaching of classical Indian medicine. In fact they do not belong to the fundamental doctrines of the latter, which invoke only those causes of diseases that are purely natural, except in the case of infantile and psychic troubles. They derive their inspiration from another current of ideas, attested since the Veda, and which has imposed itself on Indian doctors, even though they had mainly sought to constitute a rational system of explaining the diseases. Their effort to bring the case of possession back to their ordinary natural explanations, while supposing that the demons are only one cause among others for disturbing the organic elements, appears only later.[1] Exactly like diagnosis by observing presages, the diagnosis of "seizure" by the demons or gods is not an integral and primitive part of the Indian medical system. They are admitted here and more largely than the divinatory prognoses, but they are not incorporated therein more intimately.

Moreover, there are certain analogies of detail between Accadian and Indian diagnoses of demoniac "seizure" of children. These analogies are sufficiently close between the 40th tablet of the Accadian manual and texts like the *Kumāra-tantra*. On both sides, a certain number of described symptoms are the same; this can be sufficiently explained by the fact that it is a case of morbid phenomena actually observed among sick infants, but at the same time on both sides diagnosis often depends on the age, in days or in months, of the infant at the time of the attack and a "seizing female spirit" is denounced as being responsible for this trouble. On the Indian side, the mention of the "seizing female spirit" *(grāhi)* goes much higher than the medical texts which describe the symptoms of its presence; it is already found in the *Ṛgveda* (X, 161, 1).[2]

Whatever be the resemblance of the Accadian manual with Indian medical data concerning possession as a cause of diseases, the idea of different types of possession shown by specific symptoms goes up much higher in India than the scientific medical texts. In the *Hippocratic Collection* the existence of similar ideas is shown by the very fact that the text *On the Sacred Diseases* gives its examples while rejecting them.[3] But here the concordance between the Greek way of posing the diagnosis of possession with the Accadian and Indian ones remains very general. It is only the 40th tablet of the Accadian text which shows special similarities, with the post-Vedic texts regarding the diagnosis of possession of infants, which has been

1 J. Filliozat, *Le Kumāratantra de Rāvaṇa*, op. cit., p. 63.
2 ibid., p. 79.
3 ed., Littré, Vol. VI, pp. 360-63; *Le Kumāratantra*, op. cit., p. 122.

pointed out by us. These similarities, the only ones having the possibility of not being simply explained in terms of universal belief in demoniac seizures, are given on the Indian side by texts of the same stratum as provide the similarities in the domain of presages obtained on the path to the patient's house or which details the mode of enumerating morbid phenomena having fatal prognostics, deliberately separated from complete clinical tables of which, in reality, they necessarily constitute a part.

One may, therefore, ask oneself if the teaching of the Accadian manual could not have been known in India and have exercised some influence on the elaboration of Indian accounts on one side regarding certain diagnoses of possession and on the other and specially regarding a special tradition of prognostication in accord with divinatory and clinical signs racapitulated apart from other morbid symptoms, as having a special prognostic value.

In its origins the Accadian manual is very ancient, its eventual passage into India could, therefore, go back very high and one could be tempted to advance the hypothesis that it could be dated in the epoch in which there used to be communication between India and Mesopotamia, from the period of the Indus civilisation. However, the concordances with the Accadian manual are seen not only in the Vedic literature, not specially Vedic, it is true, but in much later Sanskrit texts, in most of the cases later than the Christian era in the form in which they have reached us; anterior only by a few centuries to the Christian era, if one is to go back to the common stock supposed by the accounts of Bhela, Caraka and Suśruta.

Thus, on the Indian side, these concordances show themselves first of all in a period quite near that during which on their side the Hippocratic texts have concordances with Accadian prognostics and chiefly during that later period when the Greek manuals on the veterinary art in their turn present some. If the influence of the Mesopotamian tradition, and not chance, is the cause of all these concordances, then this influence must have been exercised in the East and West during the last period of its existence.

Everything agrees in showing us precisely that it could have been most easily exercised during this epoch.

First of all, we are sure that this system was current during the Achaemenid period and in their empire itself, as one of the tablets of the manual is dated in the eleventh year of Artaxerxes. It is also certain that parts of Greek and Indian lands, both under the Achaemenids, intercommunicated across this empire for the despatch of medicines and medical notions of India to Greek lands. This is all the more reason why the communications of both with Mesopotamia, situated in the middle of the distance separating the two, was easy.

The passing of pepper, a product of South India, particularly of Malabar, in the hands of Greek doctors as an Indian medicine, is to be found in Hippocratic manuals, *On Woman's Diseases* and *On the Nature of Woman.*[1] The simultaneous passing of Indian medical teaching, on its side, is to be seen in the enunciation in the manual, *On Woman's Diseases*, of an Indian prescription on dentifrice alongwith a precept of alimentary hygiene.[2] These pieces of evidence, studied in relation with the facilities offered by the presence of Greek doctors in the Achaemenid court can explain, by means of the communication of doctrines creating at least some emulation, the concordances between Greek and Indian medicine during the Achaemenid period, i.e., before that of Alexander.[3]

In any case, the relations between Mesopotamian and Indian savants can be presumed to have existed by the mere fact that Persian administration employed in its satrapies and therefore in its satrapies of Gandhāra and Sindh, scribes of Babylonian culture writing in aramaic. Their reality is fully confirmed by the creation, in North-West India, of an aramaic transcription of the Indian language, a transcription made not in accordance with a summary notation of words following their consonantic frame-work, this being the principle of the Semitic alphabet, but in accordance with the learned phonological principles of Indian grammarians.[4] We can even specifically state that probably these grammarians belonged to the school of Pāṇini. In fact this author whose date, unfortunately uncertain, seems to be in the fifth century B.C., belonged to

[1] *supra.*, p. 252 ff.
[2] ibid., p. 253.
[3] ibid., pp. 160 ff.
[4] *L'inde classique*, Vol. II, appendix on Palaeography.

Śalātura[1] in Gandhāra. He must have been, then, a subject of the Achaemenids, if he did live in the fifth century B.C., because the latter ruled over Gandhāra approximately from the middle of the sixth century, during the reign of Cyrus[2], up to the end of the fourth century B.C., at the time of the conquest of Alexander.

Under these conditions it was, therefore, very easy for the Indians to have knowledge of the Mesopotamian teachings in medicine, like that of the manual published by Mr. Labat and which was in circulation, during the reign of Artaxerxes in 453 B.C. In this case, the hypothesis that the teachings regarding presages and medical prognostics having a place of its own in Sanskrit texts, and resembling that of the Accadian texts, owe this resemblance like this situation in Sanskrit medical tradition, to an influence of the Accadian manual exerted in those very centuries when this medical tradition developed into a classical system and that it is not due to a chance encounter, may be admitted as very likely. The hypothesis of chance encounter is the least likely when it is seen that an Accadian manual current among the Persians, has its counter-parts during their epoch or during the following epoch in the countries which were part of the Persian empire, i.e., Hellenic in the West and Indian in the East.

1 This is what is corroborated independently in the seventh century by Hiuen-Tsang (S. Julien, *Mémoires Sur les contrées occidentales*, Vol. I, pp. 127 ff.) and by a copper inscription (M. Winternitz, *Geschichte der indischen litterature*, Vol. III, 1920, p. 384, no. 1) without counting Hemacandra who came later.

2 Gandhāra is mentioned in the first inscription of Darius (Behistan) as one of the provinces under, or brought under, his authority after the rebellions that followed in the wake of Cyrus' death. Moreover, it is known that Cyrus had taken Kapiśī specifically on the route to Gandhāra, cf., A Foucher, *La vieille route de l'Inde*, Vol. II, Paris, 1947, pp. 192-93.

BIBLIOGRAPHY

(OF WORKS AND ARTICLES REFERRED TO IN THE BOOK)

I. CLASSIC WORKS—SANSKRIT:

1. *Ahirbudhnya-saṁhitā.*
2. *Agniveśa-saṁhitā.*
3. *Agniveśatantra.*
4. *Aitareya-brāhmaṇa.*
5. *Amarakoṣa.*
6. *Arthaśāstra* of Kauṭilya.
7. *Aṣṭādhyāyī* of Pāṇini.
8. *Aṣṭāṅgasaṁgraha* of Vāgbhaṭa:
   (i) Ed. by Ganeśaśarman.
   (ii) Tibetan Version.
9. *Aṣṭāṅgahṛdaya-saṁhitā* of Vāgbhaṭa. Bombay, 1880; with Eng. introduction, 1891.
10. *Āśvalāyana-gṛhyasūtra.*
11. (i) *Atharvaveda.*
   (ii) English transln., *Hymns of the Atharvaveda,* by M. Bloomfield, in S.B.E., XLII.
   (iii) Eng. transln. by W.D. Whitney, in H.O.S.
   (iv) French transln. by V. Henry, Paris, 1894-1916.
12. *Atharvaveda-pariśiṣṭa.*
13. *Āyurveda-dīpikā.*
14. (i) *Bhāgavata-purāṇa.*
   (ii) French transln. from a Tamil version by Maridās Poullé, 2nd edn., Rev. hist. de l'Inde Francaise, Vol. IV, Pondichery, 1920.
   (iii) French transln. by Eug. Burnouf, Vol. I, Paris, 1840-98.
15. *Bhela-saṁhitā.* Ed. Asutosh Mookerjee, *Journ. of the Dept. of Letters,* Vol. VI, Calcutta, 1921.
16. *Bower Manuscripts, The Arch. Surv. of India,* Vol. XXII, Calcutta, 1893-1912.
17. *Brahmāṇḍa-purāṇa.*
18. *Bṛhadāraṇyaka-upaniṣad.*
19. *Cakradatta-saṁgraha.*
20. *Carakasautrāmaṇi.*
21. *Caraka-saṁhitā:*
   (i) ed. by Narendranath Shastri, with the commentary of Cakrapāṇidatta, Lahore, 1929.
   (ii) ed. by Jivananda Vidyāsāgara, Calcutta, 1896.
   (iii) ed. by Śaṁkaraśāstrin, Bombay, no date.

(iv) published by Khemraj Śrīkṛṣṇadās, with a Hindi Translation, Bombay, 1898.
(v) ed. by Harināth Sarkar, with the commentary of Cakrapāṇidatta, no date (1880?).
(vi) ed. by Gaṅgādhara with his own commentary.
(vii) ed. by N.N. Sengupta and B.C. Sengupta, Calcutta, 1928.
(viii) Manuscript No. 1304, Sanskrit, of the Bibl. nationale, Paris.

22. *Chāndogya-upaniṣad.*
23. *Cikitsā-saṁgraha* of Cakradatta.
24. *Hārita-saṁhitā.*
25. (i) *Harivaṁśa,* Calcutta edition.
(ii) French translation by Langlois.
26. *Hastyāyurveda* of Pālakāpya.
27. *Jaiminīya-brāhmaṇa*, ed. by W. Caland as *Das Jaiminīya-brāhmaṇa in Auswahl,* Amsterdam, 1919.
28. *Jyotiṣavedāṅga.*
29. *Kacchapuṭa.*
30. *Kapiṣṭhala-kaṭhasaṁhitā.*
31. *Kāśikāvṛtti.*
32. *Kāṭhaka-saṁhitā,* ed. by Schroeder, Leipzig, 1909.
33. *Kauśikasūtra.*
34. *Kṣurikopaniṣad.*
35. *Mādhavanidāna.*
36. *Mahābhārata.*
37. *Mahābhāṣya* of Patañjali.
38. *Mahāvastu,* ed. by E. Senart, Paris, 1882-97.
39. *Mahāvyutpatti,* ed. by Sakaki, 2nd edn., Tokyo, 1961.
40. *Maitrāyaṇi-saṁhitā.*
41. *Matsyapurāṇa.*
42. *Nibandhasaṁgraha* of Dalhaṇa.
43. *Nyāyacandrikā* of Gayadāsa.
44. *Pañcatantra.*
45. *Pañcaviṁśabrāhmaṇa.*
46. *Praśna-upaniṣad.*
47. *Rāmāyaṇa.*
48. *Rasaratnākara* of Nityanātha, Bombay, 1897.
49. *Ṛgveda.*
(i) Commentary of Sāyaṇa.
(ii) Trnsln. into French by Langlois.
(iii) Trnsln. into English by H.H. Wilson.
(iv) Trnsln. into German by Geldner.
(v) Notes in German by Grassmann.
(vi) by H. Oldenberg, *Ṛgveda-Noten,* Berlin, 1912.
50. *Sāmaveda.*
51. *Saṁyuktaratnapiṭakasūtra* (from the Chinese as *Tsa pao tsang king*).
52. *Śāṅkhāyana-gṛhyasūtra.*
53. *Śārṅgadhara-saṁhitā.*
54. *Śatapatha-brāhmaṇa.*

55. *Sūryasiddhānta.*
56. *Suśruta-saṁhitā:*
(i) ed. by Madhusūdangupta, Calcutta, 1835.
(ii) ed. by Jivānanda Vidyāsāgara, Calcutta, 1889.
(iii) ed. by Kāliprasanna Kaviśekhara (in Bengali script) with the Commentary of Dalhaṇa and Bengali trnsln., Calcutta, 1898.
(iv) ed. by Jadavji Trikamji, with the Commentary of Dalhaṇa, Bombay, 1931.
57. *Taittirīya-saṁhitā.*
58. *Vājasaneyi-saṁhitā.*
59. *Vāsavadattā.*
60. *Vāyu-purāṇa.*
61. *Viṣṇu-purāṇa*—English trnsln. by H.H. Wilson, Vol. IV, London, 1868.
62. *Yajurveda, Kṛṣṇa,* Eng. trnsln. by A.B. Keith, as *The Veda of the Black Yajus School,* H.O.S., XVIII.
63. *Yogacūḍāmaṇyupaniṣad.*
64. *Yogasūtra* of Patañjali.
65. *Yogaśataka.*
66. *The Yoga Upaniṣad,* ed. by Mahadev Shastri, Adyar, 1920.

II. CLASSIC WORKS—NON-SANSKRIT:

1. *Alberuni's India,* trnsltd. into English by E. Sachau, London, 1910.
2. *Aməsā Spentas,* by B. Geiger.
3. Aristotle, *De partibus animalium.*
4. Arrian, *Indica,* IX, 9.
5. (i) *Avesta, transln.* by De Harlez, Paris, 1881.
(ii) Transln. by J. Darmesteter, Paris, 1893.
6. Barzoe, *Barzoes Einleitung zu dem Buche Kalila wa Dimna,* Strasburg, 1912.
7. *Bundahisn.*
8. Censorinus, *De die natali.*
9. *Dénkart,* edited by Peshotam Senjana, Vol. IV, Bombay, 1874-1928.
10. (i) *Doxographi graeci,* ed. by H. Diels, Berlin, 1879.
(ii) French trnsln. in P. Tannery, *Pour l'histoire de la science helléne,* ed. by A Diés, Paris, 1930.
11. Eusebius, *Preparatio evangelica*—.
12. *Fou la tsang yin yuan tchouan.*
13. Herodotus.
14. Hippocrates, *Oeuvres complétes,* ed. by Littré, E., Paris, 1839-69.
15. *Hippocratic Collection, The:*
(1) On Ancient Medicine.
(2) Aphorisms.
(3) On Flesh.
(4) Coan Prognoses.
(5) On Crises.
(6) On the Eight Months' Embryo.
(7) On Generation.

(8) On Diseases.
(9) On Woman's Diseases.
(10) On the Sacred Disease.
(11) On the Nature of the Child.
(12) On the Nature of Woman.
(13) On the Nature of Man.
(14) On Diet in Acute Diseases.
(15) On Breaths.
(16) On Alimentation.
(17) Airs, Waters and Places.

16. Hiuan-tsang, *Mémoires sur les contrées occidentales*, French translation by S. Julien.
17. *Huspāram-nask*.
18. I-tsing, *A Record of the Buddhist Religion*, translated by Takakusu, Oxford, 1896.
19. Justin, *Epitoma Historiarum Philippicarum*, XV.
20. *Kitāb al-Fihrist*.
21. *Nyāyiśn*.
22. *Pehlavi Texts*, translated by E.W. West, Vol. I, S.B.E. V, Oxford, 1880.
23. Ktesias, *Persica*
24. Philostratos, *Life of Apollonios of Tyana*.
25. *Periplus of the Erythrean Sea*.
26. Plato, *Works*, ed. by M.A. Rivaud, in Coll. Guillaume Budé, as *Platon*, Vol. X, Paris, 1925.
27. Plato, *Timée* (Timaeus), ed. by M.A. Rivaud.
28. Pliny, *Nat. Hist.*, VI, XXI, 5, ed. E. Littré.
29. *Rāmāt nask*.
30. *Sīróza*.
31. *Solin*.
32. *Strabo*.
33. Théophrastes, *Des Sensations*.
34. *Tsa pao tsang king*, (*Samyukta-ratna-piṭaka-sūtra*).
35. *Videvdāt* (Vendidād).
36. *Vīspered*.
37. (i) *Yasna*, Sanskrit translation by Neryosengh, ed. by Fr. Spiegel as *Neriosengh's Sanskrit Ubersetzung des Yasna*, Leipzig, 1861.
    (ii) ed. by Westergaard and Geldner.
38. *Zādsparam*.

III. Modern Works:

1. Achart, A. Dj., *Quinze cents plantes dans l'Inde*, Pondichéry, 1905.
2. Antoniadi, *L'astronomie égyptienne*, Paris, 1934.
3. Aufrecht, Th., *Lomaśātana*, *ZDMG*, Vol. XXXI, 1877.
4. Avalon, A., *Tantrik Texts*, Vol. III, Calcutta, London, 1944.
5. Barth, A., *Oeuvres*, Paris, 1914-27.
6. Benveniste, E., and Renou, L., *Vṛtra and Vṛthragna*, Paris, 1934.

7. Benveniste, E., *La doctrine médicale des Indo-Européens in Rev. hist. rel.*, July-December, 1945.
8. Bergaigne, A., *Etude sur le lexique du Ṛgveda*, Paris, 1884.
9. Bergaigne, A., *La religion védique d'aprés les hymnes du Ṛgveda*, 3 vols., Paris, 1878-83, 2nd edn., Paris, 1963.
10. Bidez, *Eos ou Platon et l'Orient*, Brussels, 1945.
11. Bloch, J., *Indo-aryen*, Paris, 1934.
12. Blochet, E., *Textes religieux pehlevis, RHR*, Vol. XXXI, Paris, 1895.
13. Bloomfield, M., *On the Meanings of the Word 'Suṣma', ZDMG*, 148.
14. Bloomfield, M., *Trita, The Scape-goat of the Gods, JAOS*, 1894.
15. Boissier, A., *Choix de textes relatifs ā la divination assyro-babylonienne*, 2 Vols, Geneva, 1905-1906.
16. Bolling, M., *Diseases and Medicine (Vedic)*, in *Hastings Encyclopaedia*, 1911.
17. Boulanger, *Orphée*.
18. Bréhier, E., *La philosophie de Plotin*, Paris, 1928.
19. Brown, G.W., *Prāṇa and Apāna, JAOS*, XXXIX.
20. Brown, G.W., *The Human Body in the Upanishads*, Jubbulpore, 1921.
21. Caland, W., *Altindisches Zauberritual*, Amsterdam, 1900.
22. Caland, W. and Henry, H., *L'Agniṣṭoma*, 2 Vols., Paris, 1906-7.
23. Caland, W., *Zur exegese und kritik der rituellen Sūtras* XXXIV, *Prāṇa und Apāna, ZDMG*, Vol. LV, 1901.
24. Casartelli, L.C., *La philosophie religieuse du mazdéisme sous les Sassanides*, Paris, 1884.
25. Casartelli, L.C., *Un traité pehlevi sur la mèdecine, Muséon*, November, 1886.
26. Chavannes, E., *Cinq cents contes et apologues extraits du Tripiṭaka chinois*, Vol. II and III, Paris, 1911; Vol. IV, Paris, 1934.
27. Chavannes, E., *Documents sur les Tou-kiue occidentaux*.
28. Christensen, A., *L'Iran sous les Sassanides*, Copenhagen, 1936.
29. Contenau, G., *La médicine en Assyrie et en Babylonie*, Paris, 1938.
30. Cordier, P., *Etude sur la médicine hindoue*, Paris, 1894.
31. Cordier, P., *L'enseignement médical dans l'Inde ancienne*, in *Bull. de la soc. franc. d'hist. de la méd.*, Paris, 1905.
32. Cordier, P., *Nāgārjuna et l'Uttaratantra de la Suśrutasaṁhitā*, Antananarivo, 1896.
33. Cordier, P., *Quelques données nouvelles á propos des traités médicaux sanscrits antérieurs au* XIII *siécle*, Calcutta, 1899.
34. Daremberg, Ch., *Fragments du Commentaire de Galien sur le Timée de Platon*, Paris, Leipzig, 1844.
35. Darmesteter, J., *Haurvatāt et Ameretāt*, Paris, 1875.
36. Darmesteter, J., *Ormazd et Ahriman*, Paris, 1877.
37. Dasgupta, S.N., *A History of Indian Philosophy*, Vol. II, Cambridge, 1932.
38. Dasgupta, S.N., *Yoga Philosophy*, Calcutta, 1930.

39. Delpeuch, A., *La goutte et le rhematisme*, Paris, 1900.
40. Deussen, P., *Allegemeine Einleitung und Philosophie des Veda*, Leipzig, 1920.
41. Diés, A., *Autour de Platon*, Paris, 1927.
42. Doreau, J.L., *Les bains dans l'Inde antique, monuments et textes médicaux*, Paris, 1936.
43. Duchesne-Guillemin, J., *Zoroastre*, Paris, 1948.
44. Dumézil, G., *Jupiter, Mars Quirinus*, Paris, 1941.
45. Dumézil, G., *Le Festin d'immortalité*, Paris, 1924.
46. Dumézil, G., *Le troisiéme souverain*, Paris, 1949.
47. Dumézil, G., *Les mythes romains*, *Tarpeia*, Paris, 1947.
48. Dumézil, G., *Naissance d'archanges*, Paris, 1945.
49. Eliade, Mircea, *Yoga*, Paris, 1936.
50. Ewing, Arthur, H., *The Hindu Conception of the Functions of Breath—A Study in Early Hindu Psychophysics*, *JAOS*, Vol. XXXII, 1901.
51. Festugiére, A.J., *Grecs et sages orientaux*, in *Rev. hist. des rel.*, Vol. CXXX, 1945.
52. Festugiére, A.J., *La Révélation d'Hermés Trismégiste*, Paris, 1944.
53. Festugiére, A.J., *Platon et l'Orient*, in *Revue de philologie*, Vol. XXI, 1947.
54. Fichtner, H., *Die Medizin im Avesta untersucht auf Grund der von Fr. Wolff besorgten Ubersetzung der heiligen Bucher der Parsen*, 1924.
55. Filliozat, J., *Etude de démonologie indienne*, *Le Kumāratantra de Rāvaṇa et les textes Parelléles*, Paris, 1937.
56. Filliozat, J., *Fragments de textes Koutchéens de médicine et magie*, Paris, 1948.
57. Filliozat, J., *La doctrine des Brahmanes d'aprés saint Hippolyte*, in *Rev. hist. des rel.*, July-December, 1945.
58. Filliozat, J., *Le Sommeil et les réves selon les médecins indiens et les physiologues grecs*, in *Journ. de psychologie*, July-September, 1947.
59. Filliozat, J., *Les échanges de l'Inde et de l'empire romain aux premiers siécles de l'ére chrétienne*, in *Rev. hist.*, January-March, 1949.
60. Filliozat, J., *Les gajaśāstra et les auteurs grecs*, *JA*, 1933.
61. Filliozat, J., *Les origines d'une technique mystique indienne*, in *Revue philosophique*, April-June, 1946.
62. Filliozat, J., *Magie et médecine*, Paris, 1948.
63. Filliozat, J., *Nāgārjuna et Agastya, médecins, chimistes et sorciers*, in *Actes du XX Congrés inter. des Orientalistes, 1938*, Brussels, 1940.
64. Filliozat, J., *Un chapitre de la Hārītasaṁhitā sur la rétribution des actes*, *JA*, July-September, 1934.
65. Fossey, Ch., *Notices sur les caractéres étrangers anciens et modernes de l'Imprimerie nationale*, Paris, 1948.

66. Foucher, A., *La Nicée d'Afghanistan*, in *C.r. de l'Académie des Inscriptions et Belles-Lettres*, Paris, 1938.

67. Foucher, A., *Les Satrapies orientales de l'empire achéménide*, in *Comptes rendus de l'Académie des Inscriptions et Belles-Lettres*, Paris, 1938.

68. Foucher, A., and Mrs. B. Foucher, *La vieille route de l'Inde de Bactres à Taxila*, in *Mém. Déleg. Franç. en Afghanistan*, Vols.I & II, 1947.

69. Furlani, G., *La religione degli Hittiti*, Bologna, 1936.

70. Ghirshman, R., *Bégram*, Cairo, 1946.

71. Gomperz, Th., *Les penseurs de la Gréce*, French translation by A. Raymond, 3rd edition, Paris, 1928.

72. Gotze, A., *Persische Weisheit in griechischen Gewande*, in *Zeit. Fur. Ind. und Ir.*, II, 1923.

73. Gray, Louis H., *The Indian God Dhanvantari*, in *JAOS*, 1922.

74. Grohmann, V., *Medicinisches aus dem Atharva-Veda mit besonderem Bezug auf den Takman*, in *Ind. St.*, IX, Leipzig, 1865.

75. Haug, Martin, *Essays on the Sacred Language, Writings and Religion of the Parsis*, ed. E.W. West, London, no date (1878?)

76. Henry, V., *La Magie dans l'Inde antique*, Paris, 1909.

77. Henry, V., *Le Parsisme*, Paris, 1909.

78. Henry, V., *Manuel Védique*, Paris, 1890.

79. Henry, V., *Soma et Haoma*, Paris, 1906.

80. Hertel, Johannes, *Die arische Feuerlehre*, Vol. I, Leipzig, 1925.

81. Hertel, Johannes, *Nachtrag zu Rgveda*, X-163; *Vendidad*, VIII, 35-72, in *Asia Major*, Vol. VI, 1930.

82. Herzfeld, M E., *The Aryan Myth of Naphta* in *Hist. et archéol. du pétrole*, II congres mondial du pétrole, Paris, 1937.

83. Hillebrandt, *Ritual-Litteratur (Grundriss)*, Strasburg, 1897.

84. Hoernle, *Studies in the Medicine of Ancient India*, Part I, Osteology, Oxford, 1907.

85. Hubert, H., and Mauss, M., *Esquisse d'une théorie générale de la magie*, in *Année sociologique*, Paris, 1902-3.

86. Jaeger, W., *Aristoteles*, Berlin, 1923.

87. Jaeger, W., *Diokles von Karystos*, Berlin, 1938.

88. Jolly, J., *Medicin*, Strassburg, 1901.

89. Keith, A.B., *The Religion and Philosophy of the Veda and the Upanishads*, Cambridge (Mass.), 1925.

90. Lagrange, M.J., *Les mystéres : l'orphisme*, Paris, 1937.

91. Lassen, Ch., *Indische Alterthumskunde*, 4 vols., Leipzig, 1847-61.

92 Lévi, S., *Kaniṣka et Śātavāhana*, *JA*, January-March, 1936.

93. Lévi, S., *Le tokharien B., langue de Koutcha*, *JA*, September-October, 1913.

94. Lévi, S., *L'Inde civilisatrice*, Paris, 1938.

95. Lévi, S., *Notes sur les Indo-scythes*, *JA*, November-December, 1896.

96. Liétard, Dr., *Le médicin charaka*, in *Bull. de l'Acad. de médicine*, Paris, 11 May 1897.

97. Lommel, M., *Die Yasts des Avesta*, Gottingen, 1927.
98. Luders, H., *Die magische Kraft der Wahrheit im alten Indien, ZDMG*, 1944.
99. Mackay, E., *La civilisation de l'Indus*, French Trnsln., Paris, 1936.
100. Mariadassou, P., *Le Jardin des simples de l'Inde*, Pondichéry, 1913.
101. Mauss, M., and Hubert, H., *Esquisse d'une théorie générale de la magie*, in *Année sociologique*, Paris, 1902-3.
102. Mukhopadhyāya, G.N., *History of Indian Medicine*, Vol. III, Calcutta, 1929.
103. Max Muller, F., *A History of Ancient Literature*, Allahabad, 1926.
104. Max Muller, F., *Origine et développement de la religion*, French Trnsln. by J. Darmesteter, Paris, 1879.
105. Max Muller, F., *Physical Religion*, London, 1891.
106. Muller, R.F.G., *Uber Pitta oder galle unter Bezug zur Tridoṣa-Lehere der Altindischen Medizin*, in *Janus*, 1934.
107. Muller, R.F.G., *Der Takman des Atharvaveda*, in *Artibus Asiae*, VI, 1937.
108. R. Muller, R.F.G., *Grundlagen Altindischen Medizin*, in *Nova Acta Leopoldina, neue Folge*, 11, No. 74, Halle, 1942.
109. Mus, P., *Barabuḍur*, Hanoi, 1935.
110. Nadkarni, K.N., *The Indian Materia Medica*, Bombay, no date, (about 1925).
111. Nelson, Axel, *Die Hippokratische Schrift Peri Phuson, Text und Studien*, Uppsala, 1909.
112. Nyberg, H.S., *Die Religionen des alten Iran*, Leipzig, 1938.
113. Nyberg, H.S., *Questions de cosmogonie et de cosmologie mazdéennes*, *JA*, October-December, 1931.
114. Oldenberg, H., *Die Weltanschauung der Brāhmaṇa-Texte*, Gottingen, 1919.
115. Oldenberg, H., *La Religion du Veda*, translated into French by V. Henry, Paris, 1903.
116. Pargiter, F.E,, *The Purāṇa Text of the Dynasties of the Kali Age*, Oxford, 1913.
117. Pillai, M.S.P., *Tamil Literature*, Mannirpalam, 1930.
118. Pischel, R., *Vedische Studien*, Vol. I, Stuttgartt, 1889.
119. Poussin, L. de La Vallée, *L'inde au temps des Maurya*, Paris, 1930.
120. Ray, Jogeśchandra, *The Soma Plant*, in *Indian Historical Quarterly*, XV, 1939.
121. Ray, P.C., *History of Hindu Chemistry*, Calcutta, 1911.
122. Reinaud, *Mémoire sur l'Inde*, in *Mem. de l'Académie des Inscriptions et Bells-letters*, Vol. XVIII, 2nd part, Paris, 1849.
123. Regnaud, P., *Notes d'exégése védique Détermination du sens de "tan", "tman" et "takman"*, in *Congr. Or.*, 1897.
124. Renel, Ch., *L'évolution d'un mythe Aśvins et Dioscures* in *Ann. de l'Univ. de Lyon*, Paris, 1896.
125. Renou, L., *Anthologie sanskrite*, Paris, 1947.
126. Renou, L., *Bibliographie védique*, Paris, 1931.
127. Renou, L., *Grammaire sanscrite*, Paris, 1930.

128. Renou, L., *L'hymme Aśvin de l'Ādiparvan*, Eastern and Indian Studies in Honour of P.W. Thomas.
129. Renou, L., *La "Durghaṭavṛtti"*, Vol. I, fasc. 1, Paris, 1940.
130. Renou, L., *L'ambiguité du vocabulaire du Ṛgveda*, *JA*, 1939.
131. Renou, L., *Les écoles védiques*, Paris, 1947.
132. Renou, L. and Benveniste, E., *Vṛtra et Vṛthragna*, Paris, 1934.
133. Rey. A, *La science orientale avant les Grecs*, Paris, 1930.
134. -do- , *La jeunesse de la science grecque*, Paris, 1933.
135. -do- , *La maturité de la pensée scientifique en Gréce*, Paris, 1939.
136. -do- . *L'apogée de la science technique grecque*, Paris, 1946 & 1948.
137. Ronnow, K., *Trita Āptya, eine vedische Gottheit*, Uppsala, 1927.
138. Saint-Firmin, Mme Liacre de, *Médicine et légendes bouddhiques de l'Inde*, Paris, 1916.
139. Schuhl, P.M., *Essai sur la formation de la pensée grecque*, Paris, 1949.
140. Senart, E., *Essai sur la légende du Buddha*, 2nd. ed., Paris, 1882.
141. Stein, Aurel, *On the Ephedra, the Hūm Plant and the Soma*, *BSOS*, Vol. VI, London, 1931.
142. Tannery, P., *Pour l'histoire de la science helléne*, ed. by A. Diés, 2nd. edition, Paris, 1930.
143. Tannery, P., *Recherches sur l'histoire de l'astronomie ancienne*, Paris, 1893.
144. Tassy, Garcin de, *Bagh-o-bahar*, Paris, 1878.
145. Taylor, A.E., *A Commentary on Plato's Timaeus*, Oxford, 1928.
146. Verbeke, G., *L'évolution de la doctime du pneuma du stoicisme á saint Augustin*, Paris, Louvain, 1945.
147. Voilquin, J., *Les penseurs grecs avant Socrate*, Paris, 1941.
148. Wellmann, M., *Alkmaion von Kroton*, Archeion, XI, 1929.
149. Wellmann, M., *Die Pneumatische Schule bis auf Archigenes*, Berlin, 1895.
150. Wellmann, M., *Fragments des sikelischen Ärzte*, Berlin, 1901.
151. Wieger, L., *Histoire des croyances religieuses et des opinions philosophiques en Chine*, 3rd. ed., Hien-Hien, 1927.
152. Wikander, Stig, *Vayu, Texte und Untersuchungen zur indoiranischen Religions geschichte*, Vol. I, Uppsala—Leipzig, 1940.
153 Zimmer, H., *Altindisches Leben*, Berlin, 1879.

IV. DICTIONARIES:

1. Bartholomae, *Altiranisches Worterbuch*, 2nd edn., Berlin, 1961.
2. Bloomfield, M., *A Vedic Concordance*, Cambridge (Mass.), 1906-75
3. Bohtlingk and Roth, *Sanskrit Worterbuch*, Petersburg, 1860.
4. Grassmann, H., *Worterbuch Zum Ṛgveda*, Leipzig, 1873.
5. Gupta, U.C., *Vaidyakaśabdasindhu*, Calcutta, 1894.
6. *Hastings Encyclopaedia*.
7. Jaeschke, *Tibetan Dictionary*, 3rd edn., London, 1949.
8. Keith, A.B. and Macdonell, A.A., *Vedic Index*, 2 Vols., London, 1912.
9. *Sanskrit-Tibetan Dictionary* of Tse-ring-ouang-gyal, Paris, 1930.

10. Wilson, H.H., *A Dictionary in Sanskrit and English.*

V. JOURNALS AND COLLECTIONS:

1. *Actes du Congrés Oriental*, 1897.
2. *Actes du XX Congrés international des Orientalistes, 1938*, Brussels, 1940.
3. *Annales de l'Université de Lyon.*
4. *Année sociologique.*
5. *Archeion.*
6. *Artibus Asiae.*
7. *Asia Major.*
8. *Babyloniaca.*
9. *Bulletin de l'Académie de médicine.*
10. *Bulletin de l'Ecole française de l'Extreme-Orient* (*BEFEO*).
11. *Bulletin of the School of Oriental and African Studies* (*BSOAS*).
12. *Bulletin de la société franç. de l'histoire de la médicine.*
13. *Comptes rendus de l'Academie des Inscriptions et Belles-lettres.*
14. *Gotingische Gelehrte Anzeigen.*
15. *Hermes.*
16. *Hobogirin.*
17. *Indian Historical Quarterly.*
18. *Indische Studien* (*Ind. St.*).
19. *Journal of the American Oriental Society* (*JAOS*).
20. *Journal Asiatique* (*JA*).
21. *Journal of the Department of Letters*, Calcutta University.
21. *Journal de psychologie.*
22. *Mémoirș de l'Académie des Inscriptions et Belles-lettres.*
23. *Mușeon.*
24. *Nova Acta Leopoldina*, neue Folge.
25. *Revue de l'histoire des religions* (*RHR*).
26. *Revue de philologie.*
27. *Revue philosophique.*
28. *Zeitschrift der Deutschen Morgenländischen Gessellschaft* (*ZDMG*).
29. *Zeitschrift fur Indologie uṇd Iranistik* (*Zeit. fur Ind. und Ir.*).
30. *Zeitschrift fur velgliechende-sprach-wissen-schaft, (Zeitschrift fur vergl.)*

INDEX*

*The anatomical terms are indexed on pp. 144-157; those terms are included here only where they appear elsewhere in this book.

Errata

	Read	For
p. 5, l. 35	Dhānvantara	Dhanvantara
p. 9, l. 24	Bhāradvāja	Bharadvāja
p. 1[illegible]. l. 5	After Droṇa, read[1].	This foot-note is printed on p. 17.
p. 21, l. 25	Ātreyī	Ātreya
p. 25, l. 9	Bhāradvāja	Bhardvāja
p. 43, l. 12	Dahāka	Dahāha
p. 61, l. 17	Vayu	Vāyu
p. 91, l. 20	*arta*	*ṛta*
p. 96, l. 30	*attrin*	*astrin*
p. 128, l. 25	Ślipada	Sipada
p. 147, l. 13	Neisser	*Neisser*
p. 215. l. 25	*daṇḍāpatānaka*	*daṇḍapātanaka*